Adult CCRN Exam SECRETS

Study Guide
Your Key to Exam Success

CCRN Test Review for the
Critical Care Nurses Certification
Examinations

Published by
Mometrix Test Preparation
CCRN Exam Secrets Test Prep Team

Written and edited by the CCRN Exam Secrets Test Prep Staff

Printed in the United States of America

This paper meets the requirements of ANSI/NISO Z39.48-1992 (Permanence of Paper).

Mometrix offers volume discount pricing to institutions. For more information or a price quote, please contact our sales department at sales@mometrix.com or 888-248-1219.

CCRN® is a registered trademark of the American Association of Critical-Care Nurses (AACN®), which was not involved in the production of, and does not endorse, this product.

ISBN 13: 978-1-60971-270-9
ISBN 10:1-60971-270-6

Dear Future Exam Success Story:

Congratulations on your purchase of our study guide. Our goal in writing our study guide was to cover the content on the test, as well as provide insight into typical test taking mistakes and how to overcome them.

Standardized tests are a key component of being successful, which only increases the importance of doing well in the high-pressure high-stakes environment of test day. How well you do on this test will have a significant impact on your future- and we have the research and practical advice to help you execute on test day.

The product you're reading now is designed to exploit weaknesses in the test itself, and help you avoid the most common errors test takers frequently make.

How to use this study guide

We don't want to waste your time. Our study guide is fast-paced and fluff-free. We suggest going through it a number of times, as repetition is an important part of learning new information and concepts.

First, read through the study guide completely to get a feel for the content and organization. Read the general success strategies first, and then proceed to the content sections. Each tip has been carefully selected for its effectiveness.

Second, read through the study guide again, and take notes in the margins and highlight those sections where you may have a particular weakness.

Finally, bring the manual with you on test day and study it before the exam begins.

Your success is our success

We would be delighted to hear about your success. Send us an email and tell us your story. Thanks for your business and we wish you continued success-

Sincerely,

Mometrix Test Preparation Team

Need more help? Check out our flashcards at: http://MometrixFlashcards.com/CCRN

TABLE OF CONTENTS

Top 20 Test Taking Tips

1. Carefully follow all the test registration procedures
2. Know the test directions, duration, topics, question types, how many questions
3. Setup a flexible study schedule at least 3-4 weeks before test day
4. Study during the time of day you are most alert, relaxed, and stress free
5. Maximize your learning style; visual learner use visual study aids, auditory learner use auditory study aids
6. Focus on your weakest knowledge base
7. Find a study partner to review with and help clarify questions
8. Practice, practice, practice
9. Get a good night's sleep; don't try to cram the night before the test
10. Eat a well balanced meal
11. Know the exact physical location of the testing site; drive the route to the site prior to test day
12. Bring a set of ear plugs; the testing center could be noisy
13. Wear comfortable, loose fitting, layered clothing to the testing center; prepare for it to be either cold or hot during the test
14. Bring at least 2 current forms of ID to the testing center
15. Arrive to the test early; be prepared to wait and be patient
16. Eliminate the obviously wrong answer choices, then guess the first remaining choice
17. Pace yourself; don't rush, but keep working and move on if you get stuck
18. Maintain a positive attitude even if the test is going poorly
19. Keep your first answer unless you are positive it is wrong
20. Check your work, don't make a careless mistake

Cardiovascular

Stable angina

Impairment of blood flow through the coronary arteries leads to ischemia of the cardiac muscle and angina pectoris, pain that may occur in the sternum, chest, neck, arms (especially the left) or back. The pain frequently occurs with crushing pain substernally, radiating down the left arm or both arms although this type of pain is more common in males than females, whose symptoms may appear less acute and include nausea, shortness of breath, and fatigue.

Elderly or diabetic patients may also have pain in arms, no pain at all (*silent ischemia*), or weakness and numbness in arms. Stable angina episodes usually last for <5 minutes and are fairly predictable exercise-induced episodes caused by atherosclerotic lesions blocking >75% of the lumen of the effected coronary artery. Precipitating events include exercise, decrease in environmental temperature, heavy eating, strong emotions (such as fright or anger), or exertion, including coitus. Stable angina episodes usually resolve in less than 5 minutes by decreasing activity level and administering sublingual nitroglycerin.

Unstable and variant angina

Unstable angina (also known as preinfarction or crescendo angina) is a progression of coronary artery disease and occurs when there is a change in the pattern of stable angina. The pain may increase, may not respond to a single nitroglycerin, and may persist for >5 minutes. Usually pain is more frequent, lasts longer, and may occur at rest. Unstable angina may indicate rupture of an atherosclerotic plaque and the beginning of thrombus formation so it should always be treated as a medical emergency as it may indicate a myocardial infarction.

Variant angina (also known as Prinzmetal's angina) results from spasms of the coronary arteries, can be associated with or without atherosclerotic plaques, and is often related to smoking, alcohol, or illicit stimulants. Elevation of ST segments usually occurs with variant angina. Variant angina frequently occurs cyclically at the same time each day and often while the person is at rest. Nitroglycerin or calcium channel blockers are used for treatment.

Q-wave and non-Q-wave myocardial infarctions

Myocardial infarctions (formerly classified as transmural or non-transmural) are currently classified as Q-wave or non-Q-wave:

Q-Wave
- Characterized by series of abnormal Q waves (wider and deeper) on ECG, especially in the early AM (related to adrenergic activity).
- Infarction is usually prolonged and results in necrosis.
- Coronary occlusion is complete in 80-90%.
- Q-wave MI is often, but not always, transmural.
- Peak CK levels occur in about 27 hours.
- Mortality rates are about 10%.

Non-Q Wave
- Characterized by changes in ST-T wave with ST depression (usually reversible within a few days).
- Usually reperfusion occurs spontaneously, so infarct size is smaller. Contraction necrosis related to reperfusion is common.
- Non-Q-wave MI is usually non-transmural.
- Coronary occlusion is complete in only 20-30%.
- Peak CK levels occur in 12-13 hours.
- Mortality rates are about 2-3%.
- Reinfarction is common, so 2-year survival rates are similar to Q-wave MI.

Types of myocardial infarctions

Myocardial infarctions are classified according to their location and the extent of injury. Transmural myocardial infarction involves the full thickness of the heart (the endocardium, myocardium, and epicardium), often producing a series of Q waves on ECG. An MI most frequently damages the left ventricle and the septum, but the right ventricle may be damaged, depending upon the damaged area:
- **Anterior wall infarction** occurs with occlusion in the proximal left anterior descending artery, and may damage the left ventricle.
- **Left lateral wall infarction** occurs with occlusion of the circumflex coronary artery, often causing damage to anterior wall as well.
- **Inferior wall infarction** occurs with occlusion of the right coronary artery and causes conduction malfunctions.
- **Right ventricular infarction** occurs with occlusion of the proximal section of the right coronary artery and damages the right ventricle and the inferior wall.
- **Posterior wall infarction** occurs with occlusion in the right coronary artery or circumflex artery and may be difficult to diagnose.

Clinical manifestations of myocardial infarction

Clinical manifestations of myocardial infarction may vary considerably, with males having the more "classic" symptom of sudden onset of crushing chest pain and females and those under 55 presenting with atypical symptoms. Diabetic patients may have reduced sensation of pain because of neuropathy and may complain primarily of weakness. Elderly patients may also have neuropathic changes that reduce sensation of pain. More than half of all patients present with acute MIs with no prior symptoms of cardiovascular disease. Symptoms may include:
- Angina with pain in chest that may radiate to neck or arms.
- Palpitations.
- Hypertension or hypotension
- ECG changes (ST segment and T-wave changes, tachycardia, bradycardia, and dysrhythmias).
- Dyspnea.
- Pulmonary edema, dependent edema
- Nausea and vomiting.
- Decreased urinary output.
- Pallor, skin cold and clammy, diaphoresis.
- Neurological/psychological disturbances: anxiety, light-headed, headache, visual abnormalities, slurred speech, and fear.

Myocardial infarction diagnostic procedures

Diagnosis of a myocardial infarction includes a complete physical examination and patient and family history with assessment of risk factors. Assessment may include:

- ECG obtained immediately to monitor heart changes over time. Typical changes include T-wave inversion, elevation of ST segment, and abnormal Q waves.
- Echocardiogram to evaluate ventricular function.
- Creatine kinase (CK) and isoenzyme (MB):
  - CK-MB (cardiac muscle) level increases within a few hours and peaks at about 24 hours (earlier with thrombolytic therapy or PTCA).
- Myoglobin (heme protein that transports oxygen) found in both skeletal and cardiac muscles. Levels increase in 1-3 hours after an MI and peak within 12 hours. While an increase is not specific to an MI, a failure to increase can be used to rule out an MI.
- Troponin (protein in the myocardium) and its isomers (C, I, and T) regulate contraction and levels increase as with CK-MB, but levels remains elevated for up to 3 weeks.

Fibrinolytic infusions

Fibrinolytic infusion is indicated for acute myocardial infarction under these conditions:

- Symptoms of MI, <6-12 hours since onset of symptoms.
- ≥1 mm elevation of ST in ≥2 contiguous leads.
- No contraindications and no cardiogenic shock.

Fibrinolytic agents should be administered as soon as possible, within 30 minutes is best. All agents convert plasminogen to plasmin, which breaks down fibrin, dissolving clots:

- Streptokinase & anistreplase (1st generation).
- Alteplase or tissue plasminogen activator (tPA) (second generation).
- Reteplase & tenecteplase (3rd generation).

Contraindications

- Present or recent bleeding or history of severe bleeding.
- History of intracranial hemorrhage.
- History of stroke (<3 months unless within 3 hours).
- Aortic dissection or pericarditis.
- Itracranial/intraspinal surgery or trauma within 3 months.
- Neoplasm, aneurysm, or AVM.

Relative Contraindications

- Active peptic ulcer.
- >10 minutes of CPR.
- Advanced renal or hepatic disease.
- Pregnancy.
- Anticoagulation therapy.
- Acute uncontrolled hypertension or chronic poorly controlled hypertension.
- Recent (2-4 weeks) internal bleeding.
- Noncompressible vascular punctures.

Papillary muscle rupture

The atrioventricular valves separate the atria from the ventricles with the tricuspid valve on the right and the bicuspid (mitral) valve on the left. The *papillary muscles* are located on the sides of ventricular walls and connect to the valves with fibrous bands called chordae tendineae.

During systole, the papillary muscles contract, tightening the chordae tendineae and closing the valves. One complication of an MI is papillary muscle rupture, usually on the left affecting the mitral valve, with the posteromedial papillary muscle more often affected than the anterolateral. Dysfunction of the papillary muscles occurs in about 40% of those with a posterior septal infarction, but rupture can occur with infarction of the inferior wall or an anterolateral MI.

Rupture on the right side results in tricuspid regurgitation and right ventricular failure while rupture on the left side leads to mitral regurgitation with resultant pulmonary edema and cardiogenic shock. Early identification and surgical repair is critical.

Characteristics of peripheral arterial and venous insufficiency

Arterial
- Type of Pain: Ranges from intermittent claudication to severe constant.
- Pulses: Weak or absent
- Skin of extremity: Rubor on dependency but pallor of foot on elevation. Skin pale, shiny, and cool with loss of hair on toes and foot. Nails thick and ridged
- Ulcers: Pain, deep, circular, often necrotic ulcers on toe tips, toe webs, heels, or other pressure areas.
- Extremity Edema: Minimal

Venous
- Type of Pain: Aching and cramping
- Pulses: Present
- Skin of extremity: Brownish discoloration around ankles and anterior tibial area.
- Ulcers: Varying degrees of pain in superficial, ir-regular ulcers on me-dial or lateral malleo-lus and sometimes the anterior tibial area.
- Extremity Edema: Moderate to severe.

Surgical/vascular interventions for arterial insufficiency/ulcers

The goal of management for arterial insufficiency and ulcers is to improve perfusion and save the limb, but lifestyle changes and medications may be insufficient. There are a number of indications for surgical intervention:
- Poor healing prognosis includes those with ankle brachial pressure index (ABI) < 0.5 because their perfusion is severely compromised.
- Failure to respond to conservative treatment (medications and lifestyle changes) even with an ABI > 0.5.

- Intolerable pain, such as with severe intermittent claudication, which is incapacitating and limits the patient's ability to work or carry out activities. Rest pain is an indication that medical treatment is insufficient.
- Limb-threatening condition, such as severe ischemia with increasing pain at rest, infection, and/or gangrene. Infection can cause a wound to deteriorate rapidly.

Surgical intervention is indicated only for those patients with patent distal vessels as demonstrated by radiologic imaging procedures.

Acute venous thromboembolism

Acute venous thromboembolism (VTE) is a condition that includes both deep vein thrombosis (DVT) and pulmonary emboli (PE). VTE may be precipitated by invasive procedures, lack of mobility, and inflammation, so it is a common complication in critical care units. *Virchow's triad* comprises common risk factors: blood stasis, injury to endothelium, and hypercoagulability. Some patients may be initially asymptomatic, but symptoms may include:
- Aching or throbbing pain.
- Positive Homan's sign (pain in calf when foot is dorsiflexed).
- Erythema and edema.
- Dilation of vessels.
- Cyanosis.

Diagnosis may be made by ultrasound and/or D-dimer test, which test the serum for cross-linked fibrin derivatives. CT scan, pulmonary angiogram, and ventilation-perfusion lung scan may be used to diagnose pulmonary emboli. Prophylaxis is very important, but once diagnosed; treatment involves bed rest, elevation of affected limb, anticoagulation therapy, and analgesics. Elastic stockings are worn when patient begins ambulating.

Pharmacologic measures to maximize perfusion

The primary focus of pharmacologic measures to maximize perfusion is to reduce the risk of thromboses:
- **Antiplatelet agents**, such as aspirin, Ticlid®, and Plavix®, which interfere with the function of the plasma membrane, interfering with clotting. These agents are ineffective to treat clots but prevent clot formation.
- **Vasodilators** may divert blood from ischemic areas, but some may be indicated, such as Pletal®, which dilates arteries and decreases clotting, and is used for control of intermittent claudication.
- **Antilipemic,** such as Zocor® and Questran®, slow progression of atherosclerosis.
- **Hemorrheologics,** such as Trental®, reduce fibrinogen, reducing blood viscosity and rigidity of erythrocytes; however, clinical studies show limited benefit. It may be used for intermittent claudication.
- **Analgesics** may be necessary to improve quality of life. Opioids may be needed in some cases.
- **Thrombolytics** may be injected into a blocked artery under angiography to dissolve clots.
- **Anticoagulants**, such as Coumadin® and Lovenox®, prevent blood clots from forming.

Anticoagulants

Anticoagulants are used to prevent thrombo-emboli. All pose risk of bleeding:

- **Aspirin** - Often used prophylactically to prevent clots and poses less danger of bleeding than other drugs
- **Warfarin** (Coumadin®) - Blocks utilization of vitamin K and decreases production of clotting factors and is used orally for those at risk of developing blood clots, such as those with mechanical heart valves, atrial fibrillation, and clotting disorders.
- **Heparin** - The primary intravenous anticoagulant and increases the activity of antithrombin III. It is used for those with MI and those undergoing PCI or other cardiac surgery. Monitored by aPTT.
- **Dalteparin (Fragmin®) & Enoxaparin (Lovenox®)** - Low-molecular weight heparins that increase activity of antithrombin III used for unstable angina, MI, and cardiac surgery.
- **Bivalirudin (Angiomax®)** - Direct thrombin inhibitors used for unstable angina, PCI, and for prophylaxis and treatment for thrombosis in heparin-induced thrombocytopenia [allergic response to heparin that causes a platelet count drop <150,000, usually to 30-50% of baseline, usually occurring 5l-14 days after beginning heparin].

Surgical/vascular interventions for treatment of severe arterial insufficiency

Surgical/ vascular interventions for treatment of severe arterial insufficiency include 3 different types of procedures:

- **Bypass grafts** require harvest of a section of the saphenous vein or an upper extremity vein to bypass damaged arteries and supply blood to distal vessels. Because veins have valves, they must be reversed or stripped of valves prior to attachment. Synthetic grafts are sometimes used but have a higher failure rate. The femoropopliteal (Fem-pop) bypass uses a graft to bypass blockage about the knee, with the graft extending from the femoral artery around the blockage to the popliteal artery.
- **Angioplasty** can be used if disease is not extensive (>10 in length), but arteries must be large enough to accommodate the procedure safely. Initial results are good but long-term rates have been less positive although the use of anticoagulants improves success rates.
- **Amputation** is the procedure that treatment tries to avoid, but it is sometimes required if ischemia is irreversible or if there is severe necrosis and infection that is life threatening.

Peripheral vascular disease

Transcutaneous oxygen pressure measurement (TCPO$_2$) is a non-invasive test that measures dermal oxygen, showing effectiveness of oxygen in the skin and tissues. Contact gel and electrodes are applied to the lower extremities to determine variations in oxygen tension. The electrodes are placed in special fixation rings attached to the skin to prevent environment air from affecting the readings, and then the skin is heated to increase blood flow. Two or three different sites should be tested to give a more accurate demonstration of oxygenation. This test is used for a number of purposes:

- Determining if there is enough oxygen transport for effective hyperbaric oxygen therapy treatments.
- Determining the degree of oxygenation and peripheral vascular disease.
- Establishing the degree of hypoxia in venous diseases.
- Identifying the optimum site for amputation of severely hypoxic limbs.

Test results:
- >40 mm Hg adequate oxygenation for healing.
- 20-40 mm Hg equivocal finding.
- <20 mm Hg marked ischemia, affecting healing.

Carotid artery stenosis

The common carotid artery branches from the subclavian artery and then bifurcates into the external carotid and internal carotid arteries. This point of bifurcation is a common site for development of plaques, causing carotid artery stenosis that interferes with cranial blood flow. When stenosis develops slowly, collateral vessels may form to aid circulation, but sudden occlusion can cause permanent brain damage and death. Most stenosis is caused by atherosclerosis, with increasing incidence with age. Most ischemia relates to an embolism or thrombus formation. Symptoms of occlusion include severe pain, anxiety, and those common to brain attacks (hemiparesis, confusion, aphasia, diplopia).

Treatment may include:
- **Dietary restrictions** to reduce cholesterol level <200.
- **Modification of risk factors** (stop smoking, reduce sodium intake, control diabetes and hypertension)
- **Antithrombotic therapy.**
- **Carotid endarterectomy** (recommended if stenosis >60%) poses the danger of a stroke, so the benefits must be carefully weighed.
- **Carotid stents/angioplasty** (newer non-invasive approaches).

Carotid stenosis diagnostic tests

Diagnostic tests for carotid stenosis may include:
- **Duplex ultrasound**, combing conventional ultrasound with Doppler, determines blood flow and obstruction.
- **CT scan** shows the degree of blockage.
- **Magnetic resonance angiography (MRA)** provides a 2 or 3-dimensional image of the carotid, indicating the degree of blockage.
- **Angiogram** shows the degree of blockage and blood flow.

Carotid endarterectomy involves clamping the carotids and then opening and removing the plaque that is occluding the artery. A shunt may be inserted during the procedure to ensure blood supply to the brain. Postoperative complications may include:
- Hematoma may obstruct respiration.
- Hypertension, especially in the first 48 postoperative hours, may increase neurologic impairment and hematoma.
- Hypotension usually resolves in 24-48 hours but may indicate myocardial infarction.
- Hyperperfusion syndrome caused by inadequate vasoconstriction of vessels dilated from long-term diminished blood flow can cause hemorrhage and edema, usually identified by severe unilateral headache relieved by raising head. Hemorrhage may be fatal or cause severe impairment.

Acute cardiac-related pulmonary edema

Acute cardiac-related pulmonary edema may result from MI, chronic HF, volume overload, ischemia, or mitral stenosis. Symptoms include severe dyspnea, cough with blood-tinged frothy sputum, cyanosis, and diaphoresis. Patients have obvious wheeze with rales and rhonchi present throughout lung fields. Diagnosis is by auscultation, chest x-ray, and echocardiogram. Treatment includes:

- Sitting position with 100% oxygen by mask to achieve PO_2 >60%.
- Non-invasive pressure support ventilation (BiPAP) or endotracheal intubation and mechanical ventilation, depending upon severity of condition.
- Morphine sulfate 2-8 mg (IV for severe cases), repeated every 2-4 hours as needed.
- IV diuretics (furosemide ≥40 mg or bumetanide ≥1 mg) to provide venous dilation and diuresis.
- Nitrates, such as SL nitroglycerin or isosorbide, topical nitroglycerin, or IV nitrates, OR IV nesiritide as a bolus with an infusion.
- Inhaled β-adrenergic agonists or aminophylline for bronchospasm.
- Digoxin IV for tachycardia.
- ACE inhibitors, nitroprusside to reduce afterload.

Cardiac surgical options

There are a number of different surgical options for repair of cardiac valves:

- **Valvotomy/ Valvuloplasty** is usually done through cardiac catheterization. A valvotomy/valvuloplasty may involve releasing valve leaflet adhesions interfering with functioning of the valve. In balloon valvuloplasty, a catheter with an inflatable balloon is positioned in the stenotic valve and inflated and deflated a number of times to dilate the opening.
- **Aortic valve replacement** is an open-heart procedure with cardiopulmonary bypass. Aortic valves are tricuspid (3 leaflets) and repair is usually not possible, so defective valves must be replaced with either mechanical (metal, plastic, or pyrolytic carbon) or biological (porcine or bovine xenografts).
- **Aortic homograft** uses part of a donor's aorta with the aortic valve attached to replace the recipient's faulty aortic valve and part of the ascending aorta.
- **Ross procedure** uses the patient's pulmonary artery with the pulmonary valve to replace the aortic valve and part of the aorta and then uses a donor graft to replace the pulmonary artery.

Intraaortic balloon pump

The intraaortic balloon pump (IABP) is the most commonly used circulatory assist device. It is used for a number of problems:

- After cardiac surgery to treat left ventricular failure.
- Unstable angina.
- Myocardial infarction with complications or persistent angina.
- Cardiogenic shock.
- Papillary muscle dysfunction or rupture with mitral regurgitation or ventricular septal rupture.
- Ventricular dysrhythmias that don't respond to treatment.

The IABP comprises a catheter with an inflatable balloon from the tip and lengthwise down the catheter. The catheter is usually inserted through the femoral artery but may be placed during surgery or through a cutdown. The catheter is threaded into the descending thoracis aorta, and the balloon inflates during diastole to increase circulation to the coronary arteries, and then deflates during systole to decrease afterload. IABP should be avoided in patients with aortic valve issue and large aortic aneurysms. Complications include:

- Dysrhythmias.
- Peripheral ischemia from femoral artery occlusion.
- Balloon perforation or migration.

Percutaneous coronary interventions

Percutaneous transluminal coronary angioplasty (PTCA) is a reperfusion option for patients. The decision to use PTCA versus CABG is based on multiple factors, including symptoms, severity of CAD, EF, comorbidities, number of blocked arteries, and degree of narrowing of arteries. This procedure is done to increase circulation to the myocardium by breaking through an atheroma if there is collateral circulation. Cardiac catheterization is done with a hollow catheter (sheath), usually inserted into the femoral vein or artery and fed through the vessels to the coronary arteries. When the atheroma is verified by fluoroscopy, a balloon-tipped catheter is fed over the sheath and the balloon is inflated with a contrast agent, to a specified pressure to compress the atheroma. The balloon may be inflated a number of times to ensure that residual stenosis is <20%. Laser angioplasty using the excimer laser is also used to vaporize plaque. Stents may be inserted during the angioplasty to maintain patency. Stents may be flexible plastic or wire mesh and are typically placed over the catheter, which is inflated to expand the stent against the arterial wall.

Intraoperative and postoperative complications of cardiac catheterization and PTCA

Cardiac catheterization and PTCA poses the risk of both intraoperative and postoperative complications. During the procedure, there is a risk of damage to both the coronary artery and the heart itself. The artery may dissect, perforate, or constrict with vasospasm. A myocardial infarction may occur when a clot dislodges. Ventricular tachycardia or cardiac arrest may occur. These complications may require immediate surgical repair. Postoperative complications of cardiac catheterization/PTCA include:

- **Hemorrhage or hematoma** at sheath insertion site may require pressure. Head of bed should be flat to relieve pressure.
- **Thrombus or embolus** may require further surgery and/or anticoagulation/thrombolytic treatment.
- **Arteriovenous fistula or pseudoaneurysm** from vessel trauma usually requires compression with ultrasound and surgical repair.
- **Retroperitoneal bleeding** from an arterial tear may cause back or flank pain and may require discontinuation of anticoagulants and IV fluids and/or blood transfusions.
- **Failure of angioplasty** may require repeat procedure or other surgical intervention.

Directional coronary atherectomy, rotational atherectomy, and transluminal extraction

Directional coronary atherectomy (DCA) is removal of an atheroma from an occluded coronary artery. This procedure may be more effective in some cases than angioplasty because instead of compressing an atheroma, it shaves it away. Sometimes angioplasty is the first step in DCA if the vessel is too narrow for the DCA catheter and the last step if the tissue needs smoothing. The DCA catheter is a large balloon catheter that is usually inserted over a sheath through the femoral artery. The catheter includes an open window on one side of the balloon with a rotational cutting piston that shaves the atheroma with the plaque residue pushed inside the device for removal. The procedure may require 4-20 cuts, depending upon the extent of the plaque. A similar procedure is rotational atherectomy (ROTA), which uses a catheter with a diamond-chip drill at the tip, rotating at 130,000-180,000 rpms, pulverizing the atheroma into microparticles. Transluminal extraction catheter uses a motorized cutting head with a suction device for residue.

Transmyocardial laser revascularization

Transmyocardial laser revascularization (TMR) may be done percutaneously or through a surgical procedure with a midsternal or thoracotomy incision. Percutaneously, a fiberoptic catheter is positioned inside the ventricle and against the ischemic area. Laser bursts are used to cut 20-40 channels into but not through the myocardium. The laser burns create channels and stimulate an inflammatory response, which causes new blood vessels to form (angiogenesis), improving circulation to the myocardium and reducing ischemia and pain. If the procedure is done surgically, the catheter tip is positioned on the outside of the left ventricle rather than the inside while the heart is beating without bypass. While studies indicate that these do not affect mortality, they do reduce symptoms and increase tolerance to activity, improving the quality of life. Postoperative care for the percutaneous procedure is as for PTCA while care for the surgical procedure is similar to that of coronary artery bypass graft (CABG).

Coronary artery bypass graft (CABG)

Coronary artery bypass graft (CABG) is a surgical procedure for treatment of angina that does not respond to medical treatment, unstable angina, blockage of >60% in left main coronary artery, blockage of multiple coronary arteries that include the proximal left anterior descending artery, left ventricular dysfunction, and previous unsuccessful PCIs. The surgery is performed through a midsternal incision that exposes the heart, which is chilled and placed on cardiopulmonary bypass with blood going from the right atrium to the machine and back to the body while the aorta is clamped to keep the surgical field free of blood. Bypass grafts are sutured into place to bypass areas of occluded coronary arteries. Grafts may be obtained from various sites:
- Gastroepiploic artery.
- Internal mammary artery (commonly used and superior to saphenous vein but procedure is more time-consuming).
- Radial artery.
- Saphenous vein (commonly used, especially for emergency procedures).

Minimally-invasive direct coronary artery bypass

Minimally-invasive direct coronary artery bypass (MIDCAB) applies a bypass graft on the beating heart through a 10 cm incision in the mid chest rather than midsternally, without using cardiopulmonary bypass. Because the incision must be over the bypass area, this procedure is suitable only for bypass of one or two coronary arteries, usually on the left side of the heart. A small portion or rib is removed to allow access to the heart and the internal mammary artery is used for grafting. Special instruments, such as a heart stabilizer, are used to limited movement of the heart during suturing.

Surgery usually takes 2-3 hours and recovery time is decreased as patients have less pain. Because anastomosis is difficult on a beating heart, complications such as ischemia may occur during

- 11 -

surgery so a cardiopulmonary bypass machine must be available. Early studies indicate that MIDCAB may provide longer-lasting relief than angioplasty for single vessel occlusion.

Port access coronary artery bypass graft

Port access coronary artery bypass graft is an alternative form of CABG that utilizes a number of small incisions (ports) along with cardiopulmonary bypass (CPB) and cardioplegia to do a video-assisted surgical repair. Usually 3 or more incisions are required, with one in the femoral area to allow access to the femoral artery for a multipurpose catheter that is threaded through to the ascending aorta to return blood from the CPB, block the aorta with a balloon, provide cardioplegic solution, and vent air. Another catheter is threaded through the femoral vein to the right atrium to carry blood to the CPB. An incision is also needed for access to the jugular vein for catheters to the pulmonary artery and the coronary sinus. One to three thoracotomy incisions are made for insertion of video imaging equipment and instruments. While the midsternal incision is avoided, multiple incisions pose the potential for possible morbidity.

Postoperative care of CABG and other cardiac surgeries

The postoperative care of cardiac surgery patients requires careful medical management:
- Cardiovascular support to maintain adequate cardiac output may require adjustment in HR, preload, afterload, and contractibility.
- Regulation of temperature following hypothermia induced during surgery requires warming, but not above 37°C.
- Bleeding must be monitored carefully and autotransfusion devices may be used to replace red blood cells.
- Chest tubes must be monitored for patency. "Milking" may cause less tissue damage than "stripping,"
- Cardiac tamponade may occur if blood accumulates about the heart, requiring surgical intervention.
- Respiratory care includes early extubation (usually within 4-8 hours). Supplemental oxygen as needed.
- Neurological monitoring for *postcardiotomy delirium* (disorientation progressing to agitation, hallucinations, and paranoia).
- The most effective prophylactic antibiotics for SSI associated with cardiac surgery are cephalosporins.
- Patients may need insulin infusions to maintain glucose levels between 80-150 mg/dL to lower risk of infection (Note: The results from intensive insulin therapy trials on mortality are controversial but all studies show a decrease in blood stream infection, acute renal failure and critical care polymyoneuropathy) .
- UOP should be carefully monitored/reported if <20-30 ml/hr.

Glycoprotein IIB/IIIA Inhibitors

Glycoprotein IIB/IIIA Inhibitors are drugs that are used to inhibit platelet binding and prevent clots prior to and following invasive cardiac procedures, such as angioplasty and stent placement. These medications are used in combination with anticoagulant drugs, such as heparin and aspirin for the following:
- Acute coronary syndromes (ACD), such as unstable angina or myocardial infarctions.
- Percutaneous coronary intervention (PCI), such as angioplasty and stent placement.

These medications are contraindicated in those with a low platelet count or active bleeding:

- **Abciximab** (ReoPro®): Used with both heparin and aspirin for ACS and PCI and affects platelet binding for 48 hours after administration.
- **Eptifibatide** (Integrillin®): Used with both heparin and aspirin for ACS and PCI and affects platelet binding for 6-8 hours after administration. Should not be used with renal problems.
- **Tirofiban** (Aggrastat®): Used with heparin for PCI patients, with reduced dosage for those with renal problems, and affects platelet blinding for only 4-8 hours after administration

Pericardiocentesis

Pericardiocentesis is done with ultrasound guidance to diagnose pericardial effusion or with ECG or ultrasound guidance to relieve cardiac tamponade. Pericardiocentesis may be done as treatment for cardiac arrest or with presentation of PEA with increased jugular venous pressure. Non-hemorrhagic tamponade may be relieved in 60-90% of cases, but hemorrhagic tamponade requires thoracotomy, as blood will continue to accumulate until cause of hemorrhage is corrected. Resuscitation equipment must be available, including a defibrillator, intravenous line in place and cardiac monitoring:

- Chest is elevated to 45° to bring heart closer to chest wall.
- Premedication with atropine may prevent vasovagal reactions.
- If abdominal distention present, a nasogastric tube should be inserted.
- After insertion of the needle, the obturator is removed and a syringe attached for aspiration. A sterile alligator clamp is attached from the needle to any precordial lead of the ECG for monitoring to ensure that the ventricle is not punctured.
- Post procedure chest x-ray should be done to check for pneumothorax.

Blunt cardiac trauma

Blunt cardiac trauma, including myocardial contusions, concussions and ruptures, most often occurs as the result of motor vehicle accidents, falls, or other blows to the chest, which can result in respiratory distress as well as hypovolemia from rupture of the great vessels or the heart and/or cardiac failure from cardiac tamponade or increasing intrathoracic pressure. The heart is particularly vulnerable to chest trauma, with the right atrium and right ventricle the most commonly injured because they are anterior to the rest of the heart. Cardiac trauma may be difficult to diagnose because of other injuries, but if suspected, the patient should be evaluated and an ECG should be done and if any abnormalities (dysrhythmias, ST changes, sinus tachycardia, or heart block) are present, continuous monitoring with should be done for 24-48 hours. Although the most effective test to evaluate for blunt cardiac trauma isn't agreed upon, echocardiogram in conjunction with CPK MB levels is useful in predicting complications. Decreased cardiac output and cerebral oxygenation may result in severe agitation with combative behavior, so changes in mentation should be monitored. Medications may be needed to control arrhythmias and pain.

Traumatic injury to the great vessels

Traumatic injuries to the great vessels most commonly result from severe decelerating blunt force or penetrating injuries, with aortic trauma the most common. If the aorta is torn, it will result in almost instant death, but in some cases, there is an incomplete laceration to the intimal lining (innermost membrane) of the aorta, causing an aortic hematoma or bulging. This lining, the adventitia, is quite strong and often will contain the rupture long enough to allow surgical repair. Other vessels may be injured as well, so careful examination must be done. Diagnosis is made initially with chest x-ray or CT, which may show widening of the mediastinum and a misshapen aorta. If there are indications of injury, an aortogram or a combination of CT and transesophageal echocardiogram may be used to verify the injury. Treatment requires surgical repair to avoid eventual rupture, during which other vessels are examined for clotting or internal injuries.

Penetrating cardiac injuries

The incidence of penetrating cardiac injuries has been on the rise, primarily associated with gunshot injuries and stabbings. The extent of damage caused by a stab wound is often easier to assess than gunshot wounds, which may be multiple and often result in unpredictable and widespread damage not only to the heart but other structures.

The primary complications:
- Exsanguination is frequently related to gunshot wounds, and prognosis is very poor. This may lead to hemothorax and hemorrhagic shock.
- Cardiac tamponade (compression of the heart from bleeding into the pericardial sac) is more common with knife wounds, but prognosis is fairly good with surgical repair. Cardiac tamponade often presents with three classic symptoms, known as Beck's triad that should be quickly recognized: muffled heart sounds, low arterial blood pressure, and jugular vein distention.
- Pneumothorax is an irregular amount of air coming between the lungs and chest wall that forces the lung to collapse. Small injuries will heal in time, and more complicated injuries require a tube or syringe for removal of excess air.

Mortality rates are very high in the first hour after a penetrating cardiac injury, so it is imperative the injured be taken immediately to a trauma center rather than attempts made to stabilize the person at the site. Management includes controlling bleeding, giving fluids and pressors for bp, preparing patient for surgery, and monitoring for the above mentioned complications.

Cardiogenic shock

Cardiogenic shock in adults most often is secondary to myocardial infarction damage that reduces the contractibility of the ventricles, interfering with the pumping mechanism of the heart, decreasing oxygen perfusion. Cardiogenic shock has 3 characteristics: Increased preload, increased afterload, and decreased contractibility. Together these result in a decreased cardiac output and an increase in systemic vascular resistance (SVR) to compensate and protect vital organs. This results in an increase of afterload in the left ventricle with increased need for oxygen. As the cardiac output continues to decrease, tissue perfusion decreases, coronary artery perfusion decreases, fluid backs up and the left ventricle fails to adequately pump the blood, resulting in pulmonary edema and right ventricular failure. Decreasing oxygen consumption is a major initial goal of cardiogenic shock.

Symptoms:
- Hypotension with systolic BP <90 mm Hg.
- Tachycardia > 100 beats/min with weak thready pulse and dysrhythmias.
- Decreased heart sounds.
- Chest pain.

- Tachypnea and basilar rales.
- Cool, moist skin, pallor.

Treatment:
- IV fluids.
- Inotropic agents.
- Anti-dysrhythmics.
- IAB pump or left ventricular assist device.

Hypertrophic cardiomyopathy

Hypertrophic cardiomyopathy (also known as asymmetric septal hypertrophy) is a rare genetic and occasionally idiopathic disorder that is often undetected until adolescence when the increasing symptoms become noticeable. With hypertrophic cardiomyopathy, the heart mass and size increase, especially with thickness along the septum, resulting in smaller ventricular capacity so that the ventricles fill less efficiently and the atria have to work harder. This thickening may be asymmetrical. The disease may be nonobstructive or obstructive. The increased size of the septum may pull structures, such as the mitral valve, out of alignment, causing some obstruction of the flow of blood through the valve to the aorta (idiopathic hypertrophic subaortic stenosis). The changes in the ventricles may result in increasing diastolic abnormalities although systolic function is usually normal or high. When diagnosed in young people, the disease is often more severe than in those who are diagnosed later in life.

Dilated cardiomyopathy

Dilated cardiomyopathy, the most frequently occurring type of cardiomyopathy, occurs with an increase in the size of the ventricles (without a concomitant increase in hypertrophy of the ventricular muscle) as well as systolic dysfunction. The tissue loses elasticity and areas of myocardial cells become necrotic. This loss in elasticity results in less blood being ejected during ventricular systole so that, during diastole, less blood is able to enter the partially-filled ventricles. This results in both an increase in pressure at the end of diastole but also an increase in pulmonary pressure. As the ventricles stretch, the valves may be displaced, causing regurgitation. The poor blood flow can also cause thrombus formation and emboli. Many different conditions can cause dilated cardiomyopathy, including pregnancy, alcoholism, toxic compounds, autoimmune disease, and viral infections. Progression of the disease is often very slow, so diagnosis may be delayed until the disease is advanced and the patient suffers heart failure.

Restrictive cardiomyopathy

Restrictive cardiomyopathy is the least common type of cardiomyopathy, but it is a common complication of heart transplants although, ironically, one of the treatments for this disorder is heart transplantation. The condition may be idiopathic or secondary. The disease is often related to amyloidosis, a condition in which the protein amyloid is deposited in the cells, but many times the cause is unknown. While the heart may be almost normal in size, the ventricular walls become increasingly fibrotic and rigid so that the ventricles cannot relax and fill adequately during diastole. As the disease progresses, the ventricles also are unable to contract effectively, reducing blood flow, and increasing pulmonary and peripheral and systemic edema. Because there is no cure, early diagnosis and management of symptoms is important. The condition most commonly occurs in children but can affect young adults. Medical treatment includes the use of β-blockers to allow the ventricles to fill more effectively.

Cardiac dysrhythmias

Cardiac dysrhythmias, abnormal heart beats, in adults are frequently the result of damage to the conduction system during major cardiac surgery or as the result of a myocardial infarction.

Bradydysrhythmias are pulse rates that are abnormally slow:
- Complete atrioventricular block (A-V block) may be congenital or a response to surgical trauma.
- Sinus bradycardia may be caused by the autonomic nervous system or a response to hypotension and decrease in oxygenation.
- Junctional/nodal rhythms often occur in post-surgical patients when absence of P wave is noted but heart rate and output usually remain stable, and unless there is compromise, usually no treatment is necessary.

Tachydysrhythmias are pulse rates that are abnormally fast:
- Sinus tachycardia is often caused by illness, such as fever or infection.
- Supraventricular tachycardia (200-300 BPM) may have a sudden onset and result in congestive heart failure.

Conduction irregularities are irregular pulses that often occur post-operatively and are usually not significant. Premature contractions may arise from the atria or ventricles.

Electrocardiogram (PQRSTU)

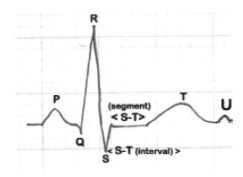

The electrocardiogram records and shows a graphic display of the electrical activity of the heart through a number of different waveforms, complexes, and intervals:
- P wave: Start of electrical impulse in the sinus node and spreading through the atria, muscle depolarization.
- QRS complex: Ventricular muscle depolarization and atrial repolarization.
- T wave: Ventricular muscle repolarization (resting state) as cells regain negative charge.
- U wave: Repolarization of the Purkinje fibers.

A modified lead II ECG is often used to monitor basic heart rhythms and dysrhythmias:

Typical placement of leads for 2-lead ECG is 3 to 5 cm inferior to the right clavicle and left lower ribcage. Typical placement for 3-lead ECG is (RA) right arm near shoulder, (LA) V$_5$ position over 5th intercostal space, and (LL) left upper leg near groin.

Administration of 12 lead ECG

The electrocardiogram provides a graphic representation of the electrical activity of the heart. It is indicated for chest pain, dyspnea, syncope, acute coronary syndrome, pulmonary embolism, and possible MI. The standard 12 lead ECG gives a picture of electrical activity from 12 perspectives through placement of 10 body leads:
- 4 limb leads are placed distally on the wrists and ankles (but may be placed more proximally if necessary),
- Precordial leads:
  - V1: right sternal border at 4th intercostal space
  - V2: left sternal border at 4th intercostal space
  - V3: Midway between V2 and V4
  - V4: Left midclavicular line at 5th intercostal space.
  - V5: Horizontal to V4 at left anterior axillary line.
  - V6: Horizontal to V5 at left midaxillary line.

In some cases, additional leads may be used: Right-sided leads are placed on the right in a mirror image of the left leads, usually to diagnose right ventricular infarction through ST elevation.

Assessment of heart sounds

Auscultation of heart sounds can help to diagnose different cardiac disorders. Areas to auscultate include the aortic area, pulmonary area, Erb's point, tricuspid area, and the apical area. The normal heart sounds represent closing of the valves.
- The first heart sound (S1) "lub" is closure of the mitral and tricuspid valves (heard at apex/left ventricular area of the heart).
- The second heart sound (S2) "dub" is closure of the aortic and pulmonic valves (heard at the base of the heart). There may be a slight splitting of the S2.

The time between S1 and S2 is systole and the time between S2 and the next S1 is diastole. Systole and diastole should be silent although ventricular disease can cause gallops, snaps, or clicks and stenosis of the valves or failure of the valves to close can cause murmurs. Pericarditis may cause a friction rub.

Additional heart sounds

Gallop rhythms: *S3* occurs after S2 in children and young adults but may indicate heart failure or left ventricular failure in older adults (heard with patient lying on left side). *S4* occurs before S1, during the contracting of the atria when there is ventricular hypertrophy, such as from coronary artery disease, hypertension, or aortic valve stenosis.

Opening snap: Unusual high-pitched sound occurring after S2 with stenosis of mitral valve from rheumatic heart disease.

Ejection click: Brief high-pitched sound occurring immediately after S1 with stenosis of the aortic valve.

Friction rub: Harsh, grating sound heard in systole and diastole with pericarditis.

Murmur: Sound caused by turbulent blood flow from stenotic or malfunctioning valves, congenital defects, or increased blood flow. Murmurs are characterized by location, timing in the cardiac cycle, intensity (rated from Grade I to Grade VI), pitch (low to high-pitched), quality (rumbling, whistling, blowing) and radiation (to the carotids, axilla, neck, shoulder, or back).

Assessing jugular venous pressure

Jugular venous pressure (neck-vein) is used to assess the cardiac output and pressure in the right heart as the pulsations relate to changes in pressure in the right atrium. This procedure is usually not accurate if pulse rate is >100. This is a non-invasive estimation of central venous pressure and waveform. Measurement should be done with the internal jugular if possible; if not, the external jugular may be used.
- Elevate the patient's head to 45° (and to 90° if necessary) with patient's head turned to the right.
- Position light at an angle to illuminate veins and shadows.
- Measure the height of the jugular vein pulsation above the sternal joint, using a ruler.
  o Normal height is ≤ 4 cm above sternal angle

Increased pressure (> 4 cm) indicates increased pressure in right atrium, and right heart failure. It may also indicate pericarditis or tricuspid stenosis. Laughing or coughing may trigger the valsalva response and also cause an increase.

Sinus bradycardia

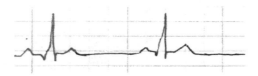

There are 3 primary types of sinus node dysrhythmias: sinus bradycardia, sinus tachycardia, and sinus arrhythmia. Sinus bradycardia (SB) is caused by a decreased rate of impulse from sinus node. The pulse and ECG usually appear normal except for a slower rate.

SB is characterized by a regular pulse <50 to 60 with P waves in front of QRS, which are usually normal in shape and duration. PR interval is 0.12 to 0.20 seconds, QRS interval 0.04 to 0.11 seconds, and P:QRS ratio of 1:1. SB may be caused by a number of factors:
- Conditions that lower the body's metabolic needs, such as hypothermia or sleep.
- Hypotension and decrease in oxygenation.
- Medications such as calcium channel blockers and β-blockers.
- Vagal stimulation that may result from vomiting, suctioning, or defecating.
- Increased intracranial pressure.
- Myocardial infarction.

Treatment involves eliminating cause if possible, such as changing medications. Atropine 0.5-1.0 mg may be given IV to block vagal stimulation.

Sinus tachycardia

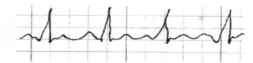

Sinus tachycardia (ST) occurs when the sinus node impulse increases in frequency. ST is characterized by a regular pulse >100 with P waves before QRS but sometimes part of preceding T wave. QRS is usually of normal shape and duration (0.04 to 0.11 seconds) but may have consistent irregularity. PR interval is 0.12-0.20 seconds and P: QRS ratio of 1:1. The rapid pulse decreases diastolic filling time and causes reduced cardiac output with resultant hypotension. Acute pulmonary edema may result from the decreased ventricular filling if untreated. ST may be caused by a number of factors:

- Acute blood loss, shock, hypovolemia, anemia.
- Sinus arrhythmia, hypovolemic heart failure.
- Hypermetabolic conditions, fever, infection.
- Exertion/exercise, anxiety.
- Medications, such as sympathomimetic drugs.

Treatment includes eliminating precipitating factors and calcium channel blockers and β-blockers to reduce heart rate.

Supraventricular tachycardia

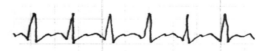

Supraventricular tachycardia (SVT) (>100 BPM may have a sudden onset and result in congestive heart failure. Rate may increase to 200 to 300 BMP. SVT originates in the atria rather than the ventricles but is controlled by the tissue in the area of the AV node rather than the SA node. Rhythm is usually rapid but regular. The P wave is present but may not be clearly defined as it may be obscured by the preceding T wave, and the QRS complex appears normal. The PR interval is 0.12 to 0.20 seconds and QRS interval 0.04 to 0.11 seconds with P: QRS ratio of 1:1. SVT may be episodic with periods of normal heart rate and rhythm between episodes of SVT, so it is often referred to as paroxysmal SVT (PSVT).

Sinus arrhythmia

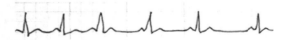

Sinus arrhythmia (SA) results from irregular impulses from the sinus node, often paradoxical (increasing with inspiration and decreasing with expiration) because of stimulation of the vagal nerve during inspiration and rarely causes a negative hemodynamic effect. These cyclic changes in the pulse during respiration are quite common in both children and young adults and often lessen with age but may persist in some adults. Sinus arrhythmia can, in some cases, relate to heart or valvular disease and may be increased with vagal stimulation for suctioning, vomiting, or defecating. Characteristics of SA include a regular pulse 50-100, P waves in front of QRS with duration (0.4 to 0.11 seconds) and shape of QRS usually normal, PR interval of 0.12 to 0.20 seconds, and P: QRS ratio of 1:1. Treatment is usually not necessary unless it is associated with bradycardia.

Premature atrial contractions

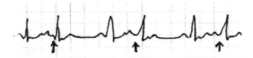

There are 3 primary types of atrial dysrhythmias, including premature atrial contractions, atrial flutter, and atrial fibrillation. Premature atrial contraction (PAC) is essentially an extra beat precipitated by an electrical impulse to the atrium before the sinus node impulse. The extra beat may be caused by alcohol, caffeine, nicotine, hypervolemia, hypokalemia, hypermetabolic conditions, atrial ischemia or infarction. Characteristics include an irregular pulse because of extra P waves, shape and duration of QRS is usually normal (0.04 to 0.11 seconds) but may be abnormal, PR interval remains between 0.12 to 0.20, and P: QRS ratio is 1:1. Rhythm is irregular with varying P-P and R-R intervals. PACs can occur in an essentially healthy heart and are not usually cause for concern unless they are frequent (>6 hr) and cause severe palpitations. In that case, atrial fibrillation should be suspected.

Atrial flutter

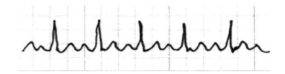

Atrial flutter (AF) occurs when the atrial rate is faster, usually 250-400 beats per minute, than the AV node conduction rate so not all of the beats are conducted into the ventricles, effectively blocked at the AV node, preventing ventricular fibrillation although some extra ventricular impulses may pass though. AF is caused by the same conditions that cause afib: coronary artery disease, valvular disease, pulmonary disease, heavy alcohol ingestion, and cardiac surgery. AF is characterized by atrial rates of 250-400 with ventricular rates of 75-150, with ventricular rate usually regular. P waves are saw-toothed (referred to as F waves), QRS shape and duration (0.4 to 0.11 seconds) are usually normal, PR interval may be hard to calculate because of F waves, and the P:QRS ratio is 2-4:1. Symptoms include chest pain, dyspnea, and hypotension.

Treatment includes: Cardioversion if condition is unstable.

Medications to slow ventricular rate and conduction through AV node: nondihydropiridine calcium channel blockers (Cardizem®, Calan®) and beta blockers.

Medications to convert to sinus rhythm: Corvert® (this is the only med approved by FDA for converting aflutter but the following are often used in practice: Cardioquin®, Norpace®, Cordarone®.)

Atrial fibrillation

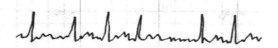

Atrial fibrillation (Afib) is rapid, disorganized atrial beats that are ineffective in emptying the atria, so that blood pools and can lead to thrombus formation and emboli.

The ventricular rate increases with a decreased stroke volume, and cardiac output decreases with increased myocardial ischemia, resulting in palpitations and fatigue. Afib is caused by coronary artery disease, valvular disease, pulmonary disease, heavy alcohol ingestion, and cardiac surgery. Afib in characterized by very irregular pulse with atrial rate of 300-600 and ventricular rate of 120-200, shape and duration (0.4 to 0.11 seconds) of QRS is usually normal. Fibrillatory (F) waves are seen instead of P waves. The PR interval cannot be measured and the P: QRS ratio is highly variable. Score as Afib during sleep with irregularly irregular ventricular rhythm and varying rapid oscillations replacing P waves.

In the patient with new onset afib, investigation into the precipitating and reversible causes of afib should be investigated and corrected. The decision tree to treat afib involves determining if the afib is paroxysmal, persistent, or permanent, as well as if the patient is symptomatic. Correcting rhythm, rate control, prevention of thromboembolism are the goals of afib care. For pharmacologic cardioversion of afib present <7 days use ibutilide, propafenone, dofetilide, or flecainide. To control ventricular rate, β-blockers, diltiazem, and verapamil (amiodarone and digoxin in patients with HF without accessory pathway) are indicated. For maintenance of rhythm current research indicates amiodarone, disopyramide, dofetilide, flecainide, procainamide, propafenone, quinidine, and sotalol (with dofetilide and sotalol, dose-adjust for kidney function and close monitoring of QT interval is indicated when initiated). For antithrombotic therapy with no risk factors: aspirin, with one moderate risk factor: aspirin or warfarin, and with high risk: warfarin. For patients on warfarin, INR range is 2.0 to 3.0. High risk factors are mitral valve stenosis, mechanical heart valve, history of CVA, TIA, or embolism. For symptomatic afib patients unable to convert to sinus rhythm with pharmacological intervention, after reversible or precipitating factors have been examined, catheter ablation is usually indicated.

Premature junctional contractions

The area around the AV node is the junction, and dysrhythmias that arise from that are called junctional dysrhythmias. Premature junctional contractions (PJCs) occur when a premature impulse starts at the AV node before the next normal sinus impulse reaches the AV node. PJCs are similar to premature atrial contractions (PACs) and generally require no treatment although they may be an indication of digoxin toxicity. The ECG may appear basically normal with an early QRS complex that is normal in shape and duration (0.4 to 0.11 seconds). The P wave may be absent, precede, be part of, or follow the QRS. The P:QRS ratio may vary from <1:1 to 1:1 (with inverted P

- 21 -

wave). Rhythm is usually regular at a heart rate of 40 to 60 BPM. Significant symptoms related to premature junctional contractions are rare.

Junctional rhythms

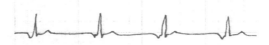

Junctional rhythms occur when the AV node becomes the pacemaker of the heart because the sinus node is depressed from increased vagal tone or a block at the AV node prevents sinus node impulses from being transmitted. While the sinus node normally sends impulses 60-100 beats per minute, the AV node junction usually sends impulses at 40-60 beats per minute. The QRS complex is of usual shape and duration (0.4 to 0.11 seconds). The P wave may be inverted and may be absent, hidden or after the QRS. If the P wave precedes the QRS, the PR interval is <0.12 seconds. The P:QRS ratio is <1:1 or 1:1. The junctional escape rhythm is a protective mechanism preventing asystole with failure of the sinus node.

An accelerated junctional rhythm is similar, but the heart rate is 60 to 100 BPM. Junctional tachycardia occurs with heart rate of >100 BPM.

AV nodal reentry tachycardia

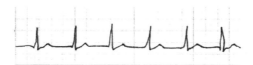

AV nodal reentry tachycardia occurs when an impulse conducts to area of the AV node, and the impulse is sent in a rapidly repeating cycle back to the same area and to the ventricles, resulting in a fast ventricular rate. The onset and cessation are usually rapid. AV nodal reentry tachycardia (also known as paroxysmal atrial tachycardia or supraventricular tachycardia if no P waves) is characterized by atrial rate of 150-250 BPM with ventricular rate of 75-250 BPM, P wave that is difficult to see or absent, QRS complex that is usually normal and a PR interval of <0.12 seconds, if a P wave is present. The P: QRS ratio is 1-2:1. Precipitating factors include nicotine, caffeine, hypoxemia, and anxiety and underlying coronary artery disease and cardiomyopathy. Cardiac output may be decreased with a rapid heart rate, causing dyspnea, chest pain, and hypotension.

Treatment may include:
- Vagal maneuvers (carotid sinus massage, gag reflex, holding breath.
- Medications (adenosine, verapamil, or diltiazem)
- Cardioversion if other methods unsuccessful.

Premature ventricular contractions

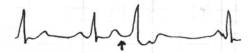

Premature ventricular contractions (PVCs) are those in which the impulse begins in the ventricles and conducts through them prior to the next sinus impulse. The ectopic QRS complexes may vary in shape, depending upon whether there is one site (unifocal) or more (multifocal) that is stimulating the ectopic beats. PVCs usually cause no morbidity unless there is underlying cardiac disease or an acute MI. PVCs are characterized by an irregular heartbeat, QRS that is >0.12 seconds and oddly shaped, P wave that may be absent or may precede or follow the QRS, a PR interval of <0.12 seconds if P wave is present, and a P: QRS rations of 0-1:1. Short-term therapy may include lidocaine, but PVCs are often not treated in otherwise healthy people. PVCs may be precipitated by caffeine, nicotine, or alcohol. Because PVCs may occur with any supraventricular dysrhythmia, the underlying rhythm (such as atrial fibrillation) must be noted as well as the PVCs.

Ventricular tachycardia

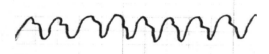

Ventricular tachycardia (VT) is ≥3 PVCs in a row with a ventricular rate of 100-200 beats per minute. Ventricular tachycardia may be triggered by the same factors as PVCs and often is related to underlying coronary artery disease. The rapid rate of contractions make VT dangerous as the ineffective beats may render the person unconscious with no palpable pulse. A detectable rate is usually regular and the QRS complex is ≥0.12 seconds and is usually abnormally shaped. The P wave may be undetectable with an irregular PR interval if P wave is present. The P: QRS ratio is often difficult to ascertain because of absence of P waves.

Narrow complex and wide complex tachycardias

Tachycardias are classified as narrow complex or wide complex. Wide and narrow refer to the configuration of the QRS complex
- **Wide complex tachycardia:** About 80% of cases of WCT are caused by ventricular tachycardia. WCT originates at some point below the AV node and may be associated with palpitations, dyspnea, anxiety, and cardiac arrest. Patients may exhibit diaphoresis. Wide complex tachycardia is diagnosed with ≥3 consecutive beats at a heart rate >100 BPM and QRS duration ≥0.12 seconds.
- **Narrow complex tachycardia:** NCT is associated with palpitations, dyspnea, and peripheral edema. NCT is generally supraventricular in origin. Narrow complex tachycardia is diagnosed with ≥3 consecutive beats at heart rate of >100 BPM and QRS duration of <0.12 seconds.

Ventricular fibrillation

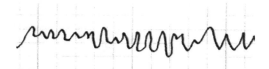

Ventricular fibrillation (VF) is a rapid, very irregular ventricular rate >300 beats per minute with no atrial activity observable on the ECG, caused by disorganized electrical activity in the ventricles. The QRS complex is not recognizable as ECG shows irregular undulations. The causes are the same as for ventricular tachycardia (alcohol, caffeine, nicotine, underlying coronary disease), and VF may result if VT is not treated. VF may also result from an electrical shock or congenital disorder, such as Brugada syndrome. VF is accompanied by lack of palpable pulse, audible pulse, and respirations and is immediately life threatening without defibrillation. After emergency defibrillation, the cause should be identified and limited. Mortality is high if VF occurs as part of a myocardial infarction.

Idioventricular rhythm

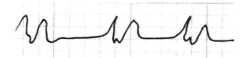

Ventricular escape rhythm (idioventricular) occurs when the Purkinje fibers below the AV node create an impulse. This may occur if the sinus node fails to fire or if there is blockage at the AV node so that the impulse does not go through. Idioventricular rhythm is characterized by a regular ventricular rate of 20-40 BPM. Rates >40 BPM are called accelerated idioventricular rhythm. The P wave is missing and the QRS complex has a very bizarre and abnormal shape with duration of ≥0.12 seconds. The low ventricular rate may cause a decrease in cardiac output, often making the patient lose consciousness. In other patients, the idioventricular rhythm may not be associated with reduced cardiac output.

Ventricular asystole

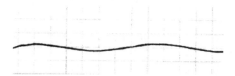

Ventricular asystole is the absence of audible heartbeat, palpable pulse, and respirations, a condition often referred to as "flatlining" or "cardiac arrest." While the ECG may show some P waves initially, the QRS complex is absent although there may be an occasional QRS "escape beat." Cardiopulmonary resuscitation is required with intubation for ventilation and establishment of an intravenous line for fluids. Without immediate treatment, the patient will suffer from severe hypoxia and brain death within minutes. Identifying the cause is critical for the patient's survival and could include hypoxia, acidosis, electrolyte imbalance, hypothermia, or drug overdose. Even with immediate treatment, the prognosis is poor and ventricular asystole is often a sign of impending death.

Sinus pause

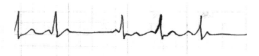

Sinus pause occurs when the sinus node fails to function properly to stimulate heart contractions and the P wave, so there is a pause on the ECG recording that may persist for a few seconds to minutes, depending on the severity of the dysfunction. A prolonged pause may be difficult to differentiate from cardiac arrest. During the sinus pause, the P wave, QRS complex and PR and QRS intervals are all absent. P: QRS ratio is 1:1 and the rhythm is irregular. The pulse rate may vary widely, usually 60 to 100 BMP. Patients frequently complain of dizziness or syncope.

Temporary transvenous pacemakers

Transvenous pacemakers, comprised of a catheter with a lead at the end, may be used prophylactically or therapeutically on a temporary basis to treat a cardiac abnormality, especially bradycardia. The catheter is inserted through a vein at the femoral or neck area and attached to an external pulse generator. Clinical uses include:
- To treat persistent dysrhythmias not responsive to medications.
- To increase cardiac output with bradydysrhythmia by increasing rate.
- To decrease ventricular or supraventricular tachycardia by "overdrive" stimulation of contractions.
- To treat secondary heart block caused by myocardial infarction, ischemia, and drug toxicity.
- To improve cardiac output after cardiac surgery.
- To provide diagnostic information through electrophysiology studies, which induce dysrhythmias for purposes of evaluation.
- To provide pacing when a permanent pacemaker malfunctions.

Complications are similar to implanted pacemakers and include increased risk of pacemaker syndrome.

Transcutaneous pacing

Transcutaneous pacing is used temporarily to treat bradydysrhythmia that doesn't respond to medications (atropine) and results in hemodynamic instability. Generally, an arterial line is placed and the patient provided oxygen before the pacing. The placement of pacing pads (large self-adhesive pads) and ECG leads varies somewhat according to the type of equipment, but usually one pacing pad (negative) is placed on the left chest, inferior to the clavicle, and the other (positive) on the left back, inferior to the scapula, so the heart is sandwiched between the two pads so that the myocardium is depolarized through the chest wall. Lead wires attach the pads to the monitor. The rate of pacing is usually set between 60 and 70 BPM. Current is increased slowly until capture occurs—a spiking followed by QRS sequence, then the current is readjusted downward if possible just to maintain capture. Both demand and fixed modes are available, but demand mode is preferred. Patients may require analgesia, especially if a higher current setting is needed.

Pacemaker syndrome

Pacemaker syndrome can occur with any type of pacemaker if there is inadequate synchronicity between the contractions of the atria and ventricles, resulting in a decrease in cardiac output, and inadequate atrial contribution to filling of ventricles. Total peripheral vascular resistance may increase to maintain blood pressure, but hypotension occurs if it decreases.

Mild
- Pulsations evident in neck and abdomen.
- Cardiac palpitations.
- Headache and feeling of anxiety.
- General malaise and unexplained weakness.
- Pain or "fullness" in jaw, chest.

Moderate
- Increasing dyspnea on exertion with accompanying orthopnea
- Dizziness, vertigo, increasing confusion.
- Feeling of choking.

Severe
- Increasing pulmonary edema with dyspnea even at rest and crackling rales.
- Syncope.
- Heart failure

Pacemaker complications

Pacemakers, transvenous and permanent, are invasive foreign bodies and as such can cause a number of different complications:
- Infection, bleeding, or hematoma may occur at the entry site of leads for temporary pacemakers or at the subcutaneous area of implantation for permanent generators.
- Puncture of the subclavian vein or internal mammary artery may cause a hemothorax.
- The endocardial electrode may irritate the ventricular wall, causing ectopic beats or tachycardia.
- Dislodgement of transvenous lead may lead to malfunction or perforation of the myocardium. This is one of the most common early complications.
- Dislocation of leads may result in phrenic nerve or muscle stimulation (which may be evidenced by hiccupping).
- Cardiac tamponade may result when epicardial wires of temporary pacing are removed.
- General malfunctioning of pacemaker may indicate dislodgement, dislocation, interference caused by electromagnetic fields, and the need for new batteries or generator.
- Pacemaker syndrome.

Cardioversion

Cardioversion is a timed electrical stimulation to the heart to convert a tachydysrhythmia (such as atrial fibrillation) to a normal sinus rhythm. Usually anticoagulation therapy is done for at least 3 weeks prior to elective cardioversion to reduce the risk of emboli and digoxin is discontinued for at least 48 hours prior to cardioversion.

During the procedure, the patient is usually sedated and/or anesthetized. Electrodes in the form of gel-covered paddles or pads are placed in the anteroposterior position, with one pad placed to the right of the sternum, about the 2nd to 3rd intercostal space and the other pad is placed between the left scapula and the spinal column, connected by leads to a computerized ECG and cardiac monitor with a defibrillator. The defibrillator is synchronized with the ECG so that the electrical current is delivered during ventricular depolarization (QRS). The timing must be precise in order to prevent ventricular tachycardia or ventricular fibrillation. Sometimes, drug therapy is used in conjunction with cardioversion; for example, antiarrhythmics (Cardizem®, Cordarone®) may be given before the procedure to slow the heart rate.

Arrythmia

Beginning Monophasic Shock:
A fib: 50-100 J
A flutter: 25-50 J
Vtach (monomorphic asymptomatic): 100-200 J

Beginning Biphasic Shock:
A fib: 25 J
A flutter: 15 J
Vtach (monomorphic asymptomatic): 50 J

Emergency defibrillation

Emergency defibrillation is nonsynchonized shock which is given to treat acute ventricular fibrillation, pulseless ventricular tachycardia, or polymorphic ventricular tachycardia with a rapid rate and decompensating hemodynamics. Defibrillation can be given at any point in the cardiac cycle. Defibrillation causes depolarization of myocardial cells, which can then repolarize to regain a normal sinus rhythm. Defibrillation delivers an electrical discharge through pads/paddles. In an acute care setting, the preferred position to place the pads is the anteroposterior position. In this position one pad is placed to the right of the sternum, about the second to third intercostal space and the other pad is placed between the left scapula and the spinal column. This decreases the chances of damaging implanted devices, such as pacemakers, and this positioning has also been shown to be more effective for external cardioversion (if indicated at some point during resuscitation).

There are two main types of defibrillator shock waveforms, monophasic and biphasic. Biphasic defibrillators deliver a shock one direction for half of the shock, and then in the return direction for the other half, making them more effective, and able to used at lower energy levels. Monophasic defibrillation is given at 200-360 J and biphasic defibrillation is given at 100-200 J.

Systolic heart failure

Systolic heart failure is the typical "left-sided" failure and reduces the amount of blood ejected from the ventricles during contraction (decreased ejection fraction), stimulating the sympathetic nervous system to produce epinephrine and norepinephrine to support the myocardium. However, this eventually causes down regulation in which beta and adrenergic receptor sites are destroyed, causing further myocardial damage. Because of reduced perfusion, the kidneys produce renin, which promotes angiotensin I, which is converted into angiotensin II, a vasoconstrictor, by the blood vessels. This in turns stimulates production of aldosterone, causing sodium and fluid

- 27 -

retention. The end result of these processes is an increase in preload and afterload, increasing the workload on the heart, especially the ventricles. The heart muscle begins to lose contractibility and blood begins to pool in the ventricles during, stretching the myocardium and enlarging the ventricles (ventricular remodeling). The heart compensates by thickening the muscle (hypertrophy) without an adequate increase in capillary blood supply because of the vasoconstriction of the coronary arteries, leading to ischemia. Symptoms include: Activity intolerance, dyspnea, edema, heart sounds S3 and S4, hepatomegaly, JVD, LOC changes, rales, and tachycardia.

Diastolic heart failure

Diastolic heart failure may be difficult to differentiate from systolic heart failure based on clinical symptoms, which are similar. With diastolic heart failure, the myocardium is unable to sufficiently relax to facilitate filling of the ventricles. This may be the end result of systolic heart failure as myocardial hypertrophy stiffens the muscles, and the causes are similar. Diastolic heart failure is more common in females >75. Typically, intracardiac pressures at rest are within normal range but increase markedly on exertion. Because the relaxation of the heart is delayed, the ventricles do not expand enough for the fill-volume, and the heart cannot increase stroke volume during exercise, so symptoms (dyspnea, fatigue, pulmonary edema) are often pronounced on exertion. Ejection fractions are usually >40-50% with increase in left ventricular end-diastolic pressure (LVEDP) and decrease in left ventricular end-diastolic volume (LVEDV). The major goal with all types of heart failure is to prevent further damage and remodeling, prevent exacerbations, and improve the patient's long term prognosis.

Acute heart failure

Acute heart failure is characterized by impairment of gas exchange and decreased cardiac output because of changes in preload, contractibility, and heart rhythm. Patients may also suffer from anxiety, decreased activity tolerance, and disturbances in sleep patterns. Medical management is aimed at increasing cardiac function, providing support, and monitoring treatment.
Treatment may include:
- Careful monitoring of fluid balance and weight to determine changes in fluid retention.
- Low sodium diet.
- Restriction of activity.
- Medications may include diuretics, vasodilators, or ACE inhibitors to decrease the heart's workload. Digoxin may be given to increase contractibility,
- Anticoagulant therapy if distended atria, enlarged ventricles, or atrial fibrillation to decrease the danger of thromboembolia.

Patient education is an important component of heart failure management in order to prevent recurrence. The patient should be an active participant in planning care as the acute condition stabilizes.

Medications for heart failure

Medications used for heart failure include:
- **ACE inhibitors:** Captopril (Capoten®), enalapril (Vasotec®), and lisinopril (Prinivil®) Decrease afterload and preload and reverse ventricular remodeling, but may cause hypotension initially and are contraindicated with renal insufficiency. Side effects include

cough, hyperkalemia, hypotension, angioedema, dizziness, and weakness. Contraindicated with pregnancy and bilateral renal artery stenosis.

- **Angiotensin receptor blockers (ARBs):** Losartan (Cozaar®) and valsartan (Diovan®) Decrease afterload and preload and reverse ventricular remodeling, causing vasodilation and reducing blood pressure. They are used for those who cannot tolerate ACE inhibitors. Side effects include cough (less common than with ACE inhibitors), hyperkalemia, hypotension, headache, dizziness, metallic taste, and rash.
- **β-Blockers:** Metoprolol (Lopressor®), carvedilol (Coreg®) and esmolol (Brevibloc®) Slow the heart rate, reduce hypertension, prevent dysrhythmias, and reverse ventricular remodeling, but should not be used during decompensation and should be monitored carefully for those with airway disease, uncontrolled diabetes, slow irregular pulse, or heart block.
- **Aldosterone agonists:** Spironolactone (Aldactone®) Decreases preload and myocardial hypertrophy and reduces edema and sodium retention but may increase serum potassium.

Vasodilators

Vasodilators may be used for arterial dilation or venous dilation in order to improve cardiac function. These drugs may be used to treat pulmonary hypertension or generalized systemic hypertension. They may be used for those who cannot tolerate ACE inhibitors or angiotensin receptor blockers. Vasodilators may dilate arteries, veins, or both:
- Arterial dilation reduces afterload, improving cardiac output.
- Venous dilation reduces preload, reducing filling pressures.

There are numerous types of vasodilators:

Smooth mucle relaxants
Decrease peripheral vascular resistance but may cause hypotension and headaches:
- Sodium nitroprusside (Nipride®) dilates both arteries and veins and is rapid in action and used for reduction of hypertension and afterload reduction for heart failure.
- Nitroglycerin (Tridil®) primarily dilates veins and is used IV to reduce preload for acute heart failure, unstable angina, and acute MI. Nitroglycerin may also be prophylactically after PCIs to prevent vasospasm.
- Hydralazine (Apresoline®) dilates arteries and is given intermittently to reduce hypertension.

Calcium channel blockers
Primarily arterial vasodilators that may affect the peripheral and/or coronary arteries. Side effects include lethargy, flushing, abdominal and peripheral edema, and indigestion:
- Dihydropyridines, such as nifedipine (Procardia®) (should be avoided in older adults) and nicardipine (Cardene®) are primarily arterial vasodilators affecting both coronary and peripheral arteries, used to treat acute hypertension.
- Benzothiazepines, such as diltiazem (Cardizem®) and phenylalkylamines, such as verapamil (Calan®, Isoptin®) dilate primarily coronary arteries and are used for angina and supraventricular tachycardias.

Angio-tensin-converting enzyme (ACE) inhibitors

Limit production of the peripheral vasoconstricting angiotensin, resulting in vasodilation, which can cause a precipitous fall in blood pressure, so use must be carefully monitored. They are often the first line of drugs to be used for acute hypertension and heart failure and are used to prevent nephropathy in patients with diabetes:

- Captopril (Capoten®) and enalapril (Vasotec®) decrease afterload and preload for heart failure.

B-type natriuretic peptide (BNP) (Nesiritide—Natrecor®)

A new type of vasodilator (non-inotropic), which is a recombinant form of a peptide of the human brain. It decreases filling pressure, vascular resistance, and increases urinary output but may cause hypotension, headache, bradycardia, and nausea. It is used short term for worsening decompensated CHF.

Alpha-adrenergic blockers

Block alpha receptors in arteries and veins, causing vasodilation but may cause orthostatic hypotension and edema from fluid retention:

- Labetalol (Normodyne®) is a combination peripheral alpha-blocker and cardiac β-blocker and is used to treat acute hypertension, acute stroke, and acute aortic dissection.
- Phentolamine (Regitine®) is a peripheral arterial dilator that reduces afterload and is used for pheochromocytoma.

Selective specific dopamine DA-1-receptor agonists Fenoldopam (Corlopam®)

A peripheral dilator affecting renal and mesenteric arteries and can be used for patients with renal dysfunction or those at risk of renal insufficiency.

Inotropic agents

Drugs used to increase cardiac output and improve contractibility of the myocardium for heart failure are the Inotropic agents. Intravenous inotropic agents may increase the risk of death, but may be used when other drugs fail. Oral forms of these drugs are less effective than intravenous. Inotropic agents include:

β-Adrenergic agonists

Dobutamine improves cardiac output, treats cardiac decompensation, and lowers blood pressure. It helps the body to utilize norepinephrine. Side effects include increased systolic blood pressure and heart rate and PVCs (5%), hypotension, and local reactions.

Dopamine improves cardiac output, blood pressure, and the excretion of urine, helping to reduce edema. Side effects include tachycardia or bradycardia, palpitations, BP changes, dyspnea, nausea and vomiting, headache, and gangrene of extremities.

Phosphodies-terase III inhibitors

Milrinone (Primacor®) increases strength of contractions and cause vasodilation. Side effects include ventricular arrhythmias, hypotension, and headaches.

Digoxin (Lanoxin®)

Increases contractibility and cardiac output and prevents arrhythmias.

Digitalis

Digitalis drugs, most commonly administered in the form of digoxin (Lanoxin®), are derived from the foxglove plant and are used to increase myocardial contractility, left ventricular output, and slow conduction through the AV node, decreasing rapid heart rates and promoting diuresis. Digoxin does not affect mortality, but increases tolerance to activity and reduces hospitalizations for heart failure. Therapeutic levels (0.5-2.0 ng/mL) should be maintained to avoid digitalis toxicity, which can occur even if digoxin levels are within therapeutic range, so observation of symptoms is critical. Potassium imbalance may cause toxicity.

Symptoms
- Early signs: Increasing fatigue, lethargy, depression, and nausea and vomiting.
- Sudden change in heart rhythm, such as regular or irregular rhythm, palpitations.
- SA or AV block, new ventricular dysrhythmias, and tachycardia (atrial, junctional, and/or ventricular).
- Bradycardia

Treatment
- Discontinue medication.
- Monitor serum levels and symptoms.
- Digoxin immune FAB (Digibind®) may be used to bind to digoxin and inactivate it if necessary.

Hypertensive crises

Hypertensive crises are marked elevations in blood pressure than can cause severe organ damage if left untreated. Hypertensive crises may be related to primary or secondary hypertension, which may result from kidney or endocrine disorders. Other diseases that may precipitate hypertensive crises include dissection of an aortic aneurysm, pulmonary edema, CNS disorders (subarachnoid hemorrhage, stroke), eclampsia, and failure to take medications properly. There are 2 classifications:
- **Hypertensive emergency** occurs when acute hypertension (1.5 x the 95th percentile), usually >120 mm Hg diastolic, must be treated immediately to lower blood pressure in order to prevent damage to vital organs, such as the heart, brain, or kidneys.
- **Hypertensive urgency** occurs when acute hypertension must be treated within a few hours but the vital organs are not in immediate danger.

Blood pressure is lowered more slowly to avoid hypotension, ischemia of vital organs, or failure of autoregulation.
- 1/3 reduction in 6 hours
- 1/3 reduction in next 24 hours
- 1/3 reduction over days 2-4

Diagnostics include ECG, Chest x-ray, CBC, BMP, Urinalysis (looking for blood and casts).

Hypertensive crisis may be managed by a variety of different medications, depending upon the cause and whether the hypertension is an emergency or urgency. In some cases, medications may be combined. Patients with hypertensive emergency receive IV medications and oxygen.

Medications include:
- Initial: Sodium nitroprusside (Nipride®) for fast-acting vasodilation.
- Short acting β-blockers (labetalol, esmolol) for dissecting aortic aneurysm.
- ACE inhibitors (enalaprilat) for heart failure.
- Nitroglycerin for chest pain.
- Dopamine-receptor agonist (fenoldopam) for renal disease to increase circulation to kidneys.
- Hydralazine for eclampsia.
- Calcium channel blocker (nicardipine) CNS disorders.
- Enalaprilat and labetalol for CNS disorders.
- Alpha-blocker (phentolamine) for pheochromocytoma.
- Diuretics, such as Lasix® and bumetanide to reduce edema.

Continuous monitoring of BP must be done and patient observed for hypotension cause by treatment. If the patient had a stroke, thrombolytic therapy (t-PA), should not be given if the systolic BP is >185 mm Hg and/or the diastolic BP is >110 mm Hg.

Hypovolemic shock/volume deficit

Hypovolemic shock occurs when there is inadequate intravascular fluid.
- The loss may be *absolute* because of an internal shifting of fluid or an external loss of fluid, as occurs with massive hemorrhage, thermal injuries, severe vomiting or diarrhea, and injuries (such as ruptured spleen or dissecting arteries) that interfere with intravascular integrity.
- Hypovolemia may also be *relative* and related to vasodilation, increased capillary membrane permeability from sepsis or injuries, and decreased colloidal osmotic pressure that may occur with loss of sodium and some disorders, such as hypopituitarism and cirrhosis.

Hypovolemic shock is classified according to the degree of fluid loss:
- Class I: <750 ml or ≤15% of total circulating volume (TCV).
- Class II: 750-100 ml or 15-30% of TCV.
- Class III: 1500-2000 ml or 30-40% of TCV.
- Class IV: >2000 ml or >40% of TCV.

Hypovolemic shock occurs when the total circulating volume of fluid decreases, leading to a fall in venous return that in turn causes a decrease in ventricular filling and preload, indicated by a decrease in right atrial pressure (RAP) and pulmonary artery occlusion pressure (PAOP). This results in a decrease in stroke volume and cardiac output. This in turn causes generalized arterial vasoconstriction, increasing afterload (increased systemic vascular resistance), causing decreased tissue perfusion.

Symptoms
- Anxiety.
- Pallor.
- Cool and clammy skin.
- Delayed capillary refill
- Cyanosis.
- Hypotension.

- 32 -

- Increasing respirations.
- Weak, thready pulse.

Treatment
- Treatment is aimed at identifying and treating the cause of fluid loss and reestablishing an adequate intravascular volume of fluid through administration of blood, blood products, autotransfusion, colloids (such as plasma protein fraction), and/or crystalloids (such as normal saline).
- Oxygen may be given through intubation and ventilation if necessary.
- Medications may include vasopressors, such as dopamine.

First degree AV block

First degree AV block occurs when the atrial impulses are conducted through the AV node to the ventricles at a rate that is slower than normal. While the P and QRS are usually normal, the PR interval is >0.20 seconds, and the P:QRS ratio is 1:1. A narrow QRS complex indicates a conduction abnormality only in the AV node, but a widened QRS indicates associated damage to the bundle branches as well. *Chronic* first-degree block may be caused by fibrosis/sclerosis of the conduction system related to coronary artery disease, valvular disease, and cardiac myopathies and carries little morbidity. *Acute* first degree block, on the other hand, is of much more concern and may be related to digoxin toxicity, β-blockers, amiodarone, myocardial infarction, hyperkalemia, or edema related to valvular surgery.

Second degree AV block, Type I

Second degree AV block occurs when some of the atrial beats are blocked. Second degree AV block is further subdivided according to the patterns of block:

Mobitz type I block (Wenckebach): Each atrial impulse in a group of beats is conducted at a lengthened interval until one fails to conduct (the PR interval progressively increases), so there are more P waves than QRS, but the QRS complex is usual of normal shape and duration. The sinus node functions at a regular rate, so the P-P interval is regular, but the R-R interval usually shortens with each impulse. The P:QRS ratio varies, such as 3:2, 4:3, 5:4. This type of block by itself usually does not cause significant morbidity unless associated with inferior wall myocardial infarction.

Second-degree AV block, Type II, and 2:1 block

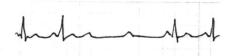

Second degree AV block and Type II (Mobitz):
Only some of the atrial impulses are conducted unpredictably through the AV node to the ventricles, and the block always occurs below the AV node in the bundle of His, the bundle branches, or the Purkinje fibers. The PR intervals are the same if impulses are conducted, and QRS complex is usually widened. The P:QRS ratio varies 2:1, 3:1, and 4:1. Type II block is more dangerous than Type I because it may progress to complete AV block and may produce Stokes-Adams syncope. Additionally, if the block is at the Purkinje fibers, there is no escape impulse. Usually a transcutaneous cardiac pacemaker and defibrillator should be at bedside. Symptoms may include chest pain if the heart block is precipitated by myocarditis or myocardial ischemia.

2:1 block: Every other atrial impulse (P:QRS ratio of 2.1) is conducted through the AV node.

Third degree AV block

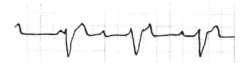

With third degree AV block, there are more P waves than QRS with no clear relationship between them and an atrial rate 2-3 times the pulse rate, so the PR interval is irregular. If the SA node malfunctions, the AV node fires at a lower rate, and if the AV node malfunctions, the pacemaker site in the ventricles takes over at a bradycardic rate; thus, with complete AV block, the heart still contracts, but often ineffectually. With this type of block, the atrial P (sinus rhythm or atrial fibrillation) and the ventricular QRS (ventricular escape rhythm) are stimulated by different impulses, so there is AV dissociation. The heart may compensate at rest but can't keep pace with exertion. The resultant bradycardia may cause congestive heart failure, fainting, or even sudden death, and usually conduction abnormalities slowly worsen. Symptoms include dyspnea, chest pain, and hypotension, which are treated with IV atropine. Transcutaneous pacing may be needed. Complete persistent AV block normally requires implanted pacemakers, usually dual chamber.

RBBB and LBBB

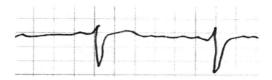

A **right bundle branch block** (RBBB) occurs when conduction is blocked in the right bundle branch that carries impulses from the Bundle of His to the ventricles. The impulse travels through the myocardium, but this causes a slight delay in contraction of the right ventricle. RBBB A left bundle branch block is characterized by normal P waves, but the QRS complex is widened and notched (rabbit-eared) although this may not be seen with minimal leads sometimes used in monitoring PR interval is normal or prolonged, and the QRS interval is > 0.12 seconds. P:QRS ratio remains 1:1 with regular rhythms, usually in the 60 to 100 range.

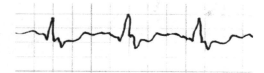

A left bundle branch block (LBBB) is characterized by normal P waves, but the QRS complex may be widened and notched (M-shaped) with interval of >0.12 seconds. The PR interval may be normal or prolonged. The P:QRS ratio is 1:1 and rhythm is regular, usually in the 60 to 100 range.

Classes of antidysrhythmics and drugs used for SVT

Antidysrhythmics include a number of drugs that act on the conduction system, the ventricles and/or the atria to control dysrhythmias. There are 4 classes of drugs that are used as well as some that are unclassified:
- Class I: 3 subtypes of sodium channel blockers (quinidine, lidocaine, procainamide)
- Class II: β-receptor blockers (Esmolol, propranolol)
- Class III: Slows repolarization (amiodarone, ibutilide)
- Class IV: Calcium channel blockers (diltiazem, verapamil)
- Unclassified (Adenosine)

Supra-ventricular tachycardia
- Adenosine affects conduction system and may cause transient flushing, decreased BP, and shortness of breath. Diltiazem (Cardizem®, Tiazac®) affects conduction system and may cause bradycardia, AV block, and decreased BP.
- Esmolol (Brevibloc®) affects the conduction system and may cause decreased BP, bradycardia, and heart failure. Propranolol (Inderal®) affects conduction system and may cause bradycardia, heart block, and heart failure.
- Procainamide affects the atria and ventricles and may cause decreased BP and ECG abnormalities (widening of QRS and QT).

Antidysrhythmics for treatment of:

Paroxysmal supraventricular tachycardia
- Adenosine.
- Digoxin (Lanoxin®) affects the conduction system and may cause bradycardia, heart block, nausea and vomiting, and CNS depression.
- Verapamil (Calan®, Verelan®) affects the conduction system and may cause decreased BP, bradycardia, and heart failure.

Sinus tachycardia
- Esmolol (Brevibloc®).

Premature ventricular contractions
- Lidocaine affects the ventricles and may cause CNS toxicity with nausea and vomiting.
- Procainamide.

Ventricular tachycardia
- Lidocaine.
- Amiodarone (Cordarone®, Pacerone®).
- Procainamide.

Ventricular fibrillation
- Lidocaine.

Atrial fibrillation
- Digoxin (Lanoxin®).
- Diltiazem (Cardizem®, Tiazac®).
- Ibutilide (Corvert®) affects the conduction system and rarely has side effects.
- Amiodarone (Cordarone®) affects the atria and ventricles and may cause decreased BP, and adverse hepatic effects.

Atrial flutter
- Digoxin (Lanoxin®).
- Diltiazem (Cardizem®, Tiazac®).
- Ibutilide (Corvert®).
- Verapamil (Calan®, Verelan®).
- Amiodarone (Cordarone®).
- Procainamide.

Dissecting aortic aneurysm

A dissecting aortic aneurysm occurs when the wall of the aorta is torn and blood flows between the layers of the wall, dilating and weakening it until it risks rupture (which has a 90% mortality). Aortic aneurysms are more than twice as common in males as females, but females have a higher mortality rate, possibly because they are often older. Different classification systems are used to describe the type and degree of dissection. Common classifications include:
- *DeBakey classification* uses anatomic location as the focal point:
  - *Type I* begins in the ascending aorta but may spread to include the aortic arch and the descending aorta (60%). This is also considered a proximal lesion or Stanford type A.
  - *Type II* is restricted to the ascending aorta (10-15%). This is also considered a proximal lesion or Stanford type A.
  - *Type III* is restricted to the descending aorta (25-30%). This is considered a distal lesion or Stanford type B.

Types I and II are thoracic and type III is abdominal.

Treatments for dissecting aortic aneurysms

Once a dissecting aortic aneurysm is identified, and the type is determined, both medical management and surgical repair may be indicated:
- **Anti-hypertensives** to reduce systolic BP, such as β-blockers (esmolol) or Alpha-β-blocker combinations (labetalol) to reduce force of blood as it leaves the ventricle to reduce pressure against aortic wall. IV vasodilators (sodium nitroprusside) may also be needed.
- **Intubation and ventilation** may be required if the patient is hemodynamically unstable.
- **Analgesia/sedation** to control anxiety and pain.

- **Diagnostic tests,** such as CT, MRI, transthoracic echocardiogram, and transesophageal echocardiograms may be needed.
- **Surgical repair:** *Type I and II* are usually repaired surgically because of the danger of *rupture and cardiac tamponade. Type III (abdominal)* is often followed medically and surgery delayed until aneurysm is >5 cm, at which point either abdominal surgical repair or endoluminal stent may be done.

Thoracic aortic aneurysm

Thoracic aortic aneurysms are usually related to atherosclerosis but may also result from Marfan syndrome, Ehlers-Danlos disease, and connective tissue disorders. The aneurysms are often asymptomatic but may cause substernal pain, back pain, dyspnea and/or stridor (from pressure on trachea), cough, distention of neck veins, and edema of neck and arms. Rupture usually does not allow time for emergent repair, so identifying and correcting before rupture is essential. Diagnosis is often made with x-ray or CT. Cardiac catheterization and echocardiogram may also be needed. Surgery is indicated for aneurysms ≥6 cm. Endovascular grafting is routinely done for aneurysms of the descending thoracic aorta. Open surgical repair is required for the ascending aorta or arch, but these surgeries are much more dangerous with higher rates of morbidity and mortality than for abdominal aorta repair. There is a 4% occurrence of paraplegia with thoracic aorta aneurysm repair and increased risk of stroke.

Abdominal aortic aneurysm

About 90% of abdominal aortic aneurysms occur below the renal arteries, but aneurysms are not usually palpable until they reach 5 cm/diameter, so they may be found incidentally. Patients may have had mild constant or intermittent pain, but rupture results in severe abdominal pain, hypotension, and a palpable mass. About 50% of patients die with rupture. Elective repair is usually advised for aneurysms >5.5 cm or those that are rapidly expanding. Ultrasound and CT are used for diagnosis with CT with contrast to show vasculature. There are two types of surgical repair:
- **Open:** An abdominal incision is made with dissection of damaged aorta and a graft is sutured in place. Aortic blood flow must be interrupted with CPB during this procedure.
- **Endovascular:** A stent graft is fed through the arteries to line the aorta and exclude the aneurysm.

Complications include myocardial infarction, renal injury can occur, and GI hemorrhage, which may occur up to years after surgery. Endo-leaks can occur with a stent graft, increasing risk of rupture.

Mitral stenosis

Mitral stenosis is caused by an autoimmune response to rheumatic fever leading to vegetative growths on the mitral valve. It can also be caused by infective endocarditis or lupus erythematosus. Over time, the leaflets thicken and calcify and the commissures (junctions) fuse, decreasing the size of the valve opening. Mitral stenosis reduces the flow of blood from the left atrium to the left ventricle. Pressure in the left atrium increases to overcome resistance, resulting in enlargement of the left atrium and increased pressure in the pulmonary veins and capillaries of the lung. Symptoms of exertional dyspnea usually occur when the valve is 50% occluded.

There are 3 mechanisms by which mitral stenosis causes pulmonary hypertension.
- Increased left atrial pressure causing backward increase in pressure of pulmonary veins.
- Hypertrophy and pulmonary artery constriction resulting from reactive left atrial and pulmonary venous hypertension.
- Thrombotic/embolitic damage to pulmonary vasculature.

Treatment includes drugs to control arrhythmias and hypertension, balloon valvuloplasty, and mitral valve replacement.

Infective endocarditis

Infective endocarditis is an infection of the lining of the heart that covers the heart valves and contains purkinje fibers, known as the endocardium. Risk factors include being over 60 years of age, being male, IV drug use, and dental infections. Staphylococcal aureus is the most common cause of infective endocarditis. Etiology includes subacute bacterial endocarditis (often related to dental procedures), prosthetic valvular endocarditis (following valve replacement, and right sided endocarditis (often related to catheter infections and IV drug use). The mitral valve is the most common valve affected, followed by aortic, tricuspid, and the pulmonary valve being the least often affected. Positive blood cultures, widened pulse pressures, ECG, murmurs, and vegetations seen on a transesophageal echocardiogram, are used to make the diagnosis. After diagnosis is made antibiotics are used for treatment, and when unsuccessful or heart failure is present valve repair may be warranted. Serious complications from endocarditis include emboli, sepsis, and heart failure. Untreated endocarditis is fatal.

Acute pericarditis

Pericarditis is inflammation of the pericardial sac sometimes leading to increased pericardial fluid. It may be an isolated process or it may be the effect of an underlying disease. If the underlying cause is autoimmune or related to malignancy of some sort, the patient usually presents with symptoms that relate to that disorder. However, in the United States most cases are related to a viral etiology, and therefore usually present with flu-like symptoms. The most common sign of pericarditis is a sharp chest pain that is worse with inspiration and is improved when the patient is leaning forward while sitting up. Pericardial effusion may be seen on imaging, a friction rub may be heard on auscultation, and new ST elevations or PR depression may be seen on ECG. In high risk patients and in patients with large effusions, pericardiocentesis or pericardial biopsy may be performed for drainage or diagnostically. In patients that have idiopathic pericarditis or viral pericarditis have a good prognosis with medication alone. Extreme physical activity can trigger pain and should be avoided until conclusion of medication treatment and symptoms have subsided (generally 6 months). NSAIDs (usually ibuprofen, aspirin, or indomethacin) are recommended for patients with pericarditis unless contraindicated to reduce inflammation and pain. Colchicine 0.5 mg every twice a day for six months is often prescribed in adjunct to NSAID therapy, as it decreases the incidence of recurrent pericarditis.

Mitral valve regurgitation

Mitral valve regurgitation may occur with mitral stenosis or independently. It can result from damage caused by rheumatic fever, myxomatous degeneration caused by a genetic defect in the valvular collagen, infective endocarditis, collagen vascular disease (Marfan's syndrome) or cardiomyopathy. Hypertrophy and dilation of the left ventricle may cause displacement of the leaflets and dilation of the valve. Regurgitation occurs when the mitral valve fails to close completely so that there is backflow into the left atrium from the left ventricle during systole, decreasing cardiac output. There are 3 phases:

- **Acute** may occur with rupture of a chordae tendineae or papillary muscle causing sudden left ventricular flooding and overload.
- **Chronic compensated** results in enlargement of the left atrium to decrease filling pressure and hypertrophy of the left ventricle to maintain stroke volume and cardiac output.
- **Chronic decompensated** occurs when the left ventricle fails to compensate for the volume overload so that stroke volume and cardiac output decrease.

Aortic stenosis

Aortic stenosis is a stricture (narrowing) of the aortic valve that controls the flow of blood from the left ventricle, causing the left ventricular wall to thicken as it increases pressure to overcome the valvular resistance, increasing afterload, and increasing the need for blood supply from the coronary arteries. This condition may result from a birth defect or childhood rheumatic fever and tends to worsen over the years as the heart grows.

Symptoms
- Chest pain on exertion and intolerance of exercise.
- Heart murmur.
- Hypotension on exertion may be associated with sudden fainting.
- Sudden death can occur.
- Tachycardia with faint pulse.
- Poor appetite.
- Increased risk for bacterial endocarditis and coronary insufficiency.
- Increases mitral regurgitation and secondary pulmonary hypertension.

Treatment
- Balloon valvuloplasty to dilate valve non-surgically.
- Surgical repair of valve or replacement of valve, depending upon the extent of stricture.

Pulmonic stenosis

Pulmonic stenosis is a stricture of the pulmonary blood that controls the flow of blood from the right ventricle to the lungs, resulting in right ventricular hypertrophy as the pressure increases in the right ventricle and decreased pulmonary blood flow. The condition may be asymptomatic or symptoms may not be evident until adulthood, depending upon the severity of the defect. Pulmonic stenosis may be associated with a number of other heart defects.

Symptoms
- Loud heart murmur
- Congestive heart murmur
- Mild cyanosis
- Cardiomegaly
- Angina
- Dyspnea
- Fainting
- Increased risk of bacterial endocarditis

Treatment
- Balloon valvuloplasty to separate the cusps of the valve for children.
- Surgical repair includes the cardiopulmonary bypass pulmonary valvotomy for older children and adults.

Hemodynamic monitoring and oxygen saturation

Hemodynamic monitoring includes monitoring oxygen saturation levels, which must be maintained for proper cardiac function. Changes in the oxygen saturation levels can indicate complications in the post-surgical patient. The central venous catheter often has an oxygen sensor at the tip to monitor oxygen saturation in the right atrium. If the catheter tip is located near the renal veins, this can cause an increase in right atrial oxygen saturation; and near the coronary sinus, a decrease:
- Increased oxygen saturation may result from left atrial to right atrial shunt, abnormal pulmonary venous return, increased delivery of oxygen or decrease in extraction of oxygen.
- Decreased oxygen saturation may be related to low cardiac output with an increase in oxygen extraction or decrease in arterial oxygen saturation with normal differences in the atrial and ventricular oxygen saturation.

Hemodynamic monitoring and mixed venous gases/SvO$_2$

Mixed venous gases (MVG), especially venous oxygen saturation (SvO$_2$), are monitored for indications of respiratory failure, reduced oxygenation, anemia, and changes in cardiac output. Mixed venous gas refers to venous blood that has returned to the heart from the superior and inferior vena cava and the coronary sinus. Obtaining a sample from the right atrium may reflect primarily blood from the superior vena cava, which usually has a lower saturation (70%) than the blood from the inferior vena cava (80%) or the coronary sinus (56%). The blood in the right ventricle and pulmonary artery is completed "mixed" and the saturation averaged. MVG are usually measured by sampling through a pulmonary artery catheter. Normal values:
- **PCO$_2$:** 41-51 mm Hg (pulmonary venous carbon dioxide pressure)
- **PvO$_2$:** 35-49 mm Hg (pulmonary venous oxygen pressure)
- **SvO$_2$:** 60-80% (pulmonary venous oxygen saturation.)

If there is a decrease in SvO$_2$, then the oxygenation is not sufficient for tissue needs.

Hemodynamic monitoring and left atrial pressure

Left atrial pressure may be monitored in the post-surgical period by way of a catheter inserted during surgery into the left atrium from the right superior pulmonary vein or through the left atrial appendage. Oxygen saturation of blood in the left atrium should be 100%.

Left atrial pressures:
- **Normal values:** 1-2 mm Hg higher than right atrial pressure (4-12 mm Hg). Pressure above 12-14 mm Hg in the post-surgical period is cause for concern.
- **Increased** pressure may indicate an increase in end-diastolic pressure of the left ventricle, a decrease in function, hypertrophy, heart failure, or an increase in left ventricular afterload. An increase may also indicate mitral valve stenosis, backflow, or thrombus obstruction, a significant right to left shunt, excessive intravascular volume, tachycardia with arrhythmias, or cardiac tamponade.
- **Decreased** pressure may indicate a decrease in intravascular fluid or insufficient preload.

Pulmonary artery pressure and pulmonary artery/capillary wedge pressure

Pulmonary artery pressure (PAP) is measured by a catheter usually fed through the right ventricle to the main pulmonary artery, measuring systolic, diastolic, and mean pressures, with the patient in supine position ≤45° elevation:

- **Normal values:** 10-20 mm Hg (mean 15 mm Hg). Postoperative rates should be <25 mm Hg. PAP is usually about 25-34% the systemic blood pressure rate. Oxygen saturation is usually about 80%.
- **Increased** pressure may indicate pulmonary obstruction or embolus, left to right shunt, left ventricular failure, pulmonary hypertension, or mitral stenosis, pneumothorax, lung/alveolar hypoplasia, hyperviscosity of blood, or increased left atrial pressure.
- **Decreased** pressure may indicate a decrease in intravascular volume or cardiac output, or obstruction of pulmonary blood flow.

The catheter may have a balloon that can be inflated in the pulmonary artery to provide a measurement of **pulmonary artery/capillary wedge pressure (PAWP/PCWP)** to evaluate pulmonary hypertension, left ventricular failure, and mitral stenosis:

- **Normal values:** 4-12 mm Hg.
- **Increased pressure** may indicate left ventricular failure, mitral insufficiency or mitral stenosis

Hemodynamic monitoring and central venous/ right atrial pressure

Hemodynamic monitoring is the monitoring of blood flow pressures. In order for effective post-surgical cardiac functioning, the correct relationship between high and low pressures must be maintained. While most catheters are placed during surgery, they are sometimes done at bedside. The most common sites are the left atrium, right atrium, and pulmonary artery or superior vena cava. Central venous pressure (CVP), the pressure in the right atrium or vena cava, is used to assess function of the right ventricles, preload, and flow of venous blood to the heart. Normal pressure ranges from 2-5 mm Hg but may be elevated after surgery to 6-8 mm Hg. Incorrect catheter placement or malfunctioning can affect readings.

- **Increased CVP** is related to overload of intravascular volume caused by decreased function, hypertrophy, or failure of the right ventricle; increased right ventricular afterload, tricuspid valve stenosis, regurgitation, or thrombus obstruction; or shunt from left ventricle to right atrium. It can also be caused by arrhythmias or cardiac tamponade.
- **Decreased CVP** is related to low intravascular volume, decreased preload, or vasodilation.

Hemodynamic monitoring and aortic blood flow

Aortic blood flow is assessed with esophageal Doppler monitoring (EDM) for evaluation of hypoperfusion (hypovolemia or septic shock), major organ dysfunction (renal or liver failure), hypotension, heart failure, cardiogenic shock, ruptures within the heart, mitral regurgitation, or tamponade. EDM may be used before, during, or after cardiac surgery. An esophageal probe is inserted through the patient's mouth while the patient is sedated, and Doppler ultrasound technology is used to monitor both the function of the left ventricle and the patient's fluid status. The probe may be left in place if the patient can tolerate it, but the patient should be monitored carefully for mucosal irritation. EDM can show the flow time; peak velocity (PV) and minute distance (MD) while stroke volume and cardiac output can be calculated.

Normal ranges include:
- Corrected flow time (FTc): 330-360 milliseconds
- Peak Velocity (PV):
  - (20 years) 90-120 cm/sec.
  - (40 years) 80-110 cm/sec.
  - (60 years) 60-90 cm/sec.
  - (80 years) 40-70 cm/sec.

Hemodynamic monitoring and intraarterial blood pressure monitoring/MAP

Intraarterial blood pressure monitoring is done for systolic, diastolic, and mean arterial pressure (MAP) for conditions that decrease cardiac output, tissue perfusion, or fluid volume. A catheter is inserted into an artery, such as the radial (most frequently used), dorsalis pedis, femoral, or axillary, percutaneously or through a cut-down. Before catheter insertion, collateral circulation must be assessed by Doppler or the Allen test (used for the hand). In the Allen test, both the radial and ulnar artery are compressed and the patient is asked to clench the hand repeatedly until it blanches, and then one artery is released, and the tissue on that side should flush. Then the test is repeated again, releasing the other artery. The MAP is most commonly used to evaluate perfusion as it shows pressure throughout the cardiac cycle. Systole is one-third and diastole two-thirds of the normal cardiac cycle. The MAP for a blood pressure of 120/60 (Normal range 70-100 mm Hg):

$$\frac{[(Diastole \times 2) + (Systole \times 1)]}{3} = MAP$$

$$(60 \times 2 = 120) + (120) = \frac{240}{3} = MAP \ of \ 80$$

Hemodynamic monitoring and implications of perfusion pressure and pulse pressure

Perfusion pressure directly affects coronary blood flow, and coronary perfusion occurs during diastole. Coronary artery perfusion pressure is equal to the diastolic blood pressure minus the pulmonary artery occlusion pressure. Normal values are 60-80 mm Hg. During the cardiac cycle, aortic pressure causes the coronaries to be perfused, while ventricular pressure compresses the coronaries during systole, decreasing perfusion. The pulse pressure is the difference between systolic and diastolic pressures, and this can be an important indicator.

For example, with a decrease in cardiac output, vasoconstriction takes place in the body's attempt to maintain the blood pressure. In this case, the MAP may remain unchanged, but the pulse pressure narrows. Necessary values for MAP include:
- >60 mm Hg to perfuse coronary arteries
- 70-90 mm Hg to perfuse the brain and other organs, such as the kidneys and to maintain cardiac patients and decrease the workload of the left ventricle.
- 90-110 mm Hg to increase cerebral perfusion after neurosurgical procedures, such as carotid endarterectomy.

Patients should be assessed for changes in pulse pressure that may be precipitated by medications, such as diuretics that alter fluid volume.

Cardiac output

Cardiac output (CO) is the amount of blood is pumped through the ventricles during a specified period. Normal cardiac output is about 5 liters per minutes at rest for an adult. Under exercise or stress, this volume may multiply 3 or 4 times with concomitant changes in the heart rate (HR) and stroke volume (SV). The basic formulation for calculating cardiac output is the heart rate (HR) per minute multiplied by the stroke volume (SR), which is the amount of blood pumped through the ventricles with each contraction. The stroke volume is controlled by preload, afterload, and contractibility.

$$CO = HR \times SV$$

The heart rate is controlled by the autonomic nervous system. Normally, if the heart rate decreases, stroke rate increases to compensate, but with cardiomyopathies, this may not occur, so bradycardia results in a sharp decline in cardiac output.

Preload and afterload

Preload refers to the amount of elasticity in the myocardium at the end of diastole when the ventricles are filled to their maximum volume and the stretch on the muscle fibers is the greatest. The preload value is based on the volume in the ventricles. The amount of preload (stretch) affects stroke volume because as stretch increases, the resultant contraction also increases (Frank-Starling Law). Preload may decrease because of dehydration, diuresis, or vasodilation. Preload may increase because of increased venous return, controlling fluid loss, transfusion, or intravenous fluids.

Afterload refers to the amount of systemic vascular resistance to left ventricular ejection of blood and pulmonary vascular resistance to right ventricular ejection of blood. Determinants of afterload include the size and elasticity of the great vessels and the functioning of the pulmonic and aortic valves. Afterload increased with hypertension, stenotic valves, and vasoconstriction.

Non-invasive hemodynamic management

Thoracic electrical bioimpedance monitoring is a non-invasive method of monitoring hemodynamics (CO, blood flow, contractibility, pre- and after-load, pulmonary artery pressure). Electrodes placed on the thorax measure changes in electrical output associated with the volume of blood through the aorta and its velocity. The monitor to which the electrodes are attached converts the signals to waveforms. The heart rate is shown on an ECG monitor. The equipment calculates the cardiac output based on the heart rate and fluid volume. A typical bioimpedence monitor has 4 sets of bioimpedance electrodes and 3 ECG electrodes. Height, weight, and length of thorax are entered into the machine. Two sets of bioimpedance electrodes are placed at the base on the neck bilaterally and then two sets on each side of the chest. The distance between the neck electrodes and the chest electrodes (on the same side) must be entered into the machine. ECG leads are placed where they consistently monitor the QRS signal (they may need to be moved to achieve this).

Important terms

Cardiac output (CO) is the amount of blood pumped through the ventricles, usually calculated in liters per minute.
Normal value at rest: 4-6 L/min.

Cardiac index (CI) is the cardiac output (CO) divided by the body surface area (BSA). This is essentially a measure of cardiac output tailored to the individual, based on height and weight, measured in liters/min per square meter of BSA.
Normal value: 2.2-4.0 L/min/m^2.

Stroke volume (SV) is the amount of blood pumped through the left ventricle with each contraction, minus any blood remaining inside the ventricle at the end of systole. Normal values 60-70 ml.
Formula: (CO in L/min) x (HR per minute) x (1000) = SV in ml.

Pulmonary vascular resistance (PVR) is the resistance in the pulmonary arteries and arterioles against which the right ventricle has to pump during contraction. It is the mean pressure in the pulmonary vascular bed divided by blood flow. If PVR increases, SV decreases. Normal value: 1.2-3.0 units or 100-250 dynes/sec/cm^5.

Pulmonary

Acute respiratory distress syndrome

Acute lung injury (ALI) comprises a syndrome of respiratory distress culminating in acute respiratory distress syndrome (ARDS). ARDS is damage to the vascular endothelium and an increase in the permeability of the alveolar-capillary membrane when damage to the lung results in toxic substances (gastric fluids, bacteria, chemicals, or toxins emitted by neutrophils as part of the inflammatory-mediated response) reducing surfactant and causing pulmonary edema as the alveoli fill with blood and protein-rich fluid and collapse. Atelectasis with hyperinflation and areas of normal tissue occur as the lungs "stiffen." The fluid in the alveoli becomes a medium for infection. Inadequate ventilation and perfusion, leads to increasing hypoxemia and tachypnea as the body tries to compensate to maintain a normal $PaCO_2$.

Symptoms are characterized by respiratory distress within 72 hours of surgery or a serious injury to a person with otherwise normal lungs and no cardiac disorder. Untreated, the condition results in respiratory failure, MODS, and a mortality rate of 5-30%. Symptoms: Crackling rales/wheezing in lungs, ↓ in pulmonary compliance which results in decreased tachypnea with expiratory grunting, cyanosis/skin mottling, hypotension and tachycardia, symptoms associated with volume overload are missing (3rd heart sound or JVD), respiratory alkalosis initally but replaced as the disease progresses with hypercarbia and respiratory acidosis, and normal X-ray initially but then diffuse infiltrates in both lungs, but the heart and vessels appear normal.

The management of acute respiratory distress syndrome (ARDS) involves providing adequate gas exchange and preventing further damage to the lung from forced ventilation. Treatment includes:
- No drug has proved effective in the clinical management or prevention of ARDS. The following are therapies that are commonly used but per the ARDS network there is insufficient evidence that they decrease mortality rates: corticosteroids (may increase mortality rates in some patient populations, though this is the most common medication given), nitrous oxide, inhaled surfactant, and anti-inflammatory medications.
- Treatment of the underlying condition is the only proven treatment, especially identifying and treating with appropriate antibiotics any infection, as sepsis is most common etiology for ARDS, but prophylactic antibiotics are not indicated.
- Conservative fluid management is indicated to reduce days on the ventilator, but does not reduce overall mortality.
- Pharmacologic preventive care: enoxaparin 40 mg subcutaneously QD, sucralfate 1 g NGT four times daily or omeprazole 40 mg IV QD, and enteral nutrition support within 24 hours of ICU admission or intubation.
- O_2 therapy by nasal prongs/cannula or mask may be sufficient in very mild cases to maintain oxygen saturation above 90%. Oxygen should be administered at 100% because of the mismatch between ventilation (V) and perfusion (Q), which can result in hypoxia on position change.
- ARDS oxygenation goal is PaO_2 55-80 mmHg or SpO_2 88-95%.
- Many times endotracheal intubation may be needed if SpO_2 falls or CO_2 levels rise.
- The ARDS Network recommends low tidal volumes (6 mL/kg) and higher PEEP (12 cm H_2O or more).

- The low tidal volume ventilation described above is referred to as lung protective ventilation, and it has been shown to reduce mortality in patients with ARDS.
- For patients with severe ARDS, trials placing patient in prone position 18-24 hours/day with chest and pelvis supported and abdomen unsupported allows the diaphragm to move posteriorly, increasing functional residual capacity (FRC) in many patients.

Acute pulmonary embolism

Acute pulmonary embolism occurs when a pulmonary artery or arteriole is blocked by a blood clot originating in the venous system or the right heart. While most pulmonary emboli are from thrombus formation, other causes may be air, fat, or septic embolus (from bacterial invasion of a thrombus). Common originating sites for thrombus formation are the deep veins in the legs, the pelvic veins, and the right atrium. Causes include stasis related to damage to endothelial wall and changes in blood coagulation factors. Atrial fibrillation poses a serious risk because blood pools in the right atrium, forming clots that travel directly through the right ventricle to the lungs. The obstruction of the artery/arteriole causes an increase in alveolar dead space in which there is ventilation but impairment of gas exchange because of the ventilation/perfusion mismatching or intrapulmonary shunting. This results in hypoxia, hypercapnia, and the release of mediators that cause bronchoconstriction. If more than 50% of the vascular bed becomes excluded, pulmonary hypertension occurs.

Clinical manifestations of acute pulmonary embolism (PE) vary according to the size of the embolus and the area of occlusion.

Symptoms
- Dyspnea with tachypnea.
- Tachycardia.
- Anxiety and restlessness.
- Chest pain.
- Fever.
- Rales.
- Cough (sometimes with hemoptysis).
- Hemodynamic instability.

Diagnostic tests
- ABG analysis may show hypoxemia (Decreased PaO_2), hypocarbia (Decreased $PaCO_2$) and respiratory alkalosis (Increased pH).
- D-dimer (will show elevation with PE).
- ECG may show sinus tachycardia or other abnormalities.
- Echocardiogram can show emboli in the central arteries and can assess the hemodynamic status of the right side of the heart.
- Chest x-ray is of minimal value.
- Spiral CT may provide definitive diagnosis.
- V/Q scintigraphy can confirm diagnosis.
- Pulmonary angiograms also can confirm diagnosis.

Medical management of pulmonary embolism

Medical management of pulmonary embolism starts with preventive measures for those at risk, including leg exercises, elastic compression stockings, and anticoagulation therapy (Coumadin®). Most pulmonary emboli present as medical emergencies, so the immediate task is to stabilize the patient. Medical management may include:

- **Oxygen** to relieve hypoxemia.
- **Intravenous infusions**: Dobutamine (Dobutrex®) or dopamine (Intropin®) to relieve hypotension.
- **Cardiac monitoring** for dysrhythmias and issues related to right sided heart failure.
- **Medications** as indicated: digitalis glycosides, diuretic, and antiarrhythmics.
- **Intubation and mechanical ventilation** may be required.
- **Analgesia** (such as morphine sulfate) or sedation to relieve anxiety.
- **Anticoagulants** to prevent recurrence (although it will not dissolve clots already present), including heparin and warfarin (Coumadin®).
- **Placement of percutaneous venous filter** (Greenfield) in the inferior vena cava to prevent further emboli from entering the lungs may be done if anticoagulation therapy is contraindicated.
- **Thrombolytic therapy,** recombinant tissue-type plasminogen activator (rt-PA) or streptokinase, for those severely compromised, but these treatments have limited success and pose the danger of bleeding.

Symptoms of acute respiratory failure

The cardinal signs of respiratory failure include:

- Tachypnea.
- Tachycardia.
- Anxiety and restlessness.
- Diaphoresis.

Symptoms may vary according to the cause. An obstruction may cause more obvious respiratory symptoms than other disorders. Early signs may include changes in the depth and pattern of respirations with flaring nares, sternal retractions, expiratory grunting, wheezing, and extended expiration as the body tries to compensate for hypoxemia and increasing levels of carbon dioxide. Cyanosis may be evident. Central nervous depression, with alterations in consciousness occurs with decreased perfusion to the brain. As the hypoxemia worsens, cardiac arrhythmias, including bradycardia, may occur with either hypotension or hypertension. Dyspnea becomes more pronounced with depressed respirations. Eventually stupor, coma, and death can occur if the condition is not reversed.

Nursing Interventions to help prevent respiratory issues: turn, position, ambulate, cough, deep breathe, vibration and percussion treatments, hydrate the patient to help hydrate the airways, and incentive spirometry.

Hypoxemic and hypercapnic respiratory failure

Hypoxemic respiratory failure occurs suddenly when gaseous exchange of oxygen for carbon dioxide cannot keep up with demand for oxygen or production of carbon dioxide:
- PaO_2 <60 mm Hg
- $PaCO_2$ >40 mm Hg
- Arterial pH <7.35

Hypoxemic respiratory failure can be the result of low inhaled oxygen, as at high elevations or with smoke inhalation. The following ventilatory mechanisms may be involved:
- Alveolar hypotension
- Ventilation-perfusion mismatch (the most common cause)
- Intrapulmonary shunts
- Diffusion impairment

Hypercapnic respiratory failure results from an increase in $PaCO_2$ >45-50 mm Hg associated with respiratory acidosis and may include:
- Reduction in minute ventilation, total volume of gas ventilated in one minute (often related to neurological, muscle, or chest wall disorders, drug overdoses, obstruction of upper airway.
- Increased dead space with wasted ventilation (related to lung disease or disorders of chest wall, such as scoliosis).
- Increased production of CO_2 (usually related to infection, burns, or other causes of hypermetabolism).

Underlying causes for respiratory failure

There are a number of underlying causes for respiratory failure:
- Airway obstruction: Obstruction may result from an inhaled object, such as a peanut or piece of meat, or from an underlying disease process, such as cystic fibrosis, asthma, pulmonary edema, or infection.
- Inadequate respirations: This is a common cause among adults, especially related to obesity and sleep apnea.
- Neuromuscular disorders: Those disorders that interfere with the neuromuscular functioning of the lungs or the chest wall, such as muscular dystrophy or spinal cord injuries can prevent adequate ventilation.
- Pulmonary abnormalities: Those abnormalities of the lung tissue, found in pulmonary fibrosis, burns, ARDS, and reactions to drugs, can lead to failure.
- Chest wall abnormalities: Disorders that impact lung parenchyma, such as severe scoliosis or chest wounds can interfere with lung functioning.

Management of respiratory failure

Respiratory failure must be treated immediately before severe hypoxemia causes irreversible damage to vital organs.
- Identifying and treating the underlying cause should be done immediately because emergency medications or surgery may be indicated. Medical treatments will vary widely depending upon the cause; for example, cardiopulmonary structural defects may require

surgical repair, pulmonary edema may require diuresis, inhaled objects may require surgical removal, and infections may require aggressive antimicrobials.
- Intravenous lines/ central lines are inserted for testing, fluids and medications.
- Oxygen therapy should be initiated to attempt to reverse hypoxemia; however, if refractory hypoxemia occurs, then oxygen therapy alone will not suffice. Oxygen levels must be titrated carefully.
- Intubation and mechanical ventilation are frequently required to maintain adequate ventilation and oxygenation. Positive end expiratory pressure (PEEP) may be necessary with refractory hypoxemia and collapsed alveoli.
- Respiratory status must be monitored constantly, including arterial blood gases and vital signs.

Acute respiratory tract infections (Pneumonia)

Pneumonia is inflammation of the lung parenchyma, filling the alveoli with exudate. It is common throughout childhood and adulthood. Pneumonia may be a primary disease or may occur secondary to another infection or disease, such as lung cancer. Pneumonia may be caused by bacteria, viruses, parasites, or fungi. Common causes for community-acquired pneumonia (CAP) include:
- Streptococcus pneumoniae.
- Legionella species.
- Haemophilus influenzae.
- Staphylococcus aureus.
- Mycoplasma pneumoniae.
- Viruses.

Pneumonia may also be caused by chemical damage. Pneumonia is characterized by location:
- Lobar involves one or more lobes of the lungs. If lobes in both lungs are affected, it is referred to as "bilateral" or "double" pneumonia.
- Bronchial/lobular involves the terminal bronchioles and exudate can involve the adjacent lobules. Usually the pneumonia occurs in scattered patches throughout the lungs.
- Interstitial involves primarily the interstitium and alveoli where white blood cells and plasma fill the alveoli, generating inflammation and creating fibrotic tissue as the alveoli are destroyed.

Hospital-acquired pneumonia (HAP)

Hospital-acquired pneumonia (HAP) is defined as pneumonia that did not appear to already be present on admission that occurs at least 48 hours after admission to a hospital. Healthcare-associated pneumonia (HCAP) is defined as pneumonia that occurs in a patient within 90 days of being hospitalized for 2 or more days at an acute care hospital or LTAC. Ventilator-associated pneumonia (VAP) is one type of hospital acquired pneumonia that a patient acquires more than 48 hours after having an ETT.

The most common way that the patient is infected is via aspiration of bacteria that is colonized in the upper respiratory tract. It is estimated that close to 75% of patients that are critically ill will be colonized with multidrug resistant bacteria within 48 hours of entering an ICU. Aspiration occurs at a rate of about 45% in patients with no health problems and the rate is much higher in the ill. Combining this with the colonization of the critically ill, leads to high rates of HAP, HCAP, and VAP.

The frequency of patients developing these types of pneumonia is increasing, with those at highest risk being those with immunosuppression, septic shock, currently hospitalized for more than five days, and those who have had antibiotics for another infection within the previous three months. These types of pneumonia should be considered if a patient already hospitalized has purulent sputum or a change in respiratory status such as deoxygenating, in combination with a worsening or new chest x-ray infiltrate.

Treatment includes:
- Antibiotic therapy.
- Using appropriate isolation and precautions with infected patients.
- Preventive measures include maintaining ventilated patients in 30° upright positions, frequent oral care for vent patients, and changing ventilator circuits as per protocol.

Antibiotic treatment options for HAP, HCAP, and VAP should take into account many factors, including culture data (when available), patient's comorbidities, flora in the unit, any recent antibiotics by the patient, and whether the patient is at high risk for having multidrug resistant bacteria. As most critical care patients are at high risk, due to factors such as being in an ICU setting, ventilators, and comorbidities, antibiotic recommendations to follow are for coverage for patients with risk factors for multidrug resistant bacteria.

One of the following:
Ceftazidime 2 g q 8 hours IV **OR**
Cefepime 2 g q 8 hours IV **OR**
Imipenem 500 mg q 6 hours IV **OR**
Pipercillin-tazobactam 4.5 g q 6 hours IV

AND:

Ciprofloxacin 400 mg q 8 hours IV **OR**
Levaquin 750 mg QD IV

Bronchiolitis

Bronchiolitis in adults is different from that in infants. Adult bronchiolitis results in inflammation of the small airways, which are 1-2 mm in diameter, sometimes affecting adjacent alveoli and causing fibrotic changes. The cause of adult bronchiolitis is unclear but may be precipitated by infection or chronic rejection response after transplantation. Classifications include:
- Cellular: Inflammation of the bronchioles.
- Follicular: Inflammation causes hyperplasia of lymphoid tissue along bronchioles and smaller airways.
- Mineral dust: Inflammation extends into alveolar ducts and causing fibrotic changes in bronchiole walls.
- Cigarette smoke: Fibrotic, edematous, distorted bronchioles.
- Diffuse pan-: chronic inflammation affecting respiratory bronchioles, alveoli, and alveolar ducts.
- Constrictive: Chronic inflammation with fibrotic scarring and sometimes obliteration of bronchioles.

- Obliterans: Inflammation causes intraluminal polyps and hyperplasia that obstruct bronchioles, extending into alveolar ducts and distal alveoli. Associated with bone marrow and heart-lung/lung transplants as well as infection.

Symptoms usually include increasing cough, malaise, fever, flu-like symptoms, and dyspnea. Treatment also varies and may include antibiotics (macrolides) and/or immunosuppressants.

Air leak syndromes

Air leak syndromes may result in significant respiratory distress. Leaks may occur spontaneously or secondary to some type of trauma (accidental, mechanical, iatrogenic) or disease. As pressure increases inside alveoli, the alveolar wall pulls away from the perivascular sheath and subsequent alveolar rupture allows air to follow the perivascular planes and flow into adjacent areas. There are two categories
- **Pneumothorax**:
  o Air in the pleural space causes a lung to collapse.
- **Barotrauma/volutrauma** with air in the interstitial space (usually resolve over time):
  o Pneumoperitoneum is air in the peritoneal area, including the abdomen and occasionally the scrotal sac of male infants.
  o Pneumomediastinum is air in the mediastinal area between the lungs.
  o Pneumopericardium is air in the pericardial sac that surrounds the heart.
  o Subcutaneous emphysema is air in the subcutaneous tissue planes of the chest wall.
  o Pulmonary interstitial emphysema (PIE) is air trapped in the interstitium between the alveoli.

Pneumothorax

Pneumothorax occurs when there is a leak of air into the pleural space, resulting in complete or partial collapse of a lung:

Symptoms
- Vary widely depending on the cause and degree of the pneumothorax and whether or not there is underlying disease: Acute pleuritic pain (95%), usually on the affected side.
- Decreased breath sounds.
- Tension pneumothorax: tracheal deviation and hemodynamic compromise.

Diagnosis
- Clinical findings. Radiograph: 6-foot upright posterior-anterior. Ultrasound may detect traumatic pneumothorax.

Treatment
- Chest-tube thoracostomy with underwater seal drainage is the most common treatment for all types of pneumothorax.
- Tension pneumothorax: Immediate needle decompression and chest tube thoracostomy.
- Small pneumothorax: Oxygen administration (3-4 L/min) and observation for 3-6 hours. If no increase shown on repeat x-ray, patient may be discharged with another x-ray in 24-48 hours.
- Primary spontaneous pneumothorax: catheter aspiration or chest tube thoracostomy.

Aspiration pneumonitis/pneumonia

Aspiration pneumonitis/pneumonia may occur as the result of any type of aspiration, including foreign objects. The aspirated material creates an inflammatory response, with the irritated mucous membrane at high risk for bacterial infection secondary to the aspiration, causing pneumonia. Gastric contents and oropharyngeal bacteria are commonly aspirated. Gastric contents can cause a severe chemical pneumonitis with hypoxemia, especially if the pH is <2.5. Acidic food particles can cause severe reactions. With acidic damage, bronchospasm and atelectasis occur rapidly with tracheal irritation, bronchitis, and alveolar damage with interstitial edema and hemorrhage. Intrapulmonary shunting and V/Q mismatch may occur. Pulmonary artery pressure increases. Non-acidic liquids and food particles are less damaging, and symptoms may clear within 4 hours of liquid aspiration or granuloma may form about food particles in 1-5 days. Depending upon the type of aspiration, pneumonitis may clear within a week, ARDS or pneumonia may develop, or progressive acute respiratory failure may lead to death.

There are a number of risk factors that can lead to aspiration pneumonitis/pneumonia:
- Altered level of consciousness related to illness or sedation.
- Depression of gag, swallowing reflex.
- Intubation or feeding tubes.
- Ileus or gastric distention.
- Gastrointestinal disorders, such as gastroesophageal reflux disorders (GERD).

Diagnosis is based on clinical findings, ABGs showing hypoxemia, infiltrates observed on x-ray, and increased WBC if infection present.

Symptoms
- Symptoms are similar to other pneumonias, depending upon the site of inflammation:
- Cough often with copious sputum
- Respiratory distress, dyspnea.
- Cyanosis.
- Tachycardia.
- Hypotension.

Treatment
- Suctioning as needed to clear upper airway.
- Supplemental oxygen.
- Antibiotic therapy as indicated after 48 hours if symptoms not resolving.
- Symptomatic respiratory support.

Management of foreign body aspiration

Foreign body aspiration can cause obstruction of the pharynx, larynx or trachea, leading to acute dyspnea or asphyxiation and the object may be drawn distally into the bronchial tree. With adults, most foreign bodies migrate more readily down the right bronchus. Food is the most frequently aspirated, but other small objects, such as coins or needles, may also be aspirated. Sometimes the object causes swelling, ulceration, and general inflammation that hamper removal.

Symptoms
- Initial: Severe coughing, gagging, sternal retraction, wheezing. Objects in the larynx may cause inability to breathe or speak and lead to respiratory arrest. Objects in the bronchus cause cough, dyspnea, and wheezing.
- Delayed: Hours, days, or weeks later, an undetected aspirant may cause an infection distal to the aspirated material. Symptoms depend on the area and extent of the infection.

Treatment
- Removal with laryngoscopy or bronchoscopy (rigid is often better than flexible).
- Antibiotic therapy for secondary infection.
- Surgical bronchotomy (rarely required).
- Symptomatic support.

Chronic bronchitis

Chronic bronchitis is a pulmonary airway disease characterized by severe cough with sputum production for at least 2 consecutive years. Irritation of the airways (often from smoke or pollutants) causes an inflammatory response, increasing the number of mucus-secreting glands and goblet cells while ciliary function decreases so that the extra mucus plugs the airways. Additionally, the bronchial walls thicken and alveoli near the inflamed bronchioles become fibrotic, and alveolar macrophages cannot function properly, increasing susceptibility to infections. Chronic bronchitis is most common in those >45 and occurs twice as frequently in females as males.

Symptoms
- Persistent cough with increasing sputum.
- Dyspnea.
- Frequent respiratory infections.

Treatment
- Bronchodilators.
- Long term continuous oxygen therapy or supplemental oxygen during exercise may be needed.
- Pulmonary rehabilitation to improve exercise and breathing.
- Antibiotics during infections.
- Corticosteroids may be used for acute episodes.

Emphysema

Emphysema, the primary component of COPD, is characterized by abnormal distention of air spaces at the ends of the terminal bronchioles, with destruction of alveolar walls so that there is less and less gaseous exchange and increasing dead space with resultant hypoxemia and hypercapnia and respiratory acidosis. The capillary bed is damaged as well, increasing pulmonary blood flow and raising pressure in the right atrium (cor pulmonale) and pulmonary artery, leading to cardiac failure. Complications include respiratory insufficiency and failure. There are 2 primary types of emphysema (and both forms may be present):
- **Centrilobular** (the most common form) involves the central portion of the respiratory lobule, sparing distal alveoli and usually affects the upper lobes. Typical symptoms include abnormal ventilation-perfusion ratios, hypoxemia, hypercapnia, and polycythemia with right-sided heart failure.

- **Panlobular** involves enlargement of all air spaces, including the bronchiole, alveolar duct, and alveoli, but there is minimal inflammatory disease. Typical symptoms include hyperextended rigid barrel chest, marked dyspnea, weight loss, and active expiration.

Chronic asthma

The 3 primary symptoms of chronic asthma are cough, wheezing, and dyspnea. In cough-variant asthma, a severe cough may be the only symptom, at least initially. Chronic asthma is characterized by recurring bronchospasm and inflammation of the airways resulting in airway obstruction. Asthma affects the bronchi and not the alveoli. While no longer considered part of COPD because airway obstruction is not constant and is responsive to treatment, over time fibrotic changes in the airways can result in permanent obstruction, especially if asthma is not treated adequately.

Symptoms of chronic asthma include nighttime coughing, exertional dyspnea, tightness in the chest, and cough. Acute exacerbations may occur, sometimes related to trigger, such as allergies, resulting in increased dyspnea, wheezing, cough, tachycardia, bronchospasm, and rhonchi. Treatment of chronic asthma includes chest hygiene, identification and avoidance of triggers, prompt treatment of infections, bronchodilators, long-acting β-2 agonists, and inhaled glucocorticoids.

Stages of chronic obstructive pulmonary disease (COPD)

Functional dyspnea, body mass index (BMI), and spirometry are used to assess the stages of COPD. Spirometry measures used are the ratio of forced expiratory volume in the 1st second of expiration (FEV_1) after full inhalation to total forced vital capacity (FVC). Normal lung function decreases after age 35; so normal values are adjusted for height, weight, gender, and age:
- **Stage 1** (mild): Minimal dyspnea with/without cough and sputum. FEV_1 is $\geq$80% of predicted rate and FEV_1: FVC = <70%
- **Stage 2** (moderate): Moderate to severe chronic exertional dyspnea with/without cough and sputum. FEV_1 is 50-80% of predicted rate and FEV_1: FVC = <70%.
- **Stage 3** (severe): As stage 2 but repeated episodes with increased exertional dyspnea and condition impacting quality of life. FEV_1 is 30-50% of predicted rate and FEV_1: FVC = <70%.
- **Stage 4** (very severe): Severe dyspnea and life-threatening episodes that severely impact quality of life. FEV_1 is 30% of predicted rate or <50% with chronic respiratory failure and FEV_1: FVC = <70%.

Management of chronic obstructive pulmonary disease (COPD)

COPD is not reversible, so management aims at slowing progressing, relieving symptoms, and improving quality of life:
- Smoking cessation is the primary means to slow progression and may require smoking cessation support in the form of classes or medications, such as Zyban®, nicotine patches or gum, clonidine, or nortriptyline.
- Bronchodilators, such as albuterol (Ventolin®) and salmeterol (Serevent), relieve bronchospasm and airway obstruction.
- Corticosteroids, both inhaled (Pulmicort®, Vanceril®) and oral (prednisone) may improve symptoms but are used most for associated asthma.
- Oxygen therapy may be long term continuous or used during exertion.
- Bullectomy (for bullous emphysema) to remove bullae (enlarged airspaces that do not ventilate).

- Lung volume reduction surgery may be done if involvement in lung is limited; however, mortality rates are high.
- Lung transplantation is a definitive high-risk option.
- Pulmonary rehabilitation includes breathing exercises, muscle training, activity pacing, and modification of activities.

Pulmonary arterial hypertension

Pulmonary arterial hypertension (PAH) may involve multiple processes. Usually the pulmonary vasculature adjusts easily to accommodate blood volume from the right ventricle. If there is increased blood flow, the low resistance causes vasodilation and *vice versa*.

However, sometimes the pulmonary vascular bed is damaged or obstructed, and this can impair the ability to handle changing volumes of blood. In that case, an increase in flow will increase the pulmonary arterial pressure, increasing pulmonary vascular resistance (PVR). This in turn, increases pressure on the right ventricle (RV) with increased RV workload, and eventual RV hypertrophy with displacement of the intraventricular septum and tricuspid regurgitation. Over time, this leads to right heart failure and death. Pulmonary hypertension is usually diagnosed by right-sided heart catheterization and is indicated by systolic pulmonary artery pressure >30 mm Hg and mean pulmonary artery pressure >25 mm Hg. Non-invasive testing may include echocardiogram to look for cardiac changes.

Pulmonary hypertension or pulmonary arterial hypertension (PAH) is a progressive disease of the pulmonary arteries that can severely compromise cardiovascular patients. PAH may be classified as primary (idiopathic) or secondary.
- **Primary (idiopathic) PAH** may result from changes in immune responses, pulmonary emboli, sickle cell disease, collagen diseases, Raynaud's, and the use of contraceptives. The cause may be unknown or genetic.
- **Secondary PAH** may result from pulmonary vasoconstriction brought on by hypoxemia related to COPD, sleep-disordered breathing, kyphoscoliosis, obesity, smoke inhalation, altitude sickness, interstitial pneumonia, and neuromuscular disorders. It may also be caused by a decrease in pulmonary vascular bed of 50-75%, which may result from pulmonary emboli, vasculitis, tumor emboli, and interstitial lung disease, (such as sarcoidosis). Primary cardiac disease, such as congenital defects in infants, and acquired disorders, such as rheumatic valve disease, mitral stenosis, and left ventricular failure may also contribute to PAH.

Treatment options for pulmonary arterial hypertension

Medical treatment for pulmonary arterial hypertension (PAH) aims to identify and treat any underlying cardiac or pulmonary disease, control symptoms, and prevent complications:
- **Oxygen therapy** may be needed, especially supplemental oxygen during exercise.
- **Calcium channel blockers** may provide vasodilation for some patients.
- **Pulmonary vascular dilators**, such as IV epoprostenol (Flolan®) and subcutaneous treprostinil sodium (Remodulin®) and oral bosentan (Tracleer®) help to control symptoms and prolong life.

- **Anticoagulants**, such as warfarin (Coumadin®) are an important part of therapy because of recurrent pulmonary emboli. Studies have shown that anticoagulation increases survival rates.
- **Diuretics**, such as furosemide (Lasix®) may be needed to relieve edema and restrict fluids, especially with right ventricular hypertrophy.

In some patients who cannot be managed adequately through medical treatment, a heart-lung transplant may be considered as the only effective treatment for long-term survival.

Pathophysiology of status asthmaticus

Status asthmaticus is a severe acute attack of asthma that does not respond to conventional therapy. An acute attack of asthma is precipitated by some stimulus, such as an antigen that triggers an allergic response, resulting in an inflammatory cascade that causes edema of the mucous membranes (swollen airway), contraction of smooth muscles (bronchospasm), increased mucus production (cough and obstruction), and hyperinflation of airways (decreased ventilation and shunting). Mast cells and T lymphocytes produce cytokines, which continue the inflammatory response through increased blood flow coupled with vasoconstriction and bronchoconstriction, resulting in fluid leakage from the vasculature. Epithelial cells and cilia are destroyed, exposing nerves and causing hypersensitivity. Sympathetic nervous system receptors in the bronchi stimulate bronchodilation.

Clinical symptoms of status asthmaticus

The person with status asthmaticus will often present in acute distress, non-responsive to inhaled bronchodilators:
- Airway obstruction.
- Sternal and intercostal retractions.
- Tachypnea and dyspnea with increasing cyanosis.
- Forced prolonged expirations.
- Cardiac decompensation with increased left ventricular afterload and increased pulmonary edema resulting from alveolar-capillary permeability. Hypoxia may trigger and an increase in pulmonary vascular resistance with increased right ventricular afterload.
- Pulsus paradoxus (decreased pulse on inspiration and increased on expiration) with extra beats on inspiration detected through auscultation but not detected radially. Blood pressure normally decreases slightly during inspiration, but this response is exaggerated. Pulsus paradoxus indicates increasing severity of asthma.
- Hypoxemia (with impending respiratory failure).
- Hypocapnia followed by hypercapnia (with impending respiratory failure).
- Metabolic acidosis.

Indications for mechanical ventilation for treatment of status asthmaticus

Mechanical ventilation (MV) for status asthmaticus should be avoided if possible because of the danger of increased bronchospasm as well as barotrauma and decreased circulation. Aggressive medical management with β-adrenergic agonists, corticosteroids, and anticholinergics should be tried prior to ventilation. However, there are some absolute indications for the use of intubation and ventilation and a number of other indications that are evaluated on an individual basis.

Absolute indications for MV
- Cardiac and/or pulmonary arrest.
- Markedly depressed mental status (obtundation).
- Severe hypoxia and/or apnea.
- Bradycardia

Relative indications for MV
- Exhaustion/ muscle fatigue from exertion of trying to breathe.
- Sharply diminished breath sounds and no audible wheezing.
- Pulse paradoxus >20-40 mm Hg. If pulse paradoxus is absent, this is an indication of imminent respiratory arrest.
- PaO_2 <70 mm Hg on 100% oxygen.
- Deteriorating mental status.
- Dysphonia.
- Central cyanosis.
- Increased hypercapnia.
- Metabolic/respiratory acidosis: pH <7.20.

In this patient population, ventilator goal is to minimize airway pressures while oxygenating the patient. Vent settings include: low tidal volume (6-8 ml/kg), low respiratory rate (10-14 respirations/minute), and high inspiratory flow rate (80-100 L/min).

Pharmacological agents used for asthma

Numerous pharmacological agents are used for control of asthma, some long acting to prevent attacks and others that are short-acting to provide relief for acute episodes. Listed with each are the standard med and dosage used for urgent care:
- **β-Adrenergic agonists** include both long-acting and short-acting preparations used for relaxation of smooth muscles and bronchodilation, reducing edema and aiding clearance of mucus. Medications include salmeterol (Serevent), sustained release albuterol (Volmax ER®) and short-acting albuterol (Proventil®) and levalbuterol (Xopenex®). Standard dose: Albuterol 2.5 to 5 mg q 20 minutes x 3 doses by nebulizer.
- **Anticholinergics** aid in preventing bronchial constriction and potentiate the bronchodilating action of β-Adrenergic agonists. The most-commonly used medication is ipratropium bromide (Atrovent®) 500 mcg q 20 minutes x 3 doses by nebulizer.
- **Corticosteroids** provide anti-inflammatory action by inhibiting immune responses, decreasing edema, mucus, and hyper-responsiveness. Because of numerous side effects, glucocorticosteroids are usually administered orally or parentally for >5 days (prednisone, prednisolone, methylprednisolone) and then switched to inhaled steroids. If a person receives glucocorticoids for more than 5 days, then dosages are tapered. Methylprednisone 60 to 125 mg IV is the standard dose for respiratory failure.
- **Methylxanthines** are used to improve pulmonary function and decrease need for mechanical ventilation. Medications include aminophylline and theophylline.
- **Magnesium sulfate** is used to relax smooth muscles and decrease inflammation. If administered intravenously, it must be given slowly to prevent hypotension and bradycardia. Inhaled, it potentiates the action of albuterol. Standard dosage: 2 g (8 mmol) IV x 1 dose over 20 minutes.

- **Heliox** (helium-oxygen) is administered to decrease airway resistance with airway obstruction, thereby decreasing respiratory effort. Heliox improves oxygenation of those on mechanical ventilation.
- **Leukotriene inhibitors** are used to inhibit inflammation and bronchospasm for long-term management. Medications include montelukast (Singulair®).

Thoracic surgery

Lung volume reduction surgery (LVRS) usually involves removing about 20-35% of lung tissue that is not functioning adequately in order to reduce the lung size so that the lungs work more effectively. This procedure is most commonly used with adult emphysematous COPD patients. In adults, surgery is usually bilateral; however, some patients are not candidates for bilateral surgery because of cardiac disease or emphysema affecting only one lung. Unilateral surgery has been shown to be effective. Surgical removal of part of the lung improves ventilation and gas exchange and does not require the immunosuppressant therapy required for lung transplantation. Studies have shown that those with low risk for the surgery and with emphysematous changes in the upper lobes can benefit from the surgery, but high risk patients with more wide spread emphysematous changes have increased mortality rates. The surgery may be done through an open-chest thoracotomy or through a less invasive video-assisted thoracotomy.

Pneumonectomy is surgical removal of one of the lungs. There are 2 surgical procedures:
- **Simple**: removal of just the lung
- **Extrapleural**: removal not only of the lung but also part of the diaphragm on the affected side and the pericardium on that same side.

During the operative procedure, much care must be taken to prevent contamination of the remaining lung, including the use of bronchus blockers or prone position during surgery.

Removal of the lung is indicated for a number of conditions, including:
- Severe bronchiectasis from chronic suppurative pneumonia, resulting in dilation of terminal bronchioles.
- Severe hypoplasia.
- Unilateral lung destruction with pulmonary hypertension.
- Pulmonary hemorrhage.
- Lobar emphysema.
- Cancerous lesions (the most common reason for surgery).
- Chronic pulmonary infections with destruction of lung tissue.

Because the lung capacity is reduced, persistent shortness of breath may occur with exertion even many months after surgery.

Lobectomy removes one or more lobes of a lung (which has 2 on the left and 3 on the right) and is usually done for lesions or trauma that is confined to one lobe, such as tubercular lesions, abscesses or cysts, cancer (usually non-small cell in early stages), traumatic injury, or bronchiectasis. Surgery is usually done through an open thoracotomy or video-assisted thoracotomy. Complications can include hemorrhage, post-operative infection with or without abscess formation, and pneumothorax. Usually 1-2 chest tubes are left in place in the immediate post-surgical period to remove air and/or fluid.

Segmental resection removes a bronchovascular segment and is used for small lesions in the periphery, bronchiectasis or congenital cysts or blebs.

Wedge resection removes a small wedged-shape portion of the lung tissue and is used for small peripheral lesions, granulomas, or blebs.

Bronchoplastic (sleeve) reconstruction removes part of bronchus and lung tissue with reanastomosis of bronchus and is used for small lesions of the carina or bronchus.

Management of pulmonary trauma (Pulmonary hemorrhage)

Pulmonary hemorrhage is an acute life-threatening injury that often results in death prior to arrival at the hospital; however, those presenting with traumatic pulmonary hemorrhage, as from a blunt or penetrating injury, requires immediate surgical repair. Even with immediate surgery, survival after serious injury to a major pulmonary vessel is rare. It is important that a large bore IV be immediately inserted and fluid replacement begun while blood is typed and cross matched. The patient should be evaluated for shock and treatment, including colloid solutions, crystalloids, or blood, provided as indicated. Pulmonary hemorrhage may result in hemothorax. In some cases, pneumothorax may also be present, resulting in mediastinal shift that increases the difficulty of identifying and repairing the bleeding vessel. If the patient is stabilized, computed tomography may provide accurate diagnosis to isolate the area of hemorrhage.

Management of pulmonary trauma (Tracheal perforation/injury)

Tracheal perforation/injury may result from external injury, such as from trauma from a vehicle accident or from an assault, such as a gunshot or knife wound or in some cases a laceration as a complication of percutaneous dilation tracheostomy (PDT) or other endotracheal tubes. In some cases, an inhaled foreign object may become lodged in the trachea and eventually erode the tissue. If the injury is severe, respiratory failure may cause death in a very short period of time, so rapid diagnosis and treatment is critical.

Symptoms
- Severe respiratory distress.
- Hemoptysis.
- Strider with progressive dysphonia.
- Pneumothorax, pneumomediastinum.
- Subcutaneous emphysema from air leaking from the pleural space into the tissues of the chest wall, neck, face, and even into the upper extremities.

Treatment
- Intubation and non-surgical healing for small lacerations.
- Surgical repair for larger wounds or severe respiratory distress.

Management of thoracic trauma

Pulmonary contusion is the result of direct force to the lung, resulting in parenchymal injury and bleeding and edema that impact the capillary-alveoli juncture, resulting in intrapulmonary shunting as the alveoli and interstitium fill with fluid. Parenchymal injury reduces compliance and impairs ventilation. Diagnosis may be more difficult if other injuries, such as fractured ribs or pneumothorax are also present because they may all contribute to respiratory distress. CT scans provide the best diagnostic tool.

Symptoms
- Symptoms vary widely depending upon the degree of injury but may include:
- Mild dyspnea.
- Severe progressive dyspnea.
- Hemoptysis.
- Acute respiratory failure.

Treatment
- Treatment varies according to the injury but can include:
- Close monitoring of arterial blood gases and respiratory status.
- Supplemental oxygen.
- Intubation and mechanical ventilation with positive-end expiratory pressure (PEEP) for more severe respiratory distress.
- Fluid management and diuretics to control pulmonary edema.
- Respiratory physiotherapy to clear secretions.

Fractured ribs are usually the result of severe trauma, such as blunt force from a motor vehicle accident or physical abuse. Underlying injuries should be expected according to the area of fractures:
- Upper 2 ribs: Injuries to trachea, bronchi, or great vessels.
- Right-sided ≥rib 8: Trauma to liver.
- Left-sided ≥ rib 8: Trauma to spleen.

Pain, often localized or experienced on respirations or compression of chest way may be the primary symptom of rib fractures, resulting in shallow breathing that can lead to atelectasis or pneumonia. Diagnostics: Chest x-ray or CT scan.

Treatment is primarily supportive as rib fractures usually heal in about 6 weeks: however, preventing pulmonary complications (pneumothorax, hemothorax) often necessitates adequate pain control. Underlying injuries are treated according to the type and degree of injury:
- Supplemental oxygen.
- Analgesia may include NSAIDs, intercostal nerve blocks, and narcotics.
- Pulmonary physiotherapy.
- Rib Belts
- ORIF
- Splinting

Hemothorax occurs with bleeding into the pleural space, usually from major vascular injury such as tears in intercostal vessels, lacerations of great vessels, or trauma to lung parenchyma. A small bleed may be self-limiting and seal, but a tear in a large vessel can result in massive bleeding, followed quickly by hypovolemic shock. The pressure from the blood may result in inability of the lung to ventilate and a mediastinal shift. Often a hemothorax occurs with a pneumothorax, especially in severe chest trauma. Further symptoms include severe respiratory distress, decreased breath sounds, and dullness on auscultation. Treatment includes placement of a chest tube to drain the hemothorax, but with large volumes, the pressure may be preventing exsanguination, which can occur abruptly as the blood drains and pressure is reduced, so a large bore intravenous line should be in place and typed and cross-matched blood immediately available. Autotransfusion may be used, contraindicated if wound is older than three hours, possibility of bowel/stomach contamination, liver failure, and malignancy.

Thoracotomy may be indicated after chest tube insertion if there is still hemodynamic instability, tension hemothorax, more than 1500 mL blood initially on insertion, or bleeding continues at a rate of >300 ml/hr.

The diagnostic procedures and tools used during assessment of pulmonary and thoracic trauma/disease will vary according to the type and degree of injury/disease, but may include:
- **Thorough physical examination** including cardiac and pulmonary status, assessing for any abnormalities.
- **Electrocardiogram** to assess for cardiac arrhythmias.
- **Chest x-ray** should be done for all those with injuries to check for fractures, pneumothorax, major injuries, and placement of intubation tubes. X-rays can be taken quickly and with portable equipment so they can be completed quickly during the initial assessment.
- **Computerized tomography** may be indicated after initial assessment, especially if there is a possibility of damage to the parenchyma of the lungs.
- **Oximetry and atrial blood gases** as indicated.
- **12-lead electrocardiogram** may be needed if there are arrhythmias for more careful observation.
- **Echocardiogram** should be done if there is apparent cardiac damage.

Agents used for pulmonary pharmacology

There are a wide range of agents used for pulmonary pharmacology, depending upon the type and degree of pulmonary disease. Agents include:
- **Opioid analgesics:** Use to provide both pain relief and sedation for those on mechanical ventilation to reduce sympathetic response. Medications may include fentanyl (Sublimaze®) or morphine sulfate (MS Contin®).
- **Neuromuscular blockers:** Used for induced paralysis of those who have not responded adequately to sedation, especially for intubation and mechanical ventilation. Medications may include pancuronium (Pavulon®) and vecuronium (Norcuron®). However, there is controversy about the use as induced paralysis has been linked to increased mortality rates, sensory hearing loss (pancuronium), atelectasis, and ventilation-perfusion mismatch.
- **Human B-type natriuretic peptides:** Used to reduce pulmonary capillary wedge pressure. Medications include nesiritide (Natrecor®).

Pulmonary pharmacology

Agents used for pulmonary pharmacology:
- **Vasopressors/Inotropic agents:** Used to increase cardiac output. Dopamine (Intropin®) increases renal output and blood pressure. Dobutamine (Dobutrex®) increases cardiac contractibility and blood pressure.
- **Surfactants:** Reduces surface tension to prevent collapse of alveoli. Beractant (Survanta®) is derived from bovine lung tissue and calfactant (Infasurf®) from calf lung tissue. They are administered as inhalants.

- **Alkalinizers:** Used to treat metabolic acidosis and ↓ pulmonary vascular resistance by achieving an alkaline pH. Medications include sodium bicarbonate and tromethamine (THAM).
- **Pulmonary vasodilator (inhaled nitric oxide):** Used to relax the vascular muscles and produce pulmonary vasodilation. Some studies show it reduces need for extracorporeal membrane oxygenation (ECMO) although this is not supported by other studies.
- **Methylxanthines:** Used to stimulate muscle contractions of chest and stimulate respirations. Medications include aminophylline (Aminophylline®), caffeine citrate (Cafcit®), and doxapram (Dopram®).
- **Diuretics:** Used to reduce pulmonary edema. Medications include loop diuretics such as furosemide (Lasix®) and metolazone (Mykrox®).
- **Nitrates:** Used for vasodilation to reduce preload and afterload to reduce myocardial need for oxygen. Medications include nitroglycerin (Nitro-Bid®) and nitroprusside sodium (Nitropress®).
- **Antibiotics:** Used for treatment of respiratory infections, including pneumonia. Medications are used according to the pathogenic agent and may include macrolides, such as azithromycin (Zithromax®), erythromycin (E-Mycin®).
- **Antimycobacterials:** Used for treatment of TB and other mycobacterial diseases. Medications include isoniazid (Laniazid®, Nydrazid®), ethambutol (Myambutol®), rifampin (Rifadin®), streptomycin sulfate, and pyrazinamide.
- **Antivirals:** Used to inhibit replication of virus early in a viral infection. Effectiveness decreases as time passes because replication process has already begun. Medications include ribavirin (Virazole®) and zanamivir (Relenza®).

Pulse oximetry

Pulse oximetry, continuous or intermittent, utilizes an external oximeter that attaches to the patient's finger or earlobe to measure arterial oxygen saturation (SPO_2), the percentage of hemoglobin that is saturated with oxygen. The oximeter also usually attaches to a machine that emits a beep with each heartbeat and indicates the current heart rate. BP monitoring is also done. The oximeter uses light waves to determine oxygen saturation (SPO_2). Oxygen saturation should be maintained >95% although some patients with chronic respiratory disorders, such as COPD may have lower SPO_2. Results may be compromised by impaired circulation, excessive light, poor positioning, and nail polish. If SPO_2 falls, the oximeter should be repositioned, as incorrect position is a common cause of inaccurate readings. Oximetry is often used postsurgically and when patients are on mechanical ventilation. Oximeters do not provide information about carbon dioxide levels, so they cannot monitor carbon dioxide retention. Oximeters cannot differentiate between different forms of hemoglobin, so if hemoglobin has picked up carbon monoxide, the oximeter may interpret it as oxygen.

Arterial blood gases (ABGs)

Arterial blood gases are monitored to assess effectiveness of oxygenation, ventilation, and acid-base status, and to determine oxygen flow rates. Partial pressure of a gas is that exerted by each gas in a mixture of gases, proportional to its concentration, based on total atmospheric pressure of 760 mm Hg at sea level. Normal values include:
- Acidity/alkalinity (pH): 7.35-7.45.
- Partial pressure of carbon dioxide ($PaCO_2$): 35-45 mm Hg.
- Partial pressure of oxygen (PaO_2): ≥80 mg Hg.

- Bicarbonate concentration (HCO_3-): 22-26 mEq/L.
- Oxygen saturation (SaO_2): ≥95%.

The relationship between these elements, particularly the $PaCO_2$ and the PaO_2 indicates respiratory status. For example, $PaCO_2$ >55 and the PaO_2 <60 in a patient previously in good health indicates respiratory failure. There are many issues to consider. Ventilator management may require a higher $PaCO_2$ to prevent barotrauma and a lower PaO_2 to reduce oxygen toxicity.

Respiratory acidosis

Respiratory acidosis is precipitated by inadequate ventilation of alveoli, interfering with gaseous exchange so that carbon dioxide increases and oxygen decreases, causing excess carbonic acid (H_2CO_3) levels. The body maintains a normal pH by balancing bicarbonate (renal) with $PaCO_2$ (pulmonary) in a 20:1 ratio. If the pH alters, the system (renal or pulmonary) that is not causing the problem compensates. Respiratory acidosis is most common in acute respiratory disorders, such as pulmonary edema, pneumothorax, sleep apnea syndrome, atelectasis, aspiration of foreign objects, severe pneumonia, ARDS, administration of oxygen to treat chronic hypercapnia, or mechanical ventilation. Diseases with respiratory muscle impairment may also cause respiratory acidosis, such as muscular dystrophy, severe Guillain-Barre, and myasthenia gravis. Respiratory acidosis may be acute or chronic:
- **Acute**: Increased $PaCO_2$ with decreased pH caused by sudden decrease in ventilation.
- **Chronic**: Increased $PaCO_2$ with normal pH and serum bicarbonate (HCO_3-) >30 mm Hg with renal compensation.

ABG values in respiratory acidosis:
- pH <7.35.
- $PaCO_2$ >42 mm Hg.

Symptoms for acute respiratory acidosis:
- Increased heart rate.
- Tachypnea. Hypertension.
- Confusion and pressure in head related to cerebrovascular vasodilation, especially if $PaCO_2$ > 60 mm Hg.
- Increased intracranial pressure with papilledema.
- Ventricular fibrillation.
- Hyperkalemia.

Symptoms for acute respiratory acidosis:
Symptoms may be subtler with chronic respiratory acidosis because of the compensatory mechanisms. If the $PaCO_2$ remains >50 mm Hg for long periods, the respiratory center becomes increasingly insensitive to CO_2 as a respiratory stimulus, replaced by hypoxemia, so supplemental oxygen administration should be monitored carefully to ensure that respirations are not depressed.

Treatment
- Improving ventilation. Mechanical ventilation may be used with care.
- Medications as indicated (depending on cause): bronchodilators, anticoagulation therapy, diuretics, and antibiotics.
- Pulmonary hygiene.

Respiratory alkalosis

Respiratory alkalosis results from hyperventilation, during which extra CO_2 is excreted, causing a decrease in carbonic acid (H_2CO_3) concentration in the plasma. Respiratory alkalosis may be acute or chronic. Acute respiratory alkalosis is precipitated by anxiety attacks, hypoxemia, salicylate intoxication, bacteremia (Gram-negative), and incorrect ventilator settings. Chronic respiratory alkalosis may result from chronic hepatic insufficiency, cerebral tumors, and chronic hypocapnia.

Characteristics
Decreased $PaCO_2$. Normal or decreased serum bicarbonate (HCO_3-) as kidneys conserve hydrogen and excrete HCO_3-. Increased pH.

Symptoms
- Vasoconstriction with decreased cerebral blood flow resulting in lightheadedness, alterations in mentation, and/or unconsciousness.
- Numbness and tingling. Tinnitus.
- Tachycardia and dysrhythmias.

Treatment
Identifying and treating underlying cause. If respiratory alkalosis is related to anxiety, breathing in a paper bag may increase CO_2 level. Some people may require sedation. ABG values in respiratory alkalosis:
- pH >7.45.
- $PaCO_2$ < 38 mm Hg.
- Decreased H_2CO_3.

Airway management

Tracheostomy, surgical tracheal opening, may be utilized for mechanical ventilation. Tracheostomy tubes are inserted into the opening to provide a conduit and maintain the opening. Tracheostomy tubes are usually silastic or plastic, most lacking an inner cannula because they are non-adherent. The tube is secured with ties around the neck. Because the air entering the lungs through the tracheostomy bypasses the warming and moistening affects of the upper airway, air is humidified through a room humidifier or through delivery of humidified air through a special mask or mechanical ventilation. The patient with a tracheostomy must have continuous monitoring of vital signs and respiratory status to ensure patency of tracheostomy.

Regular suctioning is needed, especially initially, to remove secretions:
- Suction catheter should be 50% the size of the tracheostomy tube to allow ventilation during suctioning.
- Vacuum pressure: 80-100 mm Hg.
- Catheter should only be inserted ≤ 0.5 cm beyond tube to avoid damage to tissues or perforation
- Catheter should be inserted without suction and intermittent suction on withdrawal.

Ensuring that a facemask is the correct fit and type is important for adequate ventilation, oxygenation, and prevention of aspiration. Difficulties in management of facemask ventilation relate to risk factors: >55 years, obesity, beard, edentulous, and history of snoring. In some cases, if dentures are adhered well, they may be left in place during induction. The facemask is applied by lifting the mandible (jaw thrust) to the mask and avoiding pressure on soft tissue. Oral or nasal airways may be used, ensuring that the distal end is at the angle of the mandible. There are a number of steps to prevent mask airway leaks:

- Increasing or decreasing the amount of air to the mask to allow better seal.
- Securing the mask with both hands while another person ventilates.
- Accommodating a large nose by using the mask upside down.
- Utilizing a laryngeal mask airway if excessive beard prevents seal.

A nasal cannula can be used to deliver supplemental oxygen to a patient, but it is only useful for flow rates ≤ 6 L/min as higher rates are drying of the nasal passages. As it is not an airtight system, some ambient air is breathed in as well so oxygen concentration ranges from about 24-44%. The nasal cannula does not allow for control of respiratory rate, so the patient must be able to breathe independently.

A non-rebreather mask can be used to deliver higher concentrations (60-90%) of oxygen to those patients who are able to breathe independently. The mask fits over the nose and mouth and is secured by an elastic strap. A 1.5 L reservoir bag is attached and connects to an oxygen source. The bag is inflated to about 1 liter at a rate of 8-15 L/min before the mask is applied as the patient breathes from this reservoir. A one-way exhalation valve prevents most exhaled air from being rebreathed.

High and low flow oxygen delivery

High flow oxygen delivery devices provide oxygen at flow rates higher than the patient's inspiratory flow rate at specific medium to high FIO_2, up to 100%. However a flow of 100% oxygen actually provides only 60 to 80% FIO_2 to the patient because the patient also breathes in some room air, diluting the oxygen. The actual amount of oxygen received depends on the type of interface or mask. Additionally, the flow rate is actually less than the inspiratory flow rate upon actual delivery. High flow oxygen delivery is usually not used in the sleep center. Humidification is usually required because the high flow is drying.

Low flow oxygen delivery devices provide 100% oxygen at flow rates lower than the patient's inspiratory flow rate, but the oxygen mixes with room air, so the FIO_2 varies. Humidification is usually only required if flow rate is >3L/min. Much oxygen is wasted with exhalation, so a number of different devices to conserve oxygen are available. Interfaces include transtracheal catheters and cannulae with reservoirs.

Oxygen interfaces

A number of different oxygen interfaces are used for the delivery of oxygen to the patient:

Nasal prongs (cannulae): This is the most common delivery system for oxygen because of ease of use, providing FIO_2 of 24-40% with flows ≤6 LPM. Humidification is needed for flow rates >4 LPM.

Oxygen mask: This covers the nose and mouth, delivering FIO_2 of 30-60%, but flow of oxygen should be maintained between 6 and 12 to prevent rebreathing. Because of the higher flow rate, humidification should be used. Oxygen masks are usually used short-term when higher rates of oxygen are needed.

Venturi mask: Oxygen entrainment masks come with different size color-coded nozzles to more accurately control the FIO_2, with different sizes providing different FIO_2, usually ranging from 24 to 50% although FIO_2 >35% is not always reliable. Flow rate is 12 to 15 LPM. Air-entrainment humidifiers may be used to add humidification. Oxygen entrainment masks are often used with COPD patients.

Therapeutic gases

Carbon dioxide is a potent stimulator of respirations, but it is rarely used therapeutically because it can depress respirations if hypercarbia or respiratory acidosis is present. CO_2 may be administered at times as part of anesthesia, but it is most commonly used for insufflation for laparoscopic/endoscopic procedures.

Nitric oxide (NO) is used as a pulmonary vessel dilator to improve oxygenation by decreasing pulmonary artery pressure and pulmonary vascular resistance. NO is FDA-approved for use for neonatal PPH but is sometimes used for adults, although studies have not shown it an effective treatment for RDS. NO should be delivered at 0.1 to 50 ppm to avoid toxicity that can occur over 50 ppm. Toxic reactions include methemoglobinemia and platelet inhibition with resultant bleeding.

Helium is mixed with oxygen (Heliox) and used to reduce airway resistance during mechanical ventilation and for pulmonary function tests. Heliox may also be used to treat respiratory obstruction and is used during laser surgery on the airway because it readily conducts heat away from the surgical site, reducing tissue damage. Heliox is sometimes used for COPD patients as it increases hyperventilation and reduces carbon dioxide levels.

Ventilator management

There are many types of ventilators now in use, and the specific directions for use of each type must be followed carefully, but there are general principles that apply to all ventilator management. The following should be monitored:
- **Type of ventilation:** volume-cycled, pressure-cycled, negative-pressure, HFJV, HFOV, CPAP, Bi-PAP.
- **Control mode:** controlled ventilation, assisted ventilation, synchronized intermittent mandatory [allows spontaneous breaths between ventilator controlled inhalation/exhalation], positive-end expiratory pressure (PEEP) [positive pressure at end of expiration], CPAP, Bi-PAP.
- **Tidal volume** (TV) range should be set in relation to respiratory rate.
- **Inspiratory-expiratory ratio** (I: E) usually ranges from 1:2-1:5, but may vary.
- **Respiratory rate** will depend upon TV and $PaCO_2$ target.
- **Fraction of inspired oxygen** (FiO_2) [percentage of oxygen in the inspired air], usually ranging from 21-100%, usually maintained <40% to avoid toxicity.
- **Sensitivity** determines the effort needed to trigger inspiration.
- **Pressure** controls the pressure exerted in delivering TV.
- **Rate of flow** controls the L/min speed of TV.

Positive pressure ventilators

Positive pressure ventilators assist respiration by applying pressure directly to the airway, inflating the lungs, forcing expansion of the alveoli, and facilitating gas exchange. Generally, endotracheal intubation or tracheostomy is necessary to maintain positive pressure ventilation for extended periods. There are 3 basic kinds of positive pressure ventilators:

- **Pressure cycled:** This type of ventilation is usually used for short-term treatment in adolescents or adults. The IPPB machine is the most common type. This delivers a flow of air to a preset pressure and then cycles off.   Airway resistance or changes in compliance can affect volume of air and may compromise ventilation.
- **Time cycled**: This type of ventilation regulates the volume of air the patient receives by controlling the length of inspiration and the flow rate.
- **Volume cycled**: This type of ventilation provides a preset flow of pressurized air during inspiration and then cycles off and allows passive expiration, providing a fairly consistent volume of air.

Non-invasive positive pressure ventilators

Non-invasive positive pressure ventilators provide air through a tight-fitting nasal or facemask, usually pressure cycled, avoiding the need for intubation and reducing the danger of hospital-acquired infection and mortality rates. It can be used for acute respiratory failure and pulmonary edema. There are 2 types of non-invasive positive pressure ventilators:

- **CPAP (Continuous positive airway pressure)** provides a steady stream of pressurized air throughout both inspiration and expiration. CPAP improves breathing by decreasing preload for patients with congestive heart failure. It reduces the effort required for breathing by increasing residual volume and improving gas exchange.
- **Bi-PAP (Bi-level positive airway pressure)** provides a steady stream of pressurized air as CPAP but it senses inspiratory effort and increases pressure during inspiration. Bi-PAP pressures for inspiration and expiration can be set independently. Machines can be programmed with a backup rate to ensure a set number of respirations per minute.

High frequency jet ventilation

High frequency jet ventilation (HFJV) (Life Pulse®) directs a high velocity stream of air into the lungs in a long spiraling spike that forces carbon dioxide against the walls, penetrating dead space and providing gas exchange by using small tidal volumes of 1-3 ml/kg, much smaller than with conventional mechanical ventilation. Because the jet stream technology is effective for short distances, the valve and pressure transducer must be placed by the person's head. Inhalation is controlled while expiration is passive, but the rate of respiration is up to 11 per second ("panting" respirations). HFJV may be used in conjunction with low-pressure conventional ventilation to increase flow to alveoli. HFJV reduces barotrauma because of the low tidal volume and low pressure. HFJV is used for numerous conditions, including evolving chronic lung disease, pulmonary interstitial emphysema, bronchopulmonary dysplasia, and hypoxemic respiratory failure. It reduces mean airway pressure (MAP) and the oxygenation index. Treatment with HFJV may reduce the need for ECMO.

High frequency oscillatory ventilation

High frequency oscillatory ventilation (HFOV) provides pressurized ventilation with tidal volumes approximately equal to dead space at about 150 breaths per minutes (BPM). Pressure is usually higher with HFOV than HFJV in order to maintain expansion of the alveoli and to keep the airway open during gas exchange. Oxygenation is regulated separately. HFOV has both an active inspiration and expiration, so the respiratory cycle is completely controlled. HFOV reduces pulmonary vascular resistance and improves ventilation-perfusion matching and oxygenation

- 67 -

without injuring the lung, reducing the risk of barotrauma. HFOV is used for respiratory distress syndrome, persistent pulmonary hypertension, more commonly for infants and children, but there is increasing interest in using HFOV with adults because of the smaller tidal volume that prevents overinflation of the lungs and atelectasis of those with ARDS.

Ventilation-induced lung injury

Ventilation-induced lung injury (VILI) is damage caused by mechanical ventilation. It is common in acute distress syndrome (ARDS) but can affect any ventilation patient. VILI comprises 4 interrelated elements:
- **Barotrauma**: Damage to the lung caused by excessive pressure.
- **Volutrauma**: Alveolar damage related to high tidal volume ventilation.
- **Atelectotrauma**: Injury caused by repetitive forced opening and closing of alveoli.
- **Biotrauma**: Inflammatory response.

In VILI, essentially the increased pressure and tidal volume over-distends the alveoli, which rupture, and air moves into the interstitial tissue resulting in pulmonary interstitial emphysema. With continued ventilation, the air in the interstitium moves into the subcutaneous tissue and may result in pneumopericardium and pneumomediastinum, or rupture the pleural sac can cause tension pneumothorax and mediastinal shift, which can cause respiratory failure and cardiac arrest. VILI has caused a change in ventilation procedures with lower tidal volumes and pressures used as well as newer forms of ventilation, HFJV and HFOV, preferred to traditional mechanical ventilation for many patients.

Chronic ventilatory failure

Chronic ventilatory failure occurs when alveolar ventilation fails to increase in response to increasing levels of carbon dioxide, usually associated with chronic pulmonary diseases, such as asthma and COPD, drug overdoses, or diseases that impair respiratory effort, such as Guillain-Barré and myasthenia gravis. Normally, the ventilatory system is able to maintain PCO_2 and pH levels within narrow limits, even though PO_2 levels may be more variable, but with ventilatory failure, the body is not able to compensate for the resultant hypercapnia, and pH falls, resulting in respiratory acidosis. Symptoms include increasing dyspnea with tachypnea, gasping respirations, and use of accessory muscles. Patients may become confused as hypercapnia causes increased intracranial pressure. If pH is <7.2, cardiac arrhythmias, hyperkalemia, and hypotension can occur as pulmonary arteries constrict and the peripheral vascular system dilates. Diagnosis is per symptoms, ABGs consistent with respiratory acidosis (PCO_2 >50 and pH <7.35), pulse oximetry, and chest x-ray. Treatment can include non-invasive PPV, endotracheal mechanical ventilation, corticosteroids, and bronchodilators.

Criteria for ventilator weaning

Ventilator weaning has 3 phases: removal of the ventilator, extubation, and finally removal of supportive oxygen. Criteria for ventilator weaning include:
- Vital capacity 10 to 15 mL/kg.
- Maximum (negative) inspiratory pressure of at least -20 cm H_2O.
- Tidal volume (TV) of 7 to 9 mL/kg.
- Minute ventilation of about 6L/min (Respiratory rate x TV).
- Rapid shallow breath index <100 breaths/m/L.

- PaO_2 >60 mm Hg.
- FiO_2 <40%.

If these criteria are met and the patient passes a SBT, then extubation can be done. Various protocols are followed in weaning patients off of ventilators, including the use of intermittent mandatory ventilation (IMV) and synchronized intermittent mandatory ventilation (SIMV), which can be used with pressure support ventilation (PSV). Criteria for oxygen weaning:
- FiO_2 reduced until PaO_2 70 to 100 mm Hg on room air.
- Supplemental O_2 necessary with PaO_2 < 70 mm Hg (Medicare requires PaO_2 55 mm Hg for reimbursement for home oxygen use).

Preventing ventilator complications

Methods to prevent complications from mechanical ventilation include:
- Elevate patient's head and chest to 30° to prevent aspiration and ventilation-associated pneumonia.
- Reposition patient every 2 hours.
- Provide DVT prophylaxis, such as external compression support and/or heparin (5000 u sq 2-3 times daily).
- Administer famotidine (20 mg BID per NG tube or IV) or sucralfate (1 gram per NG tube QID) to prevent gastrointestinal bleeding.
- Decrease and eliminate sedation/analgesia as soon as possible.
- Follow careful protocols for pressure settings to prevent barotrauma. Tidal volumes are usually maintained at 8 to 12 mL/kg PBW (per AACN guidelines), but in incidences of high probability of ARDS, volumes should be less (6 mL/kg) to avoid lung injury.
- Monitor for pneumothorax or evidence of barotrauma.
- Conduct nutritional assessment (including lab tests) to prevent malnutrition.
- Monitor intake and output carefully and administer IV fluids to prevent dehydration.
- Do daily spontaneous breathing trials and discontinue ventilation as soon as possible.

Thoracentesis

A thoracentesis (aspiration of fluid or air from pleural space) is done to make a diagnosis, relieve pressure on the lung caused by pleural effusion, or instill medications. A chest x-ray is done prior to the procedure. A sedative may be given. The patient is in sitting position, leaning onto a padded bedside stand, straddling a chair with head supported on the back of the chair, or lying on the opposite side with the head of the bed elevated 30-45° to ensure that fluid remains at the base. The patient should avoid coughing or moving during the procedure. The chest x-ray or ultrasound determines needle placement. After a local anesthetic is administered, a needle (with an attached 20-ml syringe and 3-way stopcock with tubing and a receptacle) is advanced intercostally into the pleural space. Fluid is drained, collected, examined, and measured. The needle is removed and a pressure dressing applied. A chest x-ray is done to ensure there is no pneumothorax. The patient is monitored for cough, dyspnea, and hypoxemia.

Bronchoscopy

Bronchoscopy utilizes a thin flexible fiberoptic bronchoscope to inspect the larynx, trachea, and bronchi for diagnostic purposes. It is also used to collect specimens, obtain biopsies, remove foreign bodies or secretions, treat atelectasis, and to excise lesions. The patient is in supine position during the procedure. The Mallampati classification may be used to determine difficulty of airway. The patient receives local anesthesia to the nares (lidocaine gel) and oropharynx (lidocaine gel, spray, or nebulizer), and usually receives a benzodiazepine (commonly midazolam or lorazepam), an opioid (fentanyl or meperidine), or propofol. Medications are usually given in small incremental doses through the procedure and may be combined. Oversedation may cause physiologic depression, but undersedation may result in recall and agitation with sympathetic activation. The tube is advanced through the nares and down the trachea to the bronchi. Airway patency, respiratory rate, and oxygen saturation must be constantly monitored. Complications can include bleeding, arrhythmias, obstruction, laryngospasm, and respiratory failure.

Conscious sedation

Conscious sedation is used to decrease sensations of pain and awareness caused by a surgical or invasive procedure, such a biopsy, chest tube insertion, fracture repair, and endoscopy. It is also used during presurgical preparations, such as insertion of central lines, catheters, and use of cooling blankets. Conscious sedation uses a combination of analgesia and sedation so that patients can remain responsive and follow verbal cues but have a brief amnesia preventing recall of the procedures. The patient must be monitored carefully, including pulse oximetry, during this type of sedation. The most commonly used drugs include:
- Midazolam (Versed®): This is a short-acting water-soluble sedative, with onset of 1-5 minutes, peaking in 30, and duration usually about 1 hour (but may last up to 6 hours).
- Fentanyl: This is a short-acting opioid with immediate onset, peaking in 10-15 minutes and with duration of about 20-45 minutes.

The fentanyl/midazolam combination provides both sedation and pain control. Conscious sedation usually requires 6 hours fasting prior to administration.

Tracheal intubation

Tracheal intubation is often necessary with respiratory failure for control of hypoxemia, hypercapnia, hypoventilation, and/or obstructed airway. Equipment should be assembled and tubes and connections checked for air leaks with a 10 ml syringe. The mouth and/or nose should be cleaned of secretions and suctioned if necessary. The patient should be supine with the patient's head level with the lower sternum of the clinician. With orotracheal/endotracheal intubation, the clinician holds the laryngoscope (in left hand) and inserts it into right corner of mouth, the epiglottis is lifted and the larynx exposed. A thin flexible intubation stylet may be used and the endotracheal tube (ETT) (in right hand) is inserted through the vocal cords and into the trachea, cuff inflated to minimal air leak (10 ml initially until patient stabilizes), and placement confirmed through capnometry or esophageal detection devices. The correct depth of insertion is verified: Approximately 21 cm (female), 23 cm (male). After insertion, the tube is secured.

Correct placement of endotracheal tubes

There are a number of methods to confirm correct placement of endotracheal tubes. Clinical assessment alone is not adequate.
- **Capnometry** utilizes an end-tidal CO_2 (ETCO$_2$) detector that measures the concentration of CO_2 in expired air, usually through pH sensitive paper that changes color (commonly purple to yellow). The capnometer is attached to the ETT and a bag-valve-mask (BVM) ventilator attached. The patient is provided 6 ventilations and the CO_2 concentration checked.

- **Capnography** is attached to the ETT and provides a waveform graph, showing the varying concentrations of CO_2 in real time throughout each ventilation (with increased CO_2 on expiration) and can indicate changes in respiratory status.
- **Esophageal detection devices** fit over the end of the ETT so that a large syringe can be used to attempt to aspirate. If the ETT is in the esophagus, the walls collapse on aspiration and resistance occurs whereas the syringe fills with air if the ETT is in the trachea. A self-inflating bulb (Ellick® device) may also be used.

Capnography with end-tidal CO_2 detector

Capnometry utilizes an end-tidal CO_2 (ETCO) detector that measures the concentration of CO_2 in expired air, usually through pH sensitive paper that changes color (commonly purple to yellow). Typically, the capnometer is attached to the ETT and a bag-valve-mask (BVM) ventilator attached. The capnogram provides data in the shape of a waveform that represents the partial pressure of exhaled gas. It is often used to confirm placement of endotracheal tubes as clinical assessment is not always sufficient, and it is a noninvasive mode of monitoring carbon dioxide in the respiratory cycle. Information provided by the capnogram includes:
- $PaCO_2$ level.
- Type and degree of bronchial obstruction, such as COPD (waveform changes from rectangular to a fin-like)
- Air leaks in the ventilation system.
- Rebreathing precipitated by need for new CO_2 absorber.
- Cardiac arrest.
- Hypothermia or reduced metabolism.

Sedation/analgesia with mechanical ventilation

Patients intubated for mechanical ventilation are usually given sedation and/or analgesia initially, but medications should be reduced and given in boluses rather than with continuous IV drip with a goal of stopping sedation as it prolongs ventilation time. Typical sedatives include midazolam, propofol, and lorazepam. Narcotic analgesics include fentanyl and morphine sulfate. Uses of sedation include:
- Controlling agitation and excessive movement that may interfere with ventilation.
- Reduce pain and discomfort associated with ventilation.
- Control respiratory distress.

Triglyceride levels must be checked periodically if propofol is administered for >24-48 hours. Neuromuscular blocking agents are rarely used because they may cause long-term weakness and increase length of ventilation although they may be indicated in some cases, such as with excessive shivering or cardiac arrest. Many patients are able to tolerate mechanical ventilation without sedation, and sedation should always be decreased to the minimal amount necessary as excess sedation may delay extubation.

Spontaneous breathing trial

A spontaneous breathing trial (SBT) should be used prior to extubating a patient if the patient is not agitated and has no evidence of myocardial ischemia or increased ICP. The patient should exhibit some spontaneous triggering of respirations and should not be receiving large doses of vasopressor or inotropic agent. SpO_2 should be ≥88% with FiO_2 of 0.50 and PEEP at 7.5 cm H_2O prior to the SBT.

The SBT should be done in the morning for a prescribed period (usually 30 to 120 minutes). The ventilator rate is adjusted to 0 and pressure support decreased to 0 to 7. The SBT should be discontinued if the following occur:

- Respiratory rate >35 or <8 for >5 minutes.
- Mental status changes.
- SpO_2 <88% for >15 minutes.
- Respiratory distress (HR >130 BPM or <60 BPM, marked dyspnea, diaphoresis, increased use of accessory respiratory muscles, respiratory arrest).

Patients who pass the SBT have an 85-90% chance of breathing successfully after extubation. Patients who repeatedly fail daily SBT may require tracheostomy.

Airway clearance

Airway clearance, the ability to move secretions/foreign particles from the upper airway and prevent aspiration, depends on an intact and functioning mucociliary system and the ability to cough effectively. Mucous provides barrier protection to the tissue, and the cilia mechanically move mucous and particles upward. Inflammation, asthma, COPD, CF, and mechanical ventilation can alter the viscosity of the mucous and impair its effectiveness. CF, lung transplantation, mechanical irritation, and smoking can damage cilia. Patients with tracheostomies and/or mechanical ventilation tend to retain secretions, impairing the exchange of oxygen and increasing the effort required to breathe, leading to increased inflammation and infection that further impairs lung function. Both increased and retained secretions lead to decreased FEV1 and higher mortality rates. Cough is impaired by mechanical ventilation as well as restrictive and obstructive respiratory diseases. Airway clearance measures include:

- Directed cough, chest physiotherapy (if not on ventilator).
- Positioning with head of bed elevated.
- Suctioning as needed (limited to 5 seconds in duration).
- Antibiotics for infection.
- Bronchodilators.

Airway devices

Airways are used to establish a patent airway and facilitate respirations:

- **Oropharyngeal**: This plastic airway curves over the tongue and creates space between the mouth and the posterior pharynx. It is used for anesthetized or unconscious patients to keep tongue and epiglottis from blocking the airway.
- **Nasopharyngeal** (trumpet): This smaller flexible airway is more commonly used in conscious patients and is inserted through one nostril, extending to the nasopharynx.
- **Tracheostomy tubes**: Tracheostomy may be utilized for mechanical ventilation. Tubes are inserted into the opening to provide a conduit and maintain the opening. Tracheostomy tubes are usually silastic or plastic, most lacking an inner cannula because they are non-adherent. The tube is secured with ties around the neck. Because the air entering the lungs through the tracheostomy bypasses the warming and moistening affects of the upper airway, air is humidified through a room humidifier or through delivery of humidified air through a special mask or mechanical ventilation.
- **The laryngeal-mask airway** (LMA) is an intermediate airway allowing ventilation but not complete respiratory control. The LMA consists of an inflatable cuff (the mask) with a

- 72 -

connecting tube. It may be used temporarily before tracheal intubation or when tracheal intubation can't be done. It can also be a conduit for later blind insertion of an endotracheal tube. The head and neck must be in neutral position for insertion of the LMA. If the patient has a gag reflex, conscious sedation or topical anesthesia (deep oropharyngeal) is required. The LMA is inserted by sliding along the hard palate, using the finger as a guide, into the pharynx, and the ring is inflated to create a seal about the opening to the larynx, allowing ventilation with mild positive-pressure. The ProSeal® LMA has a modified cuff that extends onto the back of the mask to improve seal. LMA is contraindicated in morbid obesity, obstructions or abnormalities of oropharynx, and non-fasting patients, as some aspiration is possible even with the cuff seal inflated.

- The **esophageal tracheal Combitube®** (ETC) is an intermediate airway that contains two lumens and can be inserted into either the trachea or the esophagus (≤91%). The twin-lumen tube has a proximal cuff providing a seal of the oropharynx and a distal cuff providing a seal about the distal tube. Prior to insertion, the Combitube® cuffs should be checked for leaks (15 ml of air into distal and 85 ml of air into proximal). The patient should be non-responsive and with absent gag reflex with head in neutral position. The tube is passed along the tongue and into the pharynx, utilizing markings on the tube (black guidelines) to determine depth by aligning the ETC with the upper incisors or alveolar ridge. Once in place the distal cuff is inflated (10-15 ml) and then placement in the trachea or esophagus should be determined, so the proper lumen for ventilation can be used. The proximal cuff is inflated (usually to 50-75 ml) and ventilation begun. Capnogram should be used to confirm ventilation.

Chest tubes

Chest tubes with a closed drainage system are usually left in place after thoracic surgery or pneumothorax to drain air or fluid:

- **Water** seal (wet suction): 3-chambered system with one chamber for collection, the middle for water seal, and the third for wet suction control. Sterile fluid must be instilled into the middle and suction chambers. The system contains both positive and negative pressure release valves and bubbles intermittently if functioning properly. Chambers must be in upright position.
- **Water seal (dry suction):** Similar 3-chambered system but sterile fluid must be instilled to 2 cm level in water seal chamber only. A regulator controls suction, and an indicator shows if suction pressure is correct. Dry suction has positive and negative release values and chambers must be in upright position.
- **Dry suction (one-way valve):** 2-chambered system with mechanical valve that allows air to leave chest but not enter. This system has a collection chamber and a dry suction control chamber. It requires no fluid instillation and need not be in upright position, so it is useful for ambulatory patients.

Interventions during insertion include ensuring the patient receives adequate pain control, attending to sterile technique, assisting physician with suturing as needed, attaching the tube to the chest tube drainage device, placing a dressing, and confirming placement.

Chest tube drainage systems have 3 major parts: sunction control, water seal, and a chamber for collection. The system should have no bubbling in the water seal area, but a subtle rise and fall of the water seal corresponding with respirations, and gentle bubbling in the suction control chamber.

Nursing interventions after chest tube is in place: In most circumstances, report drainage >100 mL/hr, assess tubing after position changes for occlusion, maintain sterile dressing, avoid stripping the tubing, and assessing the insertion site, the tubing, the patency of the entire system, and the output (including color, amount, and any other traits). The nurse should be knowledgeable about specimen collection, replacing the system, and dealing with clots.

Important terms

- **Alveolar hypoventilation** occurs when effectiveness of alveolar gas exchange reduces so PaO_2 and $PaCO_2$ both increase. The failure to eliminate carbon dioxide displaces oxygen in the alveolar sacs.
- **Dead space** occurs when a well-ventilated alveolus cannot be perfused because of blockage by an embolus, capillary compression, or other damage.
- **Intrapulmonary shunting** involves alveolar perfusion without ventilation, so the oxygenated blood reaches the alveolus but cannot exchange for carbon dioxide because the alveolus is damaged or diseased.
- **Physiologic shunting** is venous blood in the lung bypassing the alveoli and re-entering the arterial system. This normally occurs with 2-3% of venous blood but may increase with alveolar congestion related to pulmonary edema, atelectasis, or other disorder.
- **Refractory hypoxemia** occurs when there is so much loss of alveoli that oxygen administration is unable to correct the hypoxemia.
- **Ventilation-perfusion mismatch (V/Q)** occurs when well-ventilated alveoli lack adequate perfusion (creating partial dead space) or poorly-ventilated alveoli have adequate perfusion (creating partial shunts).

Endocrine

Glycemic disorders

Hyperglycemia is elevation of serum glucose ≥180 mg/dL although symptoms may not be evident until the level reaches ≥270 mg/dL. The most common cause is diabetes mellitus (associated with decreased levels of insulin), but elevations of glucose may also be related to chronic pancreatitis, acromegaly, Cushing's syndrome, and adverse reactions to drugs, such as furosemide, glucocorticoids, growth hormone, oral contraceptives, and thiazides. Symptoms of hyperglycemia are similar to symptoms found in chronic diabetes and include ketoacidosis, polyuria, polydipsia, polyphagia, weight loss, and encephalopathy. Stress-related hyperglycemia is common after stroke and myocardial infarction and increases risk of mortality. Physiological stress related to infection may also increase glucose levels. Hyperglycemia can be treated with insulin and by treatment of the underlying cause or discontinuation of drug administration. The American Diabetes Association and the American Association of Endocrinologist recommend a target blood glucose level of 140-180 mg/dL in critically ill patients, using insulin infusion when needed.

There are a number of different types of insulin with varying action times. Insulin is used to metabolize glucose for those whose pancreases do not produce insulin. People may need to take a combination of insulins (short and long-acting) to maintain glucose control. Duration of action may vary according to the individual's metabolism, intake, and level of activity:
- **Humalog** (Lispro H) is a fast acting, short duration insulin that acts within 5-15 minutes, peaking between 45-90 minutes and lasting 3-4 hours.
- **Regular** (R) is a relatively fast acting, 30 minutes, insulin that peaks in 2-5 hours and last 5-8 hours.
- **NPH** (N) or **Lente** (L)) insulin is intermediate acting with onset in 1-3 hours, peaking at 6-12 hours and lasting 16-24 hours.
- **Ultralente** (U) is long-acting insulin with onset in 4-6 hours, peaking at 8-20 hours, and lasting 24-28 hours.
- **Combined NPH/Regular** (70/30 or 50/50) has an onset of 30 minutes, peaks at 7-12 hours, and lasts 16-24 hours.

Acute hypoglycemia (hyperinsulinism) may result from pancreatic islet tumors or hyperplasia, increasing insulin production, or from the use of insulin to control diabetes mellitus. Hyperinsulinism can cause damage to the central nervous and cardiopulmonary systems, interfering with functioning of the brain and causing neurological impairment. Causes may include:
- Genetic defects in chromosome 11 (short arm)
- Severe infections, such as Gram-negative sepsis, endotoxic shock.
- Toxic ingestion of alcohol or drugs, such as salicylates.
- Too much insulin for body needs.
- Too little food or excessive exercise.

Symptoms
- Blood glucose <50-60 mg/dL.
- Central nervous system: seizures, altered consciousness, lethargy, and poor feeding with vomiting, myoclonus, respiratory distress, diaphoresis, hypothermia, and cyanosis.
- Adrenergic system: diaphoresis, tremor, tachycardia, palpitation, hunger, and anxiety.

Treatment
- Treatment depends on underlying cause and includes:
- Glucose/Glucagon administration to elevate blood glucose levels.
- Diazoxide (Hyperstat®) to inhibit release of insulin.
- Somatostatin (Sandostatin®) to suppress insulin production.
- Careful monitoring.

Diabetes insipidus

Diabetes insipidus (DI) is caused by a deficiency of the antidiuretic hormone (ADH), or vasopressin. DI may develop secondary to head trauma, primary brain tumor, meningitis, encephalitis, or surgical ablation or irradiation of the pituitary gland, or metastatic tumors. This is different from congenital nephrogenic diabetes insipidus, in which production of ADH is normal but the renal tubules do not respond; however, the symptoms are the same.

Symptoms
- Polydipsia.
- Polyuria.
- Patients may exhibit excessive thirst and may drink excessively 2-20 liters a day without relief of thirst.
- Withholding fluids results in dehydration but polyuria continues. (water deprivation test)

Treatment
- Vasopressin tannate is available in injectable (IM or SC) or nasal spray. Injectable forms may last up to 72 hours.
- Desmopressin acetate is available as a nasal spray or oral medication and is usually taken twice daily. Water intoxication can occur with overdose.
- Correct fluid deficits with hypotonic solutions.

Diagnostic tests include serum sodium levels, increased BUN, serum ADH level, and increased serum osmolality. Expect elevated serum sodium and serum osmolality with decreased urine osmolality.

Ketoacidosis

Ketoacidosis is a complication of diabetes mellitus. Inadequate production of insulin results in glucose being unavailable for metabolism, so lipolysis (breakdown of fat) produces free fatty acids (FFAs) as an alternate fuel source. Glycerol in both fat cells and the liver is converted to ketone bodies (β-hydroxybutyric acid, acetoacetic acid, and acetone), which are used for cellular metabolism less efficiently than glucose. Excess ketone bodies are excreted in the urine (ketonuria) or exhalations. Acidosis of any type causes potassium in cells to shift to the serum. The ketone bodies lower serum pH, leading to ketoacidosis. Normal values for fasting blood glucose: 60-100 mg/dL.

Symptoms
- Kussmaul respirations: hyperventilation to eliminate buildup of carbon dioxide, associated with "ketone breath."
- Fluid imbalance, including loss of potassium and other electrolytes from cellular death, resulting in dehydration and diuresis with excess thirst.
- Cardiac arrhythmias, related to potassium loss, can lead to cardiac arrest.
- Hyperglycemia: blood glucose may vary (300-800 mg/dL).

Treatment
- Insulin therapy by continuous infusion initially.
- Rehydration and electrolyte replacement.
- Glucose monitoring.
- Ketone monitoring.

Hypothyroidism

Hypothyroidism occurs when the thyroid produces inadequate levels of thyroid hormones. Conditions may range from mild to severe myxedema. There are a number of causes:
- Chronic lymphocytic thyroiditis (Hashimoto's thyroiditis).
- Excessive treatment for hyperthyroidism
- Atrophy of thyroid.
- Medications, such as lithium, iodine compounds
- Radiation to the area of the thyroid.
- Diseases that affect the thyroid, such as scleroderma
- Iodine imbalances.

Symptoms may include chronic fatigue, menstrual disturbances, hoarseness, subnormal temperature, low pulse rate, weight gain, thinning hair, thickening skin. Some dementia may occur with advanced conditions. Clinical findings may include increased cholesterol with associated atherosclerosis and coronary artery disease. Myxedema may be characterized by changes in respiration with hypoventilation and CO_2 retention resulting in coma. Treatment involves hormone replacement with synthetic levothyroxine (Synthroid®) based on TSH levels, but this increases the oxygen demand of the body, so careful monitoring of cardiac status must be done during early treatment to avoid myocardial infarction while reaching euthyroid (normal) level.

Hyperthyroidism

Hyperthyroidism (thyrotoxicosis) usually results from excess production of thyroid hormones (Graves' disease) from immunoglobulins providing abnormal stimulation of the thyroid gland. Other causes include thyroiditis and excess thyroid medications.

Symptoms
Symptoms vary and may be non-specific, especially in the elderly, and include:
- Hyperexcitability
- Tachycardia (90-160) and atrial fibrillation.
- Increased systolic (but not diastolic) BP.
- Poor heat tolerance, skin flushed and diaphoretic.
- Dry skin and pruritis (especially in the elderly).
- Hand tremor, progressive muscular weakness.

- Exopthalmos (bulging eyes).
- Increased appetite and intake but weight loss.

Treatment
- Radioactive iodine to destroy the thyroid gland. Propranolol may be used to prevent thyroid storm. Thyroid hormones are given for resultant hypothyroidism.
- Antithyroid medications, such as Propacil® or Tapazole® to block conversion of T4 to T3.
- Surgical removal of thyroid is used if patients cannot tolerate other treatments or in special circumstances, such as large goiter. Usually one-sixth of the thyroid is left in place and antithyroid medications are given before surgery.

Thyrotoxic storm

Thyrotoxic storm is a severe type of hyperthyroidism with sudden onset, precipitated by stress, such as injury or surgery, in those un-treated or inadequately treated for hyperthyroidism. If not promptly diagnosed and treated, it is fatal. Incidence has decreased with the use of antithyroid medications but can still occur with medical emer-gencies or pregnancy. Diagnostic findings are similar to hyper-thyroidism, and include increased T3 uptake and decreased TSH.

Symptoms
- Increase in symptoms of hyperthyroidism.
- Increased temperature >38.5°C.
- Tachycardia >130 with atrial fibrillation and heart failure.
- Gastrointestinal disorders, such as nausea, vomiting, diarrhea, and abdominal discomfort.
- Altered mental status with delirium progressing to coma.

Treatment
- Controlling production of thyroid hormone through antithyroid medications, such as propylthiouracil and methimazole.
- Inhibiting release of thyroid hormone with iodine therapy (or lithium).
- Controlling peripheral activity of thyroid hormone with propranolol.
- Fluid and electrolyte replacement.
- Glucocorticoids, such as dexamethasone.
- Cooling blankets.
- Treatment of arrhythmias as needed with antiarrhythmics and anticoagulation.

Parathyroid dysfunction

The parathyroid glands (usually 4) lie in the neck posterior to the thyroid gland (sometimes embedded in thyroid tissue). They produce parathormone, which regulates metabolism of calcium and phosphorus. As parathormone serum levels rise, calcium is absorbed from the kidney, intestines, and bones and serum levels of calcium increase. The serum-ionized calcium regulates the output of parathormone in a negative feedback.
- **Hyperparathyroidism** may be primary or secondary to renal failure or increased stimulation of the parathyroids. Hyperparathyroidism causes overproduction of parathormone and resultant decalcification of bones, which can cause fractures and benign giant cells osteoblastic tumors, and development of calcium containing kidney stones when calcium phosphate precipitates in the renal pelvis and parenchyma. If calcium levels >15

- 78 -

mg/dL, acute hypercalcemic crisis causes life-threatening neurologic, cardiovascular, and renal disorders.
- **Hypoparathyroidism** with deficiency of parathormone results in increased blood phosphates as excretion through kidneys decreases and hypocalcemia because of less dietary calcium absorption and decreased resorption from bones and kidneys.

Acute adrenal insufficiency

Acute adrenal insufficiency (adrenal crisis) is a sudden, life-threatening condition resulting from an exacerbation of primary chronic adrenal insufficiency (Addison's disease), often precipitated by sepsis, surgical stress, adrenal hemorrhage related to septicemia, anticoagulation complications, and cortisone withdrawal related to decreased dose or inadequate dose to compensate for stress. Acute adrenal insufficiency may occur in those who do not have Addison's disease, such as those who have received cortisone for various reasons, usually a minimum of 20 mg daily for at least 5 days.

Symptoms
- Fever
- Nausea and vomiting.
- Abdominal pain.
- Weakness and general fatigue.
- Disorientation, confusion.
- Hypotensive shock.
- Dehydration.
- Electrolyte imbalance with hyperkalemia, hypercalcemia, hypoglycemia and hyponatremia.

Treatment
- IV fluids in large volume
- Glucocorticoid
- 50% dextrose if indicated (hypoglycemia)
- Mineralocorticoid may be needed after intravenous solutions.
- The precipitating cause must be identified and treated as well.

Cushing syndrome

Cushing syndrome is caused by increased production of cortisol from a variety of etiologies:
- Excess of ACTH causing adrenal hyperplasia
- Hypersecretion of glucocorticoids usually related to neoplasms.
- Extra-pituitary neoplasms causing autonomous secretion of ACTH.
- Iatrogenic, resulting from exogenous corticosteroids.
- Treatment with corticosteroids.

Symptoms
- Changes in fat distribution with truncal obesity, supraclavicular fat pads, and fat pads on back of neck, moon face, large abdomen, weight gain.
- Increased bruising and poor wound healing.
- Hypertension.
- Hypokalemia.
- Hyperglycemia.

- Virilization with increased hirsutism and acne.
- Kyphosis with depressed linear growth.

Treatment
Treatment depends upon the cause:
- If caused by medications, such as prednisone, slow withdrawal of the medication should reverse symptoms over time.
- Giving medications in early morning on alternate days may reduce symptoms.
- In some cases, bilateral adrenalectomy and replacement hormone therapy (as for Addison's disease) is indicated.

Chvostek's sign and Trousseau's sign for tetany

Tetany is the most common manifestation of hypocalcemia and hypomagnesemia. It includes a range of neuromuscular symptoms related to spontaneous discharge in both the sensory and motor peripheral nerves. Muscle spasms and twitching may cause pain and there may be sensations of tingling in the fingers and peri-oral area. Seizures may occur. Two signs are present with tetany:
- **Chvostek's sign** is elicited by tapping the muscles enervated by the facial nerves about 2 cm in front of the earlobe just inferior to the zygomatic arch. A positive response is twitching of the muscle. A positive response may also occur with respiratory alkalosis.
- **Trousseau's sign** is elicited by applying a blood pressure cough to the upper arm and inflating it 20 mm Hg above systolic and leaving it in place for ≤5 minutes. A positive response occurs with increasing ischemia of the ulnar nerve: carpopedal spasm with the thumb adducted, the wrist and metacarpophalangeal joints flexed, and the interphalangeal joints extended with the fingers together.

Syndrome of inappropriate secretion of antidiuretic hormone

Syndrome of inappropriate secretion of antidiuretic hormone (SIADH) is related to hypersecretion of the posterior pituitary gland. This causes the kidneys to reabsorb fluids, resulting in fluid retention, and triggers a decrease in sodium levels (dilutional hyponatremia), resulting in production of only concentrated urine. This syndrome may result from central nervous systems disorders, such as brain trauma, surgery, or tumors. It may also be triggered by other disorders, such as tumors of various organs, pneumothorax, acute pneumonia, and other lung disorders. Some medications (vincristine, phenothiazines, tricyclic antidepressants, and thiazide diuretics) may also trigger SIADH.

Symptoms
- Anorexia with nausea and vomiting
- Irritability
- Stomach cramps
- Alterations of personality.
- Increasing neurological dysfunction, including stupor and seizures, related to progressive sodium depletion.

<u>Treatment</u>
- Identifying and treating underlying cause. (d/c causative drugs)
- Urine specific gravity
- Correct fluid volume excess and electrolytes
- Monitor UOP
- Seizure precautions

With SIADH expect low serum sodium and serum osmolality with high urine osmolality.

Hyperglycemic hyperosmolar nonketotic syndrome

Hyperglycemic hyperosmolar nonketotic syndrome (HHNS) occurs in people without history of diabetes or with mild type 2 diabetes but with insulin resistance resulting in persistent hyperglycemia, which causes osmotic diuresis. Fluid shift from intracellular to extracellular spaces to maintain osmotic equilibrium, but the increased glucosuria and dehydration results in hypernatremia and increased osmolarity. This condition is most common in those 50-70 years old and often is precipitated by an acute illness, such as a stroke, medications such as thiazides, or dialysis treatments. HNNS differs from ketoacidosis because, while the insulin level is not adequate, it is high enough to prevent the breakdown of fat. Onset of symptoms usually occurs over a few days.

<u>Symptoms</u>
- Polyuria.
- Dehydration.
- Hypotension.
- Tachycardia.
- Blood glucose: >600 mg/dL.
- Serum osmolality >350 mOsm/L
- Increased BUN and creatinine
- Changes in mental status, seizures, hemiparesis.

<u>Treatment</u>
Treatment is similar to that for ketoacidosis:
- Insulin
- Intravenous fluids and electrolytes.
- Monitor blood glucose and other labs.

Expect increased serum sodium, serum osmolality and urine osmolality.

Glucose and Hemoglobin A1C

Glucose is manufactured by the liver from ingested carbohydrates and is stored as glycogen for use by the cells. If intake is inadequate, glucose can be produced from muscle and fat tissue, leading to increased wasting. High levels of glucose are indicative of diabetes mellitus, which predisposes people to skin injuries, slow healing, and infection. Fasting blood glucose levels are used to diagnose and monitor:
- Normal values: 70-99 mg/dL.
- Impaired: 100-125 mg/dL.
- Diabetes: $\geq$126 mg/dL.

There are a number of different conditions that can increase glucose levels: stress, renal failure, Cushing syndrome, hyperthyroidism, and pancreas disorders. Medications, such as steroids, estrogens, lithium, phenytoin, diuretics, tricyclic antidepressants, may increase glucose levels. Other conditions, such as adrenal insufficiency, liver disease, hypothyroidism, and starvation can decrease glucose levels.

Hemoglobin AIC comprises hemoglobin A with a glucose molecule because hemoglobin holds onto excess blood glucose, so it shows the average blood glucose levels over a 3 month period and is used primarily to monitor long-term diabetic therapy:
- Normal value: <6%.
- Elevation: >7%.

Endocrine function studies

There are a wide range of endocrine function studies:
- Serum osmolality (275-295 mOsm/kg).
- **Pituitary** - Serum levels of pituitary hormones and hormones of target organs, dependent on stimulation by pituitary hormones, are measured to determine abnormalities.
- **Thyroid** - Thyroid stimulating hormone (TSH) (0.4-6.15 mU/L). Increase in TSH indicates hypothyroidism and decrease indicates hyperthyroidism
  - Free thyroxine (FT4) (0.9-1.7 ng/dL). FT4 is used to confirm TSH abnormalities. Serum T3 (17-20 ng/dL) and T4 (4.5-11.5 mcg/dL). These usually increase together, but T3 more accurately diagnoses hyperthyroidism. T3 resin uptake (25-35%). Increases with hyperthyroidism and decreases with hypothyroidism.
- **Parathyroid** - Parathormone level (20-70 mEq/L) and serum calcium levels (1.15-1.34 mg/dL). Both increase with hyperparathyroidism. Calcium level decreases with hypoparathyroidism and phosphate levels (2.4-4.1 mEq/L to 6 mEq/L) increase.
- **Adrenal** - Catecholamine (urine and serum) levels: Epinephrine (100 pg/mL) and norepinephrine (<100-550 pg/mL) elevate with pheochromocytoma.
  - Electrolyte and glucose levels.
  - ACTH and serum cortisol levels and ACTH stimulation test to evaluate for Addison's.
  - Dexamethasone suppression test for Cushing's disease.

Pathophysiology of hypothermia

Hypothermia occurs with exposure to low temperatures that cause the core body temperature to fall <95°F (35°C). Hypothermia may be associated with immersion in cold water, exposure to cold temperature, metabolic disorders (hypothyroidism, hypoglycemia, hypoadrenalism), or CNS abnormalities (head trauma, Wernicke disease). Many patients with hypothermia are intoxicated with alcohol or drugs. During hypothermia, metabolism slows and cerebral perfusion decreases approximately 6% per 10°C fall in body temperature. Autoregulation of cerebral blood flow is lost at 25°C and hypotension occurs. Platelet function is impaired and fibrinolysis increases, leading to hemorrhage related to a syndrome similar to DIC. Shivering and cardiac abnormalities, such as tachycardia, may occur. Pulse and respirations decline as the hypothermia worsens. Mobility and speech are impaired. Mental functioning declines and the patient may lapse into a coma. Deep tendon reflexes are depressed <32°C and are usually absent <26°C.

Hematology

Red blood cell (erythrocyte) values and morphology

Red blood cells (RBCs or erythrocytes) are biconcave disks that contain hemoglobin (95% of mass), which carries oxygen throughout the body. The heme portion of the cell contains iron, which binds to the oxygen. RBCs live about 120 days after which they are destroyed and their hemoglobin is recycled or excreted. Normal values of red blood cell count vary by gender:
- Males >18 years: 4.5-5.5 million/mm³.
- Females >18 years: 4.0-5.0 million/mm³.

The most common disorders of RBCs are those that interfere with production, leading to various types of anemia:
- Blood loss
- Hemolysis
- Bone marrow failure

The morphology of RBCs may vary depending upon the type of anemia:
- Size: Normocytes, microcytes, macrocytes.
- Shape: Spherocytes (round), poikilocytes (irregular), drepanocytes (sickled).
- Color (reflecting concentration of hemoglobin): Normochromic, hypochromic.

Red blood cell evaluation

A number of different tests are used to evaluate the condition and production of red blood cells in addition to the red blood cell count:

Hemoglobin
Carries oxygen and is decreased in anemia and increased in polycythemia. Normal values:
- Males >18 years: 14.0-17.46 g/dl.
- Females >18 years: 12.0-16.0 g/dl.

Hematocrit
Indicates the proportion of RBCs in a liter of blood (usually about 3 times the hemoglobin number). Normal values:
- Males >18 years: 45-52%.
- Females >18 years: 36-48%

Mean corpuscular volume (MCV)
Indicates the size of RBCs and can differentiate types of anemia. For adults, <80 is microcytic and >100 is macrocytic. Normal values:
- Males > 18 years: 84-96 μm3.
- Females >18 years: 76-96 μm³.

Reticulocyte count
Measures marrow production and should rise with anemia. Normal values:
- 0.5-1.5% of total RBCs.

WBC count and differential

White blood cell (leukocyte) count is used as an indicator of bacterial and viral infection. WBC is reported as the total number of all white blood cells. Normal WBC for adults: 4,800-10,000. Acute infection: 10,000+, 30,000 indicate a severe infection. Viral infection: 4,000 and below. The differential provides the percentage of each different type of leukocyte.

An increase in the white blood cell count is usually related to an increase in one type and often an increase in immature neutrophils, known as bands, referred to as a "shift to the left", an indication of an infectious process:

<u>Cells</u>

Immature neutrophils (bands)
- Normal value: 1-3%
- Change: Increase with infection.

Segmented neutrophils (segs)
- Normal value: 50-62%
- Change: Increase with acute, localized, or systemic bacterial infections

Eosinophils
- Normal value: 0-3%
- Change: Decrease with stress and acute infection.

Basophils
- Normal value:0-1%
- Change: Decrease during acute stage of infection.

Lympho-cytes
- Normal value: 25-40%
- Change: Increase in some viral and bacterial infections.

Monocytes
- Normal value: 3-7%
- Change: Increase during recovery stage of acute infection

C-reactive protein and erythrocyte sedimentation rate

C-reactive protein is an acute-phase reactant produced by the liver in response to an inflammatory response that causes neutrophils, granulocytes and macrophages to secrete cytokines. Thus, levels of C-reactive protein rise when there is inflammation or infection. It has been found to be helpful to measure of response to treatment for pyoderma gangrenosum ulcers:
- Normal values: 2.6-7.6 µg/dL.

Erythrocyte sedimentation rate (sed rate) measures the distance erythrocytes fall in a vertical tube of anticoagulated blood in one hour. Because fibrinogen, which increases in response to infection, slows the fall, the sed rate can be used as a non-specific test for inflammation when infection is

- 84 -

suspected. The sed rate is sensitive to osteomyelitis and may be used to monitor treatment response. Values vary according to gender and age:

- <50: Males 0-15 mm/hr. Females 0-20 mm/hr.
- >50: Males 0-20 mm/hr. Females 0-30 mm/hr.

Elements of the coagulation profile

The coagulation profile measures clotting mechanisms, identifies clotting disorders, screens preoperative patients, and diagnoses excessive bruising and bleeding. Values vary depending on lab:

- **Prothrombin time (PT)** 10 – 14 seconds. Time increases with anticoagulation therapy, vitamin K deficiency, decreased prothrombin, DIC, liver disease, and malignant neoplasm. Some drugs may shorten time.
- **Partial thromboplastin time (PTT)** 30 – 45 seconds. Increases with hemophilia A & B, von Willebrand's, vitamin deficiency, lupus, DIC, ad liver disease.
- **Activated partial thromboplastin time (aPTT)** 21 – 35 seconds. Similar to PTT, but decreases in extensive cancer, early DIC, and after acute hemorrhage. Used to monitor heparin dosage.
- **Thrombin clotting time (TCT) or Thrombin time (TT)** 7 – 12 seconds (<21) Used most often to determine dosage of heparin. Prolonged with multiple myeloma, abnormal fibrinogen, uremia, and liver disease.
- **Bleeding time** 2 – 9.5 minutes (Using Ivy method on the forearm). Increases with DIC, leukemia, renal failure, aplastic anemia, von Willebrand's, some drugs, and alcohol.
- **Platelet count** 150,000 - 400,000 per microliter. Increased bleeding <50,000 and increased clotting >750,000.

Sickle cell disease and crises

Sickle cell disease is a recessive genetic disorder of chromosome 11, causing hemoglobin to be defective so that red blood cells (RBCs) are sickle-shaped and inflexible, resulting in their accumulating in small vessels and causing painful blockage. While normal RBCs survive 120 days, sickled cells may survive only 10-20 days, stressing the bone marrow that can't produce fast enough and resulting in anemia. Different types of crises occur (aplastic, hemolytic, vaso-occlusive, and sequestrating), which cause infarctions in organs, severe pain, damage to organs, and rapid enlargement of liver and spleen. Sickle cell disease and crisis treatment includes:

- Intravenous fluids to prevent dehydration.
- Analgesics (morphine) during painful crises.
- Folic acid for anemia.
- Oxygen for congestive heart failure or pulmonary disease.
- Blood transfusions with chelation therapy to remove excess iron OR erythropheresis, in which red cells are removed and replaced with healthy cells, either autologous or from a donor.
- Hematopoietic stem cells transplantation is the only curative treatment.

Disseminated intravascular coagulation

Disseminated intravascular coagulation (DIC) (consumption coagulopathy) is a secondary disorder that is triggered by another, such as trauma, congenital heart disease, necrotizing enterocolitis, sepsis, and severe viral infections. DIC triggers both coagulation and hemorrhage through a complex series of events that includes trauma that causes tissue factor (transmembrane glycoprotein) to enter the circulation and bind with coagulation factors, triggering the coagulation cascade. This stimulates thrombin to convert fibrinogen to fibrin, causing aggregation and destruction of platelets and forming clots that can be disseminated throughout the intravascular system. These clots increase in size as platelets adhere to the clots, causing blockage of both the microvascular systems and larger vessels, and this can result in ischemia and necrosis.

Clot formation triggers fibrinolysis and plasmin to breakdown fibrin and fibrinogen, causing destruction of clotting factors, resulting in hemorrhage. Both processes, clotting and hemorrhage continue at the same time, placing the patient at high risk for death, even with treatment.

The onset of symptoms of DIC may be very rapid or a slower chronic progression from a disease. Those who develop the chronic manifestation of the disease usually have fewer acute symptoms and may slowly develop ecchymosis or bleeding wounds.

Symptoms
- Bleeding from surgical or venous puncture sites.
- Evidence of GI bleeding with distention, bloody diarrhea.
- Hypotension and acute symptoms of shock.
- Petechiae and purpura with extensive bleeding into the tissues.
- Laboratory abnormalities:
  o Prolonged prothrombin and partial prothrombin times.
  o Decreased platelet counts and fragmented RBCs.
  o Decreased fibrinogen.

Treatment
- Identifying and treating underlying cause.
- Replacement blood products, such as platelets and fresh frozen plasma.
- Anticoagulation therapy (heparin) to increase clotting time.
- Cryoprecipitate to increase fibrinogen levels.
- Coagulation inhibitors and coagulation factors.

DIC panel

Disseminated intravascular coagulation (DIC) panel includes a number of tests. Generally, test results that measure materials needed for clotting are decreased and those that measure clotting times are increased. Typical findings that indicate DIC include:
- **Activated partial thromboplastin time (aPTT)** - Increased time
- **Prothrombin time** - Findings vary, may be increased time (in 75%), normal time (25%), or shortened (25%).
- **Partial thromboplastin time** - Increased time (in 50-60%).
- **Thrombin time** - Increased.
- **D-Dimer** - Increased (usually more reliable than FSP): D-dimer is a specific polymer that results when fibrin breaks down, giving a marker to indicate the degree of fibrinolysis.
- **Fibrinogen** - Decreased.
- **Platelets** - <100,000 platelets per microliter.

- **Fibrin split products (FSP)** - Increased (in 75-100%). FSPs occur as more clots form and more breakdown of fibrinogen and fibrin occurs, interfering with blood coagulation by coating platelets and disrupting thrombin, and attaching to fibrinogen so stable clots can't form.
- **Clotting factor assays (V, VI, VII, X, XIII)** -Decreased.
- **Antithrombin III** - Decreased (in 90%).

Graft versus host disease

Graft versus host disease (GVHD) is an immunological response to "foreign" tissue (such as a transplanted organ or non-irradiated blood transfusion). GVHD is one of the major causes of morbidity and mortality after transplantations, so immunosuppression is provided before, during, and after transplantations (usually about 6 months for allogenic stem cell transplantation and life-long for solid organs). GVHD may be acute (<100 days after transplantation) or chronic (>100 days after transplantation). Symptoms may involve many organs, such as the skin, the GI tract, and the liver. Patients may experience diffuse lacy maculopapular rash, nausea, vomiting, diarrhea, sloughing of mucosal tissue, and increasing bilirubin. GVHD is staged according to severity of symptoms related to the skin, GI system, and liver, with each system graded 1 to 4 depending upon severity. Treatment includes corticosteroids to suppress the immune response.

Transfusions

Blood components that are commonly used for transfusions include:
- **Packed red blood cells:** RBCs (250-300 mL per unit) should be warmed >30° (optimal 37°) before administration to prevent hypothermia and may be reconstituted in 50-100 mL of normal saline to facilitate administration. RBCs are necessary if blood loss is about 30% (1500-2000 mL) (Hgb ≤7). (Above 30% blood loss, whole blood may be more effective.) RBCs are most frequently used for transfusions.
- **Platelet concentrates:** Transfusions of platelets are used if the platelet count is <50,000 cells/mm^3. One unit increases the platelet count by 5000-10,000 cells/mm^3. Platelet concentrates pose a risk for sensitization reactions and infectious diseases. Platelet concentrate is stored at a higher temperature (20-24°) than RBCs. This contributes to bacterial growth, so it is more prone to bacterial contamination than other blood products and may cause sepsis. Temperature increase within 6 hours should be considered an indication of possible sepsis. ABO compatibility should be observed but is not required.
- **Fresh frozen plasma** (FFP) (obtained from a unit of whole blood frozen ≤6 hours after collection) includes all clotting factors and plasma proteins, so each unit administered increases clotting factors by 2-3%. FFP may be used for deficiencies of isolated factors, excess warfarin therapy, and liver-disease related coagulopathy. It may be used for patients who have received extensive blood transfusions but continue to hemorrhage. It is also helpful for those with antithrombin III deficiency. FFP should be warmed to 37°C prior to administration to avoid hypothermia. ABO compatibility should be observed if possible, but it is not required. Some patients may become sensitized to plasma proteins. FFP is usually not given during surgery unless PTT or PT is prolonged ≥1.5 times.
- **Cryoprecipitate** is the precipitate that forms when FFP is thawed. It contains fibrinogen, factor VIII, von Willebrand, and factor XIII. This component may be used to treat hemophilia A and hypofibrinogenemia.

Transfusion-related complications

There are a number of transfusion-related complications, the reason that transfusions are given only when necessary. Complications include:

- **Infection**: Bacterial contamination of blood, especially platelets, can result in severe sepsis. A number of infective agents (viral, bacterial, and parasitic) can be transmitted although increased testing of blood has decreased rates of infection markedly. Infective agents include HIV, hepatitis C and B, human T-cell lymphotropic virus, CMV, WNV, malaria, Chagas' disease and variant Creutzfeldt-Jacob disease (from contact with mad cow disease).
- **Transfusion-related acute lung injury** (TRALI): This respiratory distress syndrome is increasingly common and occurs ≤6 hours. The cause is believed to be antileukocytic or anti-HLA antibodies in the transfusion. It is characterized by non-cardiogenic pulmonary edema (high protein level) with severe dyspnea and arterial hypoxemia. Transfusion must be stopped immediately and the blood bank notified. TRALI may result in fatality but usually resolves in 12-48 hours with supportive care.
- **Graft vs. host disease:** Lymphocytes cause immune response in immunocompromised individuals. Lymphocytes may be inactivated by irradiation, as leukocyte filters are not reliable.
- **Post-transfusion purpura:** Platelet antibodies develop and destroy the patient's platelets, so the platelet count decreases about 1 week after transfusion.
- **Transfusion-related immunosuppression:** Cell-mediated immunity is suppressed, so the patient is at increased risk of infection and, in cancer patients, transfusions may correlate with tumor recurrence. This condition relates to transfusions that include leukocytes. RBCs cause a less pronounced immunosuppression, suggesting a causative agent is in the plasma. Leukoreduction is becoming more common to reduce transmission of leukocyte-related viruses.
- **Hypothermia:** This may occur if blood products are not heated. Body temperature decrease of 0.5-1°C increases oxygen consumption by 4 times.

Autotransfusion

Autotransfusion (autologous blood transfusion) is collecting of the patient's blood and reinfusing it. This is life-saving if other donor blood is not available. Blood in trauma cases is usually collected from a body cavity, such as pleural (hemothorax with ≥1500 mL blood) or peritoneal space (rare). Autotransfusion is contraindicated if malignant lesions are present in area of blood loss, contamination of pooled blood, or wounds >4-6 hours old. Commercial collection/transfusion kits (Pleur-Evac®, Thora-Klex®) are available but blood can be collected through the chest tube into a sterile bottle, which is then disconnected and connected to IV tubing for infusion, OR the blood in the bottle may be transferred to a blood collection bag for use. Commercial kits use either a chest tube or suction tube to withdraw blood and provide specific procedures. Blood is filtered. Heparin is not routinely used but citrate phospate dextrose (CPD) (25-70 mL/500 mL blood) is often added to the aspirant to prevent clotting. Complications from autotransfusion are rare.

Plasmapheresis

Plasmapheresis is a process by which autoantibodies are removed from plasma as a treatment for autoimmune disorders, such as Guillain-Barre and myasthenia gravis. Immunosuppressants and/or anti-inflammatory drugs may be given in conjunction with plasmapheresis. Blood is removed from the patient through and intravenous line, separated to remove the plasma and then the cells are

- 88 -

then re-transfused along with heparin to prevent clotting through a second intravenous line. Replacement fluids are substituted for the plasma, and the plasma and autoantibodies discarded. Usually 6 to 10 treatments lasting several hours are given within a 2 to 10-week period with treatments one or two times weekly. Complications include hypotension (dizziness, pallor, blurring vision), bleeding (heparin-related), allergic response, and excessive immunosuppression, increasing risk of infection.

Immunosuppressant drugs

Antibodies (Monoclonal)
- Actions: Act to depress particular antigens, such a CD-3, and lowers T cell count. Used to treat acute rejection responses.
- Side effects: Marked cell-med-iated immune depression increases risk of infection and devel-opment of cancer.

Antibodies (Polyclonal)
- Actions: (Obtained from animal serum.) Inhibit T cell production and promote destruction of T cells. Used with other immunosuppressant drugs to reduce dosage. Depress cell-mediated immune response and used to prevent GVHD response
- Side effects: Allergic/anaphylactic reactions to serum, including serum sickness, fever, arthralgia, urticaria, erythema.

Azathioprine
- Actions: Inhibits cell reproduction, especially those that repli-cate quickly, such as B and T cells. Used with trans-plantations and autoimmune diseases, such as MS, Crohn's disease and restrictive lung disease.
- Side effects: Bone marrow sup-pression, increasing risk of infection. Nausea, loss of hair, malaise, and rash. Increased risk of cancer, especially skin tumors, with long-term use.

Corticosteroids
- Actions: Depress cell-mediated immune response, humoral immune response, and inflammation, reducing proliferation of T cells and B cells. Used to prevent GVHD disease.
- Side effects: Weight gain, edema, Cushing syndrome, bruising, and osteoporosis. Abruptly stopping drugs may trigger Addisonian crisis.

Ciclosporin
- Actions: Inhibit activation of T cells. Used to prevent transplantation rejection, to treat autoimmune diseases and nephrotic syndrome.
- Side effects: Tremor, excessive facial hair, gingivitis, bone marrow suppres-sion with increased risk of infection and cancer, especially skin cancer.

Intra-venous immune-globulin G (IVIG)
- Actions: Used to combat immunosuppression by increasing antibodies to prevent infection or treat acute infection, such as Guillain-Barre. Used off-label for many different disorders and infections.
- Side effects: Dermatitis, headache, renal failure, venous thrombosis. Infections can occur because IVIG is extracted from pooled plasma.

Methotrexate
- Actions: Inhibits folic acid, which interferes with RNA/DNA synthesis and cell division. Used for many different cancers and many autoimmune diseases. Also used for elective abortions.
- Side effects: Nausea, vomiting, loss of hair, bone marrow suppression with leukopenia, stomatitis, Teratogenic.

Tacrolimus
- Actions: Used after of surgery to prevent rejection of heart, kidney and liver transplants (usually in combination with azathioprine or MMF). Taken with adrenal corticosteroids.
- Side effects: (May interact with grapefruit juice.) Anaphylaxis, especially with IV infusion, tremor, headache, nausea, diarrhea, hypertension, and kidney dysfunction. Bone marrow suppression may result in increased risk of infection, bleeding, and cancer, especially skin cancer. Increases risk of developing diabetes.

Idiopathic thrombocytopenic purpura

The autoimmune disorder idiopathic thrombocytopenic purpura (ITP) causes an immune response to platelets, resulting in decreased platelet counts. It may be triggered by viral infections. ITP affects primarily children and young women although it can occur at any age. The acute form primarily occurs in children, but the chronic form affects primarily adults.

Platelet counts are usually 150,000-400,000 per cu/ml. With ITP, they may be as low as 0 or 100,000 in less severe cases. A count of about 30,000 is necessary to prevent intracranial hemorrhage, the primary concern. The cause of ITP is unclear and may be precipitated by viral infection, sulfa drugs, and conditions, such as lupus erythematosus. ITP is usually not life threatening and can be controlled.

Symptoms
- Bruising and petechiae with hematoma in some cases.
- Epistaxis.
- Increased menstrual flow in females post-puberty.

Treatment
- Corticosteroids depress immune response and increase platelet count.
- Splenectomy may be indicated for chronic conditions.
- Platelet transfusions.
- Avoiding aspirin or ibuprofen.

Heparin-induced thrombocytopenia and thrombosis syndrome

Heparin-induced thrombocytopenia and thrombosis syndrome (HITTS) occurs in patients receiving heparin for anticoagulation. There are two types:
- **Type I is** a transient condition occurring within a few days and causing depletion of platelets ($<100,000$ mm^3), but heparin may be continued as the condition usually resolves without intervention.
- **Type II** is an autoimmune reaction to heparin that occurs in 3-5% of those receiving unfractionated heparin and also occurs with low-molecular weight heparin. It is characterized by low platelets ($<50,000$ mm^3) that are $\geq50\%$ below baseline. Onset is 5-14 days but can occur within hours of reheparinization. Death rates are $\leq30\%$. Heparin-

antibody complexes form and release platelet factor 4 (PF4), which attracts heparin molecules and adheres to platelets and endothelial lining, stimulating thrombin and platelet clumping. This puts the patient at risk for thrombosis and vessel occlusion rather than hemorrhage, causing stroke, myocardial infarction, and limb ischemia with symptoms associated with the site of thrombosis. Treatment includes:

o Discontinuation of heparin.
o Direct thrombin inhibitors (lepirudin, argatroban).

ReoPro-induced coagulopathy

ReoPro® (abciximab) is used to prevent cardiac ischemia for those undergoing percutaneous cardiac intervention. It inhibits the aggregation of platelets. It is used with aspirin and/or weight-adjusted low dose heparin and potentiates the action of anticoagulants. However, its use with non-weight adjusted longer acting heparin can cause thrombocytopenia with increased risk of hemorrhage, especially with readministration of the drug, which can induce the formation of antibodies and an allergic reaction that is characterized by anaphylaxis and thrombocytopenia, referred to as Reo-Pro® induced coagulopathy. Because of the danger of hemorrhage, ReoPro® is contraindicated if there is active bleeding or a history of bleeding within the 2 years prior, history of a CVA, platelet count <100,000 mm³, or recent history of oral anticoagulation. Careful monitoring of platelet counts prior to administration and the use of weight-adjusted low dose heparin is important to prevent bleeding. Heparin should be discontinued after the PCI.

Neurology

Cerebral aneurysms

Cerebral aneurysms, weakening and dilation of a cerebral artery, are usually congenital (90%) while the remaining (10%) result from direct trauma or infection. Aneurysms usually range from 2-7 mm and occur in the Circle of Willis at the base of the brain. A rupturing aneurysm may decrease perfusion as well as increasing pressure on surrounding brain tissue. Cerebral aneurysm are classified as follows:

- **Berry/saccular:** The most common congenital type occurs at a bifurcation and grows from the base on a stem, usually at the Circle of Willis.
- **Fusiform***: Large and irregular (>2.5 cm) and rarely ruptures but causes increased intracranial pressure. Usually involves the internal carotid or vertebrobasilar artery.
- **Mycotic***: Rare type that occurs secondary to bacterial infection and aseptic emboli.
- **Dissecting***: Wall is torn apart and blood enters layers. This may occur during angiography or secondary to trauma or disease.
- **Traumatic Charcot-Bouchard (pseudoaneurysm):** small lesion resulting from chronic hypertension.

Ruptured aneurysm treatment

Surgical clipping of a ruptured aneurysm is necessary because of the danger of rebleeding, 4% in the first 24 hours and 1-2% each day for the next month. Mortality rates with rebleeding are about 70%. Surgical repair is usually done within 48 hours. Clipping may be done prophylactically to prevent rupture. Clipping is done to secure the aneurysm without impairing circulation. Typically, a craniotomy is done and an incision is made into the brain to access the site of the aneurysm. When bleeding is controlled, a small spring-like clip (or sometimes multiple clips) is placed about the neck of the aneurysm. The bulging part of the aneurysm is drained with a needle to make sure that it does not refill and angiography may be done to ensure patency of the artery that feeds the aneurysm. It is possible during surgery for a clot to break away from the aneurysm with resultant extensive hemorrhage. Neurological damage may occur related to surgical manipulation, especially if access is difficult.

Embolization is a minimally-invasive method that is an alternative to clipping for some aneurysms and is also used for AVMs. There are different types of embolization, but all use percutaneous transfemoral catheterization and fluoroscopy. The catheter is fed through the carotid artery to the area of requiring repair:

- AVM repair introducing small silastic beads or glue into the feeder vessels, allowing blood flow to carry the material to the site. This may also be done prior to surgical repair.
- AVM or aneurysm repair placing one or more detachable balloons into the aneurysm or an AVM and inflating it with a liquid polymerizing agent that solidifies.
- Aneurysm repair with endovascular coiling involves feeding very small platinum coils through the catheter to fill the aneurysm.

Results of endovascular coiling have been very positive, with risk of death or disability at one year over 22% lower than those treated with clipping although distal ischemia related to emboli is a possible complication.

Cerebral vasospasm

Cerebral vasospasm, a luminal narrowing of cerebral arteries, occurs in about 70% of patients after aneurysmal subarachnoid hemorrhage, resulting in ischemic stroke or death in about 15-20%. Onset is usually 4-12 days after initial rupture. The cause is unclear but may relate to narrowing caused by pressure of the clot on the arteries. The large arteries are usually affected, causing decreased perfusion to large cerebral areas. A number of therapies are under study, but 3 common approaches include:

- **Hypertensive hypervolemic hemodilution therapy** (HHH) involves using vasoactive drugs to increase systolic BP to 150-160 while diluting the blood with intravenous fluids and volume expanders in order to improve perfusion. However, if done prior to clipping of the aneurysm, this poses a danger of rebleeding. Cerebral edema, increased intracranial pressure, cardiac failure, and electrolyte imbalance may also occur.
- **Nimodipine** every 4 hours for 21 days reduces vasospasm.
- **Cerebral angioplasty** may be done if medical approaches fail but poses a danger of perforation, thromboembolism, and stenosis.

Determination of brain death

While each state has separate statutes that describe the legal definition of brain death, most include some variation of this description:

- Brain death has occurred if the person has "sustained irreversible cessation of circulatory and respiratory functions; or has sustained irreversible cessation of all functions of the entire brain, including the brain stem."

Some states specify the number of physicians that must make the determination and others simply say the decision must be made in accordance with accepted medical practice. Criteria for determination of brain death include coma or lack of responsiveness, apnea (without ventilation), and absence of brainstem reflexes. In many states, findings must be confirmed by at least 2 physicians. Tests used to confirm brain death include:

- Cerebral angiograms: Delayed intracerebral filling or obstruction.
- EEG: Lack of response to auditory, visual, or somatic stimuli.
- Ultrasound (transcranial): Abnormal flow.
- Cerebral scintograms: Static images at preset time intervals.

Arteriovenous malformation

Arteriovenous malformation (AVM) is a congenital abnormality within the brain consisting of a tangle of dilated arteries and veins without a capillary bed. AVMs can occur anywhere in the brain and may cause no significant problems. Usually the AVM is "fed" by one or more cerebral arteries, which enlarge over time, shunting more blood through the AVM. The veins also enlarge in response to increased arterial blood flow because of the lack of a capillary bridge between the two. Because vein walls are thinner and lack the muscle layer of an artery, the veins tend to rupture as the AVM becomes larger, causing a subarachnoid hemorrhage. Chronic ischemia that may be related to the AVM can result in cerebral atrophy.

Sometimes small leaks, usually accompanied by headache and nausea and vomiting, may occur before rupture. AVMs may cause a wide range of neurological symptoms, including changes in mentation, dizziness, sensory abnormalities, confusion, and, increasing ICP, and dementia. Treatment includes:

- Supportive management of symptoms.
- Surgical repair or focused irradiation (definitive treatments).

Surgical excision of AVM

Surgical excision of AVM is the definitive treatment for AVMs as both embolization and radiotherapy treatment pose the risk that the abnormal vessels will recur. Sometimes, 2-3 different surgeries may be required for large AVMs. Usually nonfunctioning brain tissue surrounds the AVM, so it's possible to remove the AVM without damaging brain tissue. However, reperfusion bleeding may occur as blood is diverted to surrounding arterials that had dilated because of chronic ischemia. The sudden increase in blood flow and pressure may cause leakage of blood from the vessels. There may be extensive blood loss during surgery, so constant monitoring of arterial pressure and multiple IV cannulas are important. Embolization may be done prior to surgery to reduce bleeding. Hyperventilation and mannitol are often used and β-blockers may be used to prevent hypertension and cerebral edema. Postoperatively, blood pressure is kept low to prevent reperfusion bleeding.

Anoxic encephalopathy

Anoxic encephalopathy, resulting from complete lack of oxygen to the brain, can occur with cardiac arrest, head trauma, asphyxia, increasing ICP, fat embolism, status epilepticus, and severe cerebral atherosclerosis. Biochemical changes occur in the brain within 5 minutes without oxygenation. Assessment includes:

Level of consciousness
Use verbal stimuli, shaking patient, and digital supraorbital pressure to elicit response.

Motor activity
Brainstem damage: Flaccidity and areflexia.
Mid-brain and upper pons damage: Extensor posturing.
Hemispheric damage: Flexor posturing.

Eyes
Pupillary response and elicited eye move-ments: Absence indicates severe damage.
Papilledema: May occur after cardiac arrest without increase ICP.
Horizontal movement of eyes: Can remain with damage to frontal or occipital areas if midbrain and pons intact.

Imaging
MRI provides better early information than CT.
EEG shows cortical and epileptic activity

Treatment depends on the causes, but reestablishing circulation is primary. After cardiac arrest, hypothermia (32 to 34°C) with neuro-muscular blockade should be initiated quickly with rewarming after 24 hours to reduce cerebral damage.

Hypertensive encephalopathy and cerebral edema

Hypertensive encephalopathy can occur as part of hypertensive crisis. With chronic hypertension, the brain adapts to higher pressures to regulate blood flow, but in a hypertensive crisis, autoregulation of the blood-brain barrier is overwhelmed and the capillaries leak fluid into the tissue and vasodilation takes place with resultant cerebral edema. Damage to arterioles occurs, causing increasing neurological deficits and papilledema. Hypertensive encephalopathy is relatively rare, but carries a high mortality rate and is most common in middle-aged males with long-standing hypertension.

Symptoms usually develop over 1-2 days and include:
- Non-specific neurological deficits, such as weakness and visual abnormalities.
- Alterations in mental status, including confusion.
- Headache, often constant.
- Nausea and vomiting.
- Seizures.
- Coma.

Hypertensive encephalopathy with cerebral edema requires prompt treatment in order to prevent neurological damage. Treatment includes identifying and treating the underlying causes for the hypertensive crisis and taking steps to lower the blood pressure:
- **Nitroprusside sodium (Nitropress®)** is usually used initially to lower BP.
- **Positioning** of patient to prevent obstruction of venous return from the head.
- **Monitoring blood gas** and maintaining $PaCO_2$ at 33-37 mm Hg to facilitate vasoconstriction of cerebral arteries.
- **Preventing hyperthermia** with antipyretics and cooling devices.
- **BP monitoring** and maintenance.
- **Seizure control** with phenobarbitol and/or phenytoin.
- **Lidocaine** through endotracheal tube or intravenously prior to nasotracheal suctioning.
- **Diuretics**, such as osmotic agents (mannitol) and loop diuretics (furosemide) to control fluid volume.
- **Controlling metabolic demand** by measures to increase pain control and reduce stimulation.
- **Barbiturates** (pentobarbital, thiopental) in high doses may be used if other treatments fail to decrease intracranial pressure.

Cerebral hypoxia

Cerebral hypoxia (hypoxic encephalopathy) occurs when the oxygen supply to the brain is decreased. If hypoxia is mild, the brain compensates by increasing cerebral blood flow, but it can only double in volume and cannot compensate for severe hypoxic conditions. Hypoxia may be the result of insufficient oxygen in the environment, inadequate exchange at the alveolar level of the lungs, or inadequate circulation to the brain. Brain cells may begin dying within 5 minutes if deprived of adequate oxygenation, so any condition or trauma that interferes with oxygenation can result in brain damage:
- Near-drowning.
- Asphyxia.
- Cardiac arrest.
- High altitude sickness.

- Carbon monoxide.
- Diseases that interfere with respiration, such as myasthenia gravis and amyotrophic lateral sclerosis.
- Anesthesia complications.

Symptoms include increasing neurological deficits, depending upon the degree and area of damage, with changes in mentation that range from confusion to coma. Prompt identification of the cause and increase in perfusion to the brain is critical for survival.

Metabolic encephalopathy

Metabolic encephalopathy (hepatic encephalopathy) is damage to the brain resulting from a disturbance in metabolism, primarily hepatic failure to remove toxins from the blood. There may impairment in cerebral blood flow, cerebral edema, or increased intracranial pressure. It can occur as the result of ingestion of drugs or toxins, which can have a direct toxic affect on neurons, but can also occur with liver disease, especially when stressed by co-morbidities, such as hemorrhage, hypoxemia, surgery, trauma, renal failure with dialysis, or electrolyte imbalances. Symptoms may vary:
- Irritability and agitation.
- Alterations in consciousness.
- Dysphonia.
- Lack of coordination, spasticity.
- Seizures are common and may be the presenting symptom.
- Disorientation progressing to coma.

Prompt diagnosis is important because the condition may be reversible if underlying causes are identified and treated before permanent neuronal damage occurs. Treatment varies according to the underlying cause.

Infectious encephalopathy

Infectious encephalopathy is an encompassing term describing encephalopathies caused by a wide range of bacteria, viruses, or prions. Common to all infections are altered brain function that results in alterations in consciousness and personality, cognitive impairment, and lethargy. A wide range of neurological symptoms may occur: myoclonus, seizures, dysphagia, and dysphonia, neuromuscular impairment with muscle atrophy and tremors or spasticity. Treatment depends on the underlying cause and response to treatment. Prior infections are not treatable, but bacterial infections may respond to antibiotic therapy, and viral infections may be self-limiting. HIV-related encephalopathy results from opportunistic infections as immune responses decrease, usually indicated by CD4 counts <50. Aggressive antiretroviral treatment and treatment of the infection may reverse symptoms if permanent damage has not occurred for HIV-related encephalopathy. Treatment for other infectious encephalopathies varies according to the type of infection and underlying causes.

Implications of blunt head trauma

Head trauma can occur as the result from intentional or unintentional blunt or penetrating trauma, such as from falls, automobile accidents, sports injuries, or violence. The degree of injury correlates with the impact force. The skull provides protection to the brain, but a severe blow can cause significant neurological damage. Blunt trauma can include:

- **Acceleration-deceleration injuries** are those in which a blow to the stationary head causes the elastic skull to change shape, pushing against the brain, which moves sharply backward in response, striking against the skull.
- **Bruising** can occur at the point of impact (*coup*) and the point where the brain hits the skull (*contrecoup*). So a blow to the frontal area can cause damage to the occipital region.
- **Shear injuries,** where vessels are torn, results from sudden movement of the brain.
- **Severe compression** may force the brain through the tentorial opening, damaging the brainstem.

Complications of head trauma

Head injuries that occur at the time of trauma include fractures, contusions, hematomas, and diffuse cerebral and vascular injury. These injuries may result in hypoxia, increased intracranial pressure, and cerebral edema. Open injuries may result in infection. Patients often suffer initial hypertension, which increases intracranial pressure, decreasing perfusion. Often the primary problem with head trauma is a significant increase in swelling, which also interferes with perfusion, causing hypoxia and hypercapnia, which trigger increased blood flow. This increased volume at a time when injury impairs auto-regulation increases cerebral edema, which, in turn, increases intracranial pressure and results in a further decrease in perfusion with resultant ischemia. If pressure continues to rise, the brain may herniate. Concomitant hypotension may result in hypoventilation, further complicating treatment. Treatments include:

- Monitoring ICP and CCP.
- Providing oxygen.
- Elevating head of bed and maintaining proper body alignment.
- Giving medications: Analgesics, anticonvulsants, and anesthetics.
- Providing blood/fluids to stabilize hemodynamics.
- Managing airway, providing mechanical ventilation if needed.
- Providing osmotic agents, such as mannitol and hypertonic saline solution, to reduce cerebral edema.

A variety of different injuries can occur as a result of head trauma:

- **Concussions** are the most common injury and are usually relatively transient, causing no permanent neurological damage. They may result in confusion, disorientation, and mild amnesia, which last only minutes or hours.
- **Contusions/lacerations** are bruising and tears of cerebral tissue. There may be petechial areas at the impact site (coup) or larger bruising. Contrecoup injuries are less common in children than in adults. Areas most impacted by contusions and lacerations are the occipital, frontal, and temporal lobes. The degree of injury relates to the amount of vascular damage, but initial symptoms are similar to concussion; however, symptoms persist and may progress, depending upon the degree of injury. Lacerations are often caused by fractures.

Fractures are a common cause of penetrating wounds causing cerebral lacerations. Open fractures are those in which the dura is torn, and closed is when the dura remain intact. While fractures by themselves do not cause neurological damage, force is needed to fracture the skull, often causing damage to underlying structures. Meningeal arteries lie in groves on the underside of the skull, and a fracture can cause an arterial tear and hemorrhage.

Skull fractures include:
- **Basilar**: Occurs in bones at the base of the brain and can cause severe brainstem damage.
- **Comminuted**: Skull fractures into small pieces.
- **Compound**: Surface laceration extends to include a skull fracture.
- **Depressed**: Pieces of the skull are depressed inward on the brain tissue, often producing dural tears.
- **Linear/hairline:** Skull fracture forms a thin line without any splintering.

Hydrocephalus

The ventricular system produces and circulates cerebrospinal fluid (CSF). There are right and left lateral ventricles, which open into the third ventricle at the interventricular foramen (foramen of Monro). The aqueduct of Sylvius connects the third and fourth ventricles. The fourth ventricle, anterior to the cerebellum, supplies CSF to the subarachnoid space and the spinal cord (dorsal surface). The CSF circulates and then returns to the brain and is absorbed in the arachnoid villi. Hydrocephalus occurs when there is an imbalance between production and absorption of cerebrospinal fluid in the ventricles, resulting from impaired absorption or obstruction, which may be congenital or acquired. There are 2 common types of hydrocephalus:
- **Communicating:** CSF flows (communicates) between the ventricles but is not absorbed in the subarachnoid space (arachnoid villi).
- **Noncommunicating:** CSF is obstructed (non-communicating) between the ventricles with obstruction, often stenosis of the aqueduct of Sylvius but it can occur anywhere in the system.

Symptoms of hydrocephalus depend on the age of onset. In *early infancy*, before closure of cranial sutures, head enlargement is the most common presentation, but in adults with less elasticity in the skull, neurological symptoms usually relate to increasing pressure on structures of the brain. Hydrocephalus may occur at any age, but the type that occurs in *young/middle-aged adults* is different than that common in children or those >50. Hydrocephalus in young and middle-aged adults may result from a congenital defect, hydrocephalus of infancy with shunt failure, or trauma and is characterized by:
- Headache relieved by vomiting, papilledema.
- Lack of bladder control.
- Strabismus and other visual disorders.
- Ataxia.
- Irritability.
- Lethargy.
- Confusion and impairment of cognitive abilities.

With adult-onset normal pressure hydrocephalus (>50) cerebrospinal fluid increases and dilates the ventricles, but frequently without increasing intracranial pressure. The cause is often unclear. Symptoms include gait disturbance, bladder control issues, and mild dementia. Treatment for all types of hydrocephalus involves shunting.

Hydrocephalus is diagnosed through CT and MRI, which help to determine the cause. Treatment may vary somewhat depending upon the underlying disorder, which may require treatment. For example, if obstruction is caused by a tumor, surgical excision to directly remove the obstruction is required.

Generally, however, most hydrocephalus is treated with shunts:

- **Ventricular-peritoneal shunt:** This procedure is the most common and consists of placement of a ventricular catheter directly into the ventricles (usually lateral) at one end with the other end in the peritoneal area to drain away excess CSF. There is a one-way valve near the proximal end that prevents backflow but opens when pressure rises to drain fluid. In some cases the distal end drains into the right atrium.
- **Third ventriculostomy:** A small opening is made in the base of the third ventricle so CSF can bypass an obstruction. This procedure is not common and is done with a small endoscope.

Intracranial/intraventricular hemorrhage

Subarachnoid hemorrhage (SAH) may occur after trauma but is common from rupture of a berry aneurysm or an arteriovenous malformation (AVM). However, there are a number of disorders that may be implicated: neoplasms, sickle cell disease, infection, hemophilia, and leukemia. The first presenting symptom may be complaints of severe headache, nausea and vomiting, nuchal rigidity, palsy related to cranial nerve compression, retinal hemorrhages, and papilledema. Late complications include hyponatremia and hydrocephalus. Symptoms worsen as intracranial pressure rises. SAH from aneurysm is classified as follows:

- Grade I: No symptoms or slight headache and nuchal rigidity.
- Grade II: Mod-severe headache with nuchal rigidity and cranial nerve palsy.
- Grade III: Drowsy, progressing to confusion or mild focal deficits.
- Grade IV: Stupor, with hemiparesis (mod-severe), early decerebrate rigidity, and vegetative disturbances.
- Grade V: Coma state with decerebrate rigidity.

Treatment includes:

- Identifying and treating underlying cause.
- Observing for re-bleeding.
- Anti-seizure medications (such as Dilantin®) to control seizures.
- Antihypertensives.
- Surgical repair if indicated.

Hemorrhage is always a concern with head trauma because even injuries that appear slight can result in vascular rupture, resulting in hemorrhage between the skull and the brain. There are two types of hemorrhage that often occur from head trauma: epidural and subdural. Epidural hemorrhage is bleeding between the dura and the skull, pushing the brain downward and inward. The hemorrhage is usually caused by arterial tears, so bleeding is often rapid, leading to severe neurological deficits and respiratory arrest. Initially, the body compensates by rapidly absorbing cerebrospinal fluid and decreasing blood flow, but the compensatory measure is soon overwhelmed. The most common site is the parietotemporal region, forcing the medial part of the temporal lobe under the tentorial edge, compressing nerves and vessels. This type of injury usually results from skull fractures with middle meningeal artery lacerations or venous bleeding, such as may occur with a blow to the head from a fall or motor vehicle accident.

Subdural hemorrhage is bleeding between the dura and the cerebrum, usually from tears in the cortical veins of the subdural space. It tends to develop more slowly than epidural hemorrhage and can result in a subdural hematoma. If the bleeding is acute and develops within minutes or hours of injury, the prognosis is poor. Subacute hematomas that develop more slowly cause varying degrees of injury. Subdural hemorrhage is a common injury related to trauma but it can result from coagulopathies or aneurysms. Symptoms of acute injury may occur within 24-48 hours, but subacute bleeding may not be evident for up to 2 weeks after injury. Chronic hemorrhage occurs primarily in the elderly. Symptoms vary and may include bradycardia, tachycardia, hypertension, and alterations in consciousness. Older children and adults usually require surgical evacuation of the hematoma.

Neurologic infectious diseases

West Nile virus is an RNA virus, spread by infected mosquitoes. Infection has been traced to donor organs, blood transfusions, and breast milk although the blood supply has been monitored for WNV since 2003. While WNV is more common in adult, especially the elderly, it can affect infants and children, who show symptoms more readily than adults. The incubation period ranges from 2-14 days. There are 3 types of infection:

- **Viremia**: 80%, infection but no symptoms.
- **Mild**: 20% (West Nile fever), characterized by fever, malaise, lymphadenopathy, headache, rash, nausea, and vomiting. The acute stage is usually is self-limiting within a few days, but symptoms can persist for weeks, including muscular weakness, fatigue, concentration problems, fever, and headache. About 30% require hospitalization.
- **Severe**: <1%, severe neurological symptoms with meningitis and associated symptoms being the most common in children and young adults.

There are a number of arboviruses in addition to West Nile Virus that can cause flu-like symptoms that progress to viral encephalitis, and incidence is increasing across the United States, often spread by mosquitoes. Because many people are unaware of emerging causes for diseases, the cause of the ensuing encephalitis is frequently misdiagnosed. Encephalitis is an infection of the brain tissue and usually lasts for 2-3 weeks. Symptoms vary somewhat from one type of infection to another, but they have similar characteristics.

- Onset usually involves flu-like symptoms with sore throat, headaches, muscle aches, fever and chills, myalgia. In some cases, a rash may appear.
- Progressive symptoms include photophobia, vomiting, and increased weakness.
- Advanced symptoms may include altered mental status, seizures, memory loss, coma, and death.

Encephalitis may also result from complications of Lyme disease, spread by infected ticks. One of the most common causes of viral encephalitis is the herpes simplex virus.

Bacterial meningitis

Bacterial meningitis may be caused by a wide range of bacteria, including *Streptococcus pneumoniae* and *Neisseria meningitidis*. Bacteria can enter the CNS from distant infection, surgical wounds, invasive devices, nasal colonization, or penetrating trauma. The infective process includes inflammation, exudates, WBC accumulation, and brain tissue damage with hyperemia and edema. Purulent exudate covers the brain and invades and blocks the ventricles, obstructing CSF and leading to increased intracranial pressure. Symptoms include abrupt onset, fever, chills, severe headache, nuchal rigidity, and alterations of consciousness with seizures, agitation, and irritability. Antibodies specific to bacteria don't cross the blood brain barrier, so immune response is poor. Some may have photophobia, hallucinations, and/or aggressive behavior or may become stuporous and lapse into coma. Nuchal rigidity may progress to opisthotonos. Reflexes are variable but Kernig and Brudzinski signs are often positive. Signs may relate to particular bacteria, such as rashes, sore joints, or draining ear. Diagnosis is usually based on lumbar puncture examination of cerebrospinal fluid and symptoms. Treatment includes IV antibiotics and supportive care.

Kernig's sign, Brudzinski sign, and positive jolt maneuver

Patients with bacterial meningitis may exhibit signs to help support the diagnosis. While the following are not universally present, they are specific to meningitis and are rarely positive with other disorders:
- **Kernig's sign:** Flex each hip and then try to straighten the knee while the hip is flexed. Spasm of the hamstrings makes this painful and difficult with meningitis.
- **Brudzinski sign:** With the patient lying supine, flex the neck by pulling head toward chest. The neck stiffness causes the hips and knees to pull up into a flexed position with meningitis.
- **Jolt accentuation maneuver:** (Used if nuchal rigidity is not present.) Ask patient to rapidly move his/her head from side to side horizontally. Increase in headache is positive for meningitis.

Myasthenia gravis

Myasthenia gravis (MG) is an autoimmune disorder of the neuromuscular system in which acetylcholine receptors are damaged at neural synapses, preventing transmission of impulses to contract muscles. In order for muscles to contract, there must be continuous binding of acetylcholine (from neural synapses) to receptor sites on the endplates of muscles. In MG, the receptor sites are damaged by antibodies in an autoimmune response, so there are fewer receptor sites to receive acetylcholine. This results in weakness of voluntary muscles, increasing with activity, as the need for acetylcholine is not met. Muscles initially affected include those of the eye, neck and face. Additionally, the thymus gland develops abnormalities, such as hypertrophy or thymoma in about 90% of those with MG. About 80-90% of people with MG test positive for antibodies. It is believed that, in those who test negative for antibodies, the antibodies target only selected receptor sites, not the entire complex.

Muscular dystrophy

Muscular dystrophies are genetic disorders with gradual degeneration of muscle fibers and progressive weakness and atrophy of skeletal muscles and loss of mobility. Types differ according to the muscles involved, the age of onset, and the speed of progression:
- **Facioscapulohumeral muscular dystrophy** (Landouzy-Dejerine) is a slowly-progressive autosomal recessive disorder with onset usually between 10 and 24. Typically, the shoulders angle forward, the face loses mobility, and the patient cannot raise the arms above the head because of weakness of the upper arms. The lower extremities may be affected as the disease progresses.
- **Limb-girdle muscular dystrophy** is a group of autosomal recessive or dominant disorders with onset in later childhood or adolescence, manifesting as weakness of proximal muscles of the pelvic and shoulder girdles although muscles in proximity to these (upper arms and thighs) may weaken over time. There are over a dozen forms, related to specific genetic defects. Some forms cause serious disability in a few years and others progress very slowly.

Guillain-Barré syndrome

Guillain-Barré syndrome (GBS) is an autoimmune disorder of the myelinated motor peripheral nervous system, often triggered by a viral gastroenteritis or *Campylobacter jejuni* infection. Diagnosis is by history, clinical symptoms, and lumbar puncture, which often show increased protein with normal glucose and cell count although protein may not increase for a week or more.

Symptoms
- Numbness and tingling with increasing weakness of lower extremities that may become generalized, sometimes resulting in complete paralysis and inability to breathe without ventilatory support.
- Deep tendon reflexes are typically absent and some people experience facial weakness and ophthalmoplegia (paralysis of muscles controlling movement of eyes).

Treatment
- Supportive
- Patients should be hospitalized for observation and placed on ventilator support if forced vital capacity is reduced.
- While there is no definitive treatment, plasma exchange or IV immunoglobulin shorten the duration of symptoms.

Intracranial pressure monitoring and the Monroe-Kellie hypothesis

Increasing intracranial pressure (ICP) is a frequent complication of brain injuries, tumors, or other disorders affecting the brain, so monitoring the ICP is very important. Increased ICP can indicate cerebral edema, hemorrhage, and/or obstruction of cerebrospinal fluid. The Monroe-Kellie hypothesis states that in order to maintain a normal ICP, a change in volume in one compartment must be compensated by a reciprocal change in volume in another compartment. There are 3 compartments in the brain: the brain tissue, cerebrospinal fluid (CSF), and blood.The CSF and blood can change more easily to accommodate changes in pressure than tissue, so medical intervention focuses on cerebral blood flow and drainage. Normal ICP is 0-15 mm Hg on transducer or 80-180 mm H_2O on manometer. As intracranial pressure increases, symptoms include:
- Headache.
- Alterations in level of consciousness.
- Restlessness.
- Slowly reacting or nonreacting dilated or pinpoint pupils.
- Seizures.
- Motor weakness.
- Cushing's triad (late sign):
  o Increased systolic pressure with widened pulse pressure.
  o Bradycardia in response to increased pressure.
  o Decreased respirations.

ICP monitoring devices

The intracranial pressure (ICP) monitoring device may be placed during surgery or a ventriculostomy performed in which a burr hole is drilled into the frontal area of the scalp and an intraventricular catheter threaded into the lateral ventricle. The intraventricular catheter may be used to monitor ICP and to drain excess CSF.

Other monitoring devices include:
- **Intracranial pressure monitor bolt** (subarachnoid bolt) is applied through a burr hole with the distal end of the monitor probe resting in the subarachnoid space.
- **Epidural monitors** are placed into the epidural space.
- **Fiberoptic monitors** may be placed inside the brain.

The intraventricular catheter is the most accurate. CSF may be drained continuously or intermittently and must be monitored hourly for amount, color, and character. For ICP measurement, the patient's head must be elevated to 30 to 45° and the transducer leveled to the outer canthus of the eye. Normal ICP is 0-15 mm Hg on transducer or 80-180 mm H_2O on manometer.

Lumbar puncture

The lumbar puncture (spinal tap) is done between the 3rd and 4th or 4th and 5th lumbar vertebrae. The patient is in the lateral recumbent position with knees drawn toward the chest during the procedure. A local anesthetic is applied to prevent pain when the needle is inserted into the subarachnoid space to withdraw CSF and measure CSF pressure, which should be 70 to 200 mm H_2O.

Queckenstedt's test
- Compress jugular veins on each side of the neck during the procedure.
- Note pressure and then release the veins and note pressure in 10-second intervals.
- Pressure should rise quickly with compression and fall quickly with release.
- Slower or no response indicates blockage of subarachnoid pathways.

CSF analysis

Normal values:
- Clear and colorless.
- Protein: 15-45 mg/dL.
- Glucose: 60-80 mg/dL.
- Lactic acid: <25.2 mg/dL
- Culture: Negative
- RBCs: 0
- WBCs: 0.5/mL

After a lumbar puncture, the patient should remain in the prone position for at least 3 hours to ensure that the needle puncture sites through the dural and arachnoid areas remain separate in order to reduce the chance of CSF leakage. If >20 mL of CSF is removed, then the patient should remain prone for 2 hours, side-lying (flat) for 2 or 3 hours and supine or prone for 6 additional hours. Relieving intracranial pressure by withdrawing CSF may cause herniation of the brain, so lumbar puncture should be done with care in the presence of increased ICP. The most common complaint is of spinal headache, which may occur within a few hours or several days of the procedure. Increased fluid intake may reduce risk of headache. If headache occurs, it may be treated with analgesics, fluids, and bed rest; however, if the headache is severe or persistent, an epidural blood patch may be done, with venous blood withdrawn and then injected into the epidural space at the site of the puncture to seal the leaking opening.

Hypertonic saline solution

Hypertonic saline solution (HSS) has a sodium concentration higher than 0.9% (NS) and is used to reduce intracranial pressure/cerebral edema and treat traumatic brain injury. Concentrations usually range from 2% to 23.4%. The hypertonic solution draws fluid from the tissue through osmosis. As edema decreases, circulation improves. HSS also expands plasma, increasing CPP, and counteracts hyponatremia that occurs in the brain after injury and causes increased ICP. Administration:
- Peripheral lines: HSS <3% only.
- Central lines: HSS ≥3%

HSS can be administered continuously at rates varying from 30 mL to 150 mL/hr. Rate must be carefully controlled. Fluid status must be monitored to prevent hypovolemia, which increases risk of renal failure. Boluses (typically 30 mL of 23.4%) may be administered over 15 minutes for acute increased ICP or transtentorial herniation. Laboratory monitoring includes:
- Sodium (every 6 hours): Maintain at 145 to 155 mmol/L. Higher levels can cause heart/respiratory/renal failure.
- Serum osmolality (every 12 hours): Maintain at 320 mOsmol/L. Higher levels can cause renal failure.

Mannitol

Mannitol is an osmotic diuretic that increases excretion of both sodium and water and reduces intracranial pressure and brain mass, especially after traumatic brain injury. Mannitol may also be used to shrink the cells of the blood-brain barrier in order to help other medications breach this barrier. Mannitol is administered per intravenous infusion:
- 0.25g to 2g/kg in a 15% to 25% solution over one-half to one hour.

Cerebral spinal fluid pressure should show decrease within 15 minutes. Fluid and electrolyte balances must be carefully monitored as well as I &O and body weight. Concentrations of 20% to 25% require a filter. Crystals may form if the mannitol solution is too cold and the mannitol container may require heating (in 80° C water) and shaking to dissolve crystals, but solution should be cooled to ≤body temperature prior to administration. Mannitol cannot be administered in polyvinylchloride bags as precipitates form. Side effects include fluid and electrolyte imbalance, nausea, vomiting, hypotension, tachycardia, fever, and urticaria.

Cerebral blood flow, mean arterial pressure, and cerebral perfusion pressure

Mean arterial pressure (MAP) can be calculated as diastolic BP (DBP) + 1/3 pulse pressure. MAP has a direct effect on cerebral blood flow:
- Normal: 50 to 150 mm Hg.
- <50 mm Hg: Cerebral flow decreases, resulting in ischemia.
- >60 mm Hg: Needed to perfuse coronary arteries.
- 70 to 90 mm Hg: Needed to perfuse brains and other organs.
- 90 to 110 mm Hg needed to increase cerebral perfusion after neurosurgical procedures.
- >150 mm Hg: Cerebral blood vessels become maximally constricted and the brain barrier is disrupted, resulting in cerebral edema and increased ICP.

Cerebral perfusion pressure (CPP) is the pressure required to maintain adequate blood flow to the brain. CPP is based on mean arterial pressure (MAP), intracranial pressure (ICP), and jugular venous pressure (JVP). CPP is calculated as MAP - ICP (when ICP >JVP) OR MAP – JVP (when JVP > ICP):
- Normal: 60 to 100 mm Hg.
- <100 mm Hg: Hyperperfusion occurs with increased ICP.
- <60 mm Hg: Hypoperfusion occurs with ischemia.
- <30 mm Hg: Hypoperfusion is marked and incompatible with life.

Neuromuscular blockade

Neuromuscular blockade relaxes muscles for surgical procedures, aids in intubation, reduces extreme agitation and skeletal muscle activity, facilitates mechanical ventilation, and prevents increased ICP with intracranial hypertension. Sedatives/analgesics should be given prior to and during neuromuscular blockade to prevent PTSD from recall of pain. Neuromuscular blocking agents (NMBA) may cause muscle weakness, myopathy, and bronchoconstriction from release of histamine. Apnea and airway obstruction may occur:
- **Depolarizing agents** (agonists), such as succinylcholine, bind directly to acetylcholine receptors, blocking access and activating the receptor to depolarize. Some drugs potentiate effects: Numerous antibiotics (streptomycin, tetracycline, and clindamycin), antiarrhythmics (quinidine, CCBs), lithium carbonate, and magnesium sulfate. Side effects include myalgia, malignant hyperthermia, and severe anaphylactic/anaphylactoid reactions.
- **Non-depolarizing agents** (antagonists) bind directly to acetylcholine receptors, blocking access, but do not activate the receptors, so depolarization does not occur. Non-depolarizing agents are further classified by duration of action: short acting (mivacurium, rapacuronium), intermediate acting (rocuronium, vecuronium, atracurium, cisatracurium), and long acting (pancuronium, doxacurium, pipecuronium). Non-depolarizing NMBAs have slower onset and longer duration than succinylcholine.

Sedation

Sedation may be used for drug-induced coma to treat traumatic brain injury and increased intracranial pressure. The most commonly used drugs are barbiturates (pentobarbital or thiopental) and sedatives (propofol). Barbiturates depress the reticular activating system in the brain stem, an area controlling body functions, including consciousness. Barbiturates with phenyl serve as anticonvulsants (phenobarbitol) but those with methyl (methohexital) do not. If sulfur is added to the compound to replace some oxygen, the barbiturates have increased lipid solubility (thiopental, methohexital, and thiamylal), making them useful as rapid acting anesthetics. Barbiturates have a number of systemic effects. Blood pressure falls and heart rate increases although cardiac output is usually maintained. With hypovolemia, CHF, and β-adrenergic blockade, there may be peripheral pooling of blood and myocardial depression that causes a pronounced drop in BP and cardiac output. Barbiturates reduce cerebral blood flow and decrease ICP, but cerebral oxygen consumption is also reduced. Barbiturates do not relax muscles or reduce sensation of pain.

Sedation used for drug-induced coma often includes propofol. Propofol is an IV non-opioid hypnotic anesthetic, the most common used for induction. It is also used for maintenance and postoperative sedation. Onset of action is rapid because of high lipid solubility, and propofol has a short distribution half-life and rapid clearance, so recovery is also fast. Propofol is metabolized by the liver as well as extrahepatically through the lungs. Propofol decreases cerebral blood flow, metabolic rate of oxygen consumption and ICP, similarly to thiopental. Propofol causes vasodilation with resultant hypotension, but with bradycardia rather than tachycardia. Tachycardia during induction may indicate metabolic acidosis. Propofol is a respiratory depressant, resulting in apnea after induction and decreased tidal volume, respiratory rate, and hypoxic drive during maintenance. Upper airway reflexes are more reduced than with thiopental and there is less wheezing with induction and intubation, so propofol is often used as sedation for those on mechanical ventilators. Propofol has antiemetic properties as well but does not produce analgesia.

Glasgow coma scale

The Glasgow coma scale (GCS) measures the depth and duration of coma or impaired level of consciousness and is used for post-operative assessment. The GCS measures three parameters: Best eye response, best verbal response, and best motor response, with a total possible score that ranges from 3 to 15:

Eye opening
4: Spontaneous.
3: To verbal stimuli.
2: To pain (not of face).
1: No response.

Verbal
5: Oriented.
4: Conversation confused, but can answer questions.
3: Uses inappropriate words.
2: Speech incomprehensible.
1: No response.

Motor
6: Moves on command.
5: Moves purposefully respond pain.
4: Withdraws in response to pain.
3: Decorticate posturing (flexion) in response to pain.
2: Decerebrate posturing (extension) in response to pain.
1: No response.

Injuries/conditions are classified according to the total score:
- 3-8 Coma
- ≤ 8 Severe head injury
- 9-12 Moderate head injury
- 13-15 Mild head injury.

Evacuation of hematomas

Evacuation of hematomas can be done in a number of different ways, including burr holes, needle aspiration, direct surgical craniotomy, or endoscopic craniotomy, but evacuation can pose considerable risks:

- **Epidural hematomas** are usually arterial but may be venous (20%) and are always medical emergencies and require craniotomy with evacuation before compression damage to the brain occurs. Prognosis is good if corrected early because underlying brain damage is rarely severe.
- **Subdural hematomas**, often from acceleration-deceleration accidents or abuse, involve damage to the brain tissue. Evacuation may be done if the hematoma is large and causing compression, but the brain tissue beneath hematomas is often extremely swollen. If the dura is opened, suddenly relieving the pressure may cause the brain to herniate through the opening, so aggressive therapy to reduce swelling preoperatively and careful surgical planning are necessary.

Craniotomies

Craniotomies for tumors or other surgical repair (AVMs, aneurysms) are increasingly done with micro-endoscopic equipment, but the surgical opening must be large enough to allow access and the use of necessary instruments. Procedures vary widely according to the reason for craniotomy, the type of tumor, and the age and condition of the patient. Direct craniotomies through the skull are needed in some instances, but newer approaches, including transnasal and transsphenoidal endoscopy are used when possible.

Some areas of the brain are not accessible with craniotomy, but may be accessible through stereotactic radiosurgery with Gamma Knife® or CyberKnife®. Stereotactic radiosurgery is often used as a secondary treatment after primary removal of tumor for regrowth or residual tumor. Radiosurgery may be fractionated and given in a series of treatments. These non-invasive treatments are usually done while adults are awake.

In the post-operative period immediately following a craniotomy, the patient must be observed carefully for any complications or changes in condition:

- Intracranial pressure monitoring.
- Positioning: Head is usually positioned in midline, neutral position. The head of bed is elevated 30-45° for supratentorial surgery and is flat or only slightly elevated for infratentorial surgery.
- Fluid balance (intake and output).
- Wound care includes observation for swelling, drainage, and emptying and measuring any drainage devices (such as Hemovacs®) left in place.
- Oximetry and ABGs to ensure proper oxygenation.
- Analgesia and antiemetics are usually given routinely to maintain comfort and prevent stress from vomiting.
- Corticosteroids to reduce postoperative swelling.
- Anticoagulants (heparin) to prevent clotting.
- Monitor laboratory status:
  - Complete blood count to observe for blood loss/ infection.
  - Electrolyte levels, especially observing for hyponatremia and/or hyperkalemia.
  - Blood glucose level (may elevate with corticosteroids).

- Monitor thermoregulation and prevent hyperthermia.
- Anti-thromboembolism measures: Compression stockings or intermittent pneumatic compression.

Transsphenoidal hypophysectomy

The sella turcica is a depressed area that holds the pituitary gland (which extends down from the brain on a stalk) in the sphenoid bone at the base of the skull. Pituitary tumor < 10 mm diameter is removed in a transsphenoidal hypophysectomy. In addition to general anesthesia, supplemental infraorbital blocks may provide postoperative pain relief. Vasoconstrictors (such as epinephrine) with local anesthesia are usually administered intranasally to control bleeding. Microscopic surgery is done with an incision in the gingival mucosa beneath the upper lip then through the nasal septum and through the roof of the sphenoid cavity to access the base of the sella turcica and the pituitary tumor. Endoscopic surgery is done directly through the nares with removal of mucosa but no incision. After microscopic surgery, stents are placed in the nasal septum and the nose packed. With both procedures, nasal discharge must be observed for CSF leakage and the patient cautioned not to blow the nose.

Epilepsy

Epilepsy is diagnosed based on a history of seizure activity as well as supporting EEG findings. Treatment is individualized. First line treatments include phenytoin, carbamazepine, and sodium valproate for partial and generalized tonic-clonic seizures. Usually treatment is started with one medication, but this may need to be changed, adjusted, or an additional medication added until the seizures are under control or to avoid adverse effects, which include allergic reactions, especially skin irritations, and acute or chronic toxicity. Milder reactions often subside with time or adjustment in doses. Toxic reactions may vary considerably, depending upon the medication and duration of use, so close monitoring is essential. Severe rash and hepatotoxicity are common toxic reactions that occur with many of the antiepileptic drugs. Dosages of drugs may need to be adjusted to avoid breakthrough seizures during times of stress, such as during illness or surgery. Alcohol/drug abuse and sleep deprivation may also cause breakthrough seizures. Most anticonvulsant drugs are teratogenic.

Anticonvulsants

Carbamazepine (Tegretol®)
- Use: Partial, tonic-clonic, and absence seizures. Analgesia for trigeminal neuralgia.
- Side effects: Dizziness, drowsiness, nausea, and vomiting. Toxic reactions include severe skin rash, agranulocytosis, aplastic anemia, and hepatitis

Clonazepam (Klonopin®)
- Use: Akinetic, absence, and myoclonic seizures
- Side effects: Behavioral changes, hirsutism or alopecia, headaches, and drowsiness. Toxic reactions include hepatotoxicity, thrombocytopenia, ataxia, and bone marrow failure.

Ethosuximide (Zarontin®)
- Use: Absence seizures
- Side effets: Headaches and gastrointestinal disorders. Toxic reactions include skin rash, blood dyscrasias (sometimes fatal), hepatitis and lupus erythematosus.

Felbamate (Felbatol®)
- Use: Lennox-Gastaut syndrome
- Side effects: Headache, fatigue, insomnia, and cognitive impairment. Toxic reactions include aplastic anemia and hepatic failure. It is recommended only if other medications have failed.

Fosphenytoin (Cerebyx®)
- Use: Status epilepticus. Prevention and treatment of seizures during neurosurgery
- Side effects: CNS depression, hypotension, cardiovascular collapse, dizziness, nystagmus, pruritus.

Gabapentin (Neurotonin®)
- Use: Partial seizures
- Side effects: Post-herpetic neuralgia Dizziness, somnolence, drowsiness, ataxia, weight gain, and nausea. Toxic reactions include hepatotoxicity and leukopenia.

Lamotrigine (Lamictal®)
- Use: Partial and primary generalized tonic-clonic seizures. - Lennox-Gastaut syndrome.
- Side effects: Tremor, ataxia, weight gain, dizziness, headache, and drowsiness. Toxic reactions include severe rash, which may require hospitalization.

Levetiracetam (Keppra®)
- Use: Partial onset, myoclonic, and generalized tonic-clonic seizures
- Side effects: Idiopathic generalized epilepsy. Dizziness, somnolence, irritability, alopecia, double vision, sore throat, and fatigue. Toxic reactions include bone marrow suppression and liver failure.

Oxcarbazepine (Trileptal®)
- Use: Partal seizures.
- Side effects: Double or abnormal vision, tremor, abnormal gait, GI disorders, dizziness, and fatigue. A toxic reaction is hepatotoxicity.

Phenobarbital (Luminal®)
- Use: Tonic-clonic and cortical local seizures. Acute convulsive episodes. Hypnotic for insomnia.
- Side effects: Sedation, double vision, agitation, and ataxia. Toxic reactions include anemia and skin rash.

Phenytoin (Dilantin®)
- Use: Tonic-clonic and complex partial seizures
- Side effects: Nystagmus, vision disorders, gingival hyperplasia, hirsutism, dysrhythmias, and dysarthria. Toxic reactions include collapse of cardiovascular system and CNS depression

Primidone (Mysoline®)
- Use: Grand mal, psychomotor, and focal seizures.
- Side effects: Double vision, ataxia, impotence, lethargy, and irritability. A toxic reaction is skin rash.

Tiagabine (Gabitril®)
- Use: Partial seizures
- Side effects: Concentration problems, weak knees, dysarthria, abdominal pain, tremor, dizziness, fatigue, and agitation.

Topira-mate (Topamax®)
- Use: Partial and tonic-clonic seizures. Migraines
- Side effects: Anorexia, weight loss, confusion, ataxia, and confusion. A toxic reaction includes kidney stones.

Valproate/ Valproic acid (Depakote®, Depakene®)
- Use: Complex par-tial, simple, and complex absence seizures. Bipolar disorder.
- Side effects: Weight gain, alopecia, tremor, menstrual disorders, nausea, and vomiting. It is also used to treat bipolar disorder. Toxic reactions include hepatotoxicity, severe pancreatitis, rash, blood dyscrasias, and nephritis.

Zonisamide (Zonegran®, Excegran®)
- Use: Partial seizures.
- Side effects: Anorexia, nausea, agitation, rash, headache, dizziness, and somnolence. Toxic reactions include leukopenia and hepatotoxicity.

Seizure disorders

Partial seizures are caused by an electrical discharged to a localized area of the cerebral cortex, such as the frontals, temporal, or parietal lobes with seizure characteristics related to area of involvement. They may begin in a focal area and become generalized, often preceded by an aura.
- **Simple partial:** Unilateral motor symptoms including somatosensory, psychic, and autonomic.
  o Aversive: Eyes and head turned away from focal side
  o Sylvan (usually during sleep): Tonic-clonic movements of the face, salivation, and arrested speech.
- **Special sensory:** Various sensations (numbness, tingling, prickling, or pain) spreading from one area. May include visual sensations, posturing or hypertonia.

- **Complex (Psychomotor):** No loss of consciousness, but altered consciousness and non-responsive with amnesia. May involve complex sensorium with bad tastes, auditory or visual hallucinations, feeing of déjà vu, strong fear. May carry out repetitive activities, such as walking, running, smacking lips, chewing, or drawling. Rarely aggressive. Seizure usually followed by prolonged drowsiness and confusion. Most common ages 3 through adolescence.

Generalized seizures lack a focal onset and appear to involve both hemispheres, usually presenting with loss of consciousness and no preceding aura.
- **Tonic-clonic (Grand Mal):** Occurs without warning.
  - Tonic period (10-30 seconds): Eyes roll upward with loss of consciousness, arms flexed; stiffen in symmetric tonic contraction of body, apneic with cyanosis and salivating.
  - Clonic period (10 seconds to 30 minutes, but usually 30 seconds). Violent rhythmic jerking with contraction and relaxation. May be incontinent of urine and feces. Contractions slow and then stop.

Following seizures, there may be confusion, disorientation, and impairment of motor activity, speech and vision for several hours. Headache, nausea, and vomiting may occur. Person often falls asleep and awakens conscious.

Absence (Petit Mal): Onset between 4-12 and usually ends in puberty. Onset is abrupt with brief loss of consciousness for 5-10 seconds and slight loss of muscle tone but often appears to be daydreaming. Lip smacking or eye twitching may occur.

Status epilepticus (SE) is usually generalized tonic-clonic seizures that are characterized by a series of seizures with intervening time too short for regaining of consciousness. The constant assault and periods of apnea can lead to exhaustion, respiratory failure with hypoxemia and hypercapnia, cardiac failure, and death.

Brain tumors

Any type of brain tumor can occur in adults. Brain tumors may be primary, arising within the brain, or secondary as a result of metastasis:
- **Glioblastoma:** This is the most common and most malignant adult brain tumor Treatment includes a surgery, radiation, and chemotherapy, but survival rates are very low.
- **Astrocytoma:** This arises from astrocytes, which are glial cells. It is the most common type of tumor, occurring throughout the brain. There are many types of astrocytomas, and most are slow growing. Some are operable while others are not. Radiation may be given after removal. Astrocytomas include glioblastomas, aggressively malignant tumors occurring most often in adults 45-70.
- **Brain stem glioma:** This may be fast or slow growing but is generally not operable because of location although it may be treated with radiation or chemotherapy.
- **Craniopharyngioma:** This is a congenital, slow-growing, recurrent (especially if >5 cm) and benign cystic tumor but difficult to resect, and treated with surgery and radiation.
- **Meningioma:** Slow growing recurrent tumors are usually benign and most often occur in women, ages 40 to 70; however, they can cause severe impairment/death, depending on size and location. Meningiomas are surgically removed if causing symptoms.
- **Ganglioglioma:** This can occur anywhere in the brain, usually slow growing and benign.

- **Medulloblastoma**: There are many types of medulloblastoma, most arising in the cerebellum, malignant, and fast growing. Surgical excision is done and often followed by radiation and chemotherapy although recent studies show using just chemotherapy controls recurrence with less neurological damage.
- **Oligodendroglioma**: This tumor most often occurs in the cerebrum, primarily the frontal or temporal lobes, involving the myelin sheath of the neurons. It is slow growing and most common in those 40-60.
- **Optical nerve glioma**: This slow growing tumor of the optic nerve is usually a form of astrocytoma. It is often associated with neurofibromatosis type I (NF1), occurring in 15-40%. Despite surgical, chemotherapy or radiotherapy treatment, it is usually fatal.

Strokes

Strokes (brain attacks, cerebrovascular accidents) result when there is interruption of the blood flow to an area of the brain. The two basic types are ischemic and hemorrhagic. About 80% are ischemic, resulting from blockage of an artery supplying the brain:
- **Thrombosis** in large artery, usually resulting from atherosclerosis, may block circulation to a large area of the brain. It is most common in the elderly and may occur suddenly or after episodes of transient ischemic attacks.
- **Lacunar infarct** (penetrating thrombosis in small artery) is most common in those with diabetes mellitus and/or hypertension.
- **Embolism** travels through the arterial system and lodges in the brain, most commonly in the left middle cerebral artery. An embolism may be cardiogenic, resulting from cardiac arrhythmia or surgery. An embolism usually occurs rapidly with no warning signs.
- **Cryptogenic** has no identifiable cause.

Medical management of ischemic strokes with tissue plasminogen activator (tPA) (Activase®), the primary treatment, should be initiated within 3 hours:
- **Thrombolytic,** such as tPA, which is produced by recombinant DNA and is used to dissolve fibrin clots. It is given intravenously (0.9mg/kg up to 90 mg) with 10% injected as an initial bolus and the rest over the next hour.
- **Antihypertensives** if MAP >130 mm HG or systolic BP >220.
- **Cooling** to reduce hyperthermia.
- **Osmotic diuretics** (mannitol), hypertonic saline, loop diuretics (Lasix®), and/or corticosteroids (dexamethasone) to decrease cerebral edema and intracranial pressure.
- **Aspirin/anticoagulation** may be used with embolism.
- **Stool softeners** to prevent constipation.
- Monitor and treat hyperglycemia.

Contraindications to thrombolytic therapy include:
- Evidence of cerebral or subarachnoid hemorrhage or other internal bleeding or history of intracranial hemorrhage, recent stroke, head trauma, or surgery
- Uncontrolled hypertension, seizures.
- Intracranial AVM, neoplasm, or aneurysm.
- Current anticoagulation therapy.
- Low platelet count (<100,000 mm^3).

Hemorrhagic strokes account for about 20% and result from a ruptured cerebral artery, causing not only lack of oxygen and nutrients but also edema that causes widespread pressure and damage:

- **Intracerebral** is bleeding into the substance of the brain from an artery in the central lobes, basal ganglia, pons, or cerebellum. Intracerebral hemorrhage usually results from atherosclerotic degenerative changes, hypertension, brain tumors, anticoagulation therapy, or some illicit drugs, such as crack and cocaine. Onset is often sudden and may cause death.
- **Intracranial aneurysm** occurs with ballooning cerebral artery ruptures, most commonly at the Circle of Willis.
- **Arteriovenous malformation** (AVM) is a tangle of dilated arteries and veins without a capillary bed. This is a congenital abnormality. Rupture of AVMs is a cause of brain attack in young adults.

Subarachnoid hemorrhage is bleeding in the space between the meninges and brain, resulting from aneurysm, AVM, or trauma. This type of hemorrhage compresses brain tissue.

Strokes most commonly occur in the right or left hemisphere, but the exact location and the extent of brain damage affects the type of presenting symptoms. If the frontal area of either side is involved, there tends to be memory and learning deficits. Some symptoms are common to specific areas and help to identify the area involved:

- **Right hemisphere:** This results in left paralysis or paresis and a left visual field deficit that may cause spatial and perceptual disturbances so that people may have difficulty judging distance. Fine motor skills may be impacted, resulting in trouble dressing or handling tools. People may become impulsive and exhibit poor judgment, often denying impairment. Left-sided neglect (lack of perception of things on the left side) may occur. Depression is common as well as short-term memory loss and difficulty following directions. Language skills usually remain intact.

Symptoms of strokes vary according to the area of the brain affected:

- **Left hemisphere:** This results in right paralysis or paresis and a right visual field defect. Depression is common and people often exhibit slow, cautious behavior, requiring repeated instruction and reinforcement for simple tasks. Short-term memory loss and difficulty learning new material or understanding generalizations is common. Difficulty with mathematics, reading, writing, and reasoning may occur. Aphasia (expressive, receptive, or global) is common.
- **Brain stem:** Because the brain stem controls respiration and cardiac function, a brain attack frequently causes death, but those who survive may have a number of problems, including respiratory and cardiac abnormalities. Strokes may involve motor or sensory impairment or both.
- **Cerebellum:** This area controls balance and coordination. Strokes in the cerebellum are rare but may result in ataxia, nausea and vomiting, and headaches and dizziness or vertigo.

Thrombolytics

Thrombolytics are drugs used to dissolve clots in myocardial infarction, ischemic stroke, DVT, and pulmonary embolism. Thrombolytics may be given in combination with heparin or low-weight heparin to increase anticoagulation effect. Thrombolytics should be administered within 90 minutes but may be given up to 6 hours after an event. They may increase the danger of hemorrhage and are contraindicated with hemorrhagic strokes, recent surgery, or bleeding.

Thrombolytics include:

- **Alteplase tissue-type plasminogen activator** (t-PA) (Activase®) is an enzyme that converts plasminogen to plasmin, which is a fibrinolytic enzyme. T-PA is used for ischemic stroke, MI, and pulmonary embolism and must be given IV within 3 hours or by catheter directly to the site of occlusion within 6 hours.
- **Anistreplase** (Eminase®) is used for treatment of acute MI and is given intravenously in a 30-unit dose over 2-5 minutes.
- **Reteplase** (Retavase®) is a plasminogen activator used after MI to prevent CHF (contraindicated for ischemic strokes). It is given in 2 doses, a 10-unit bolus over 2 minutes and then repeated in 30 minutes.
- **Streptokinase** (Streptase®) is used for pulmonary emboli, acute MI, intracoronary thrombi, DVT, and arterial thromboembolism. It should be given within 4 hours but can be given up to 24 hours. Intravenous infusion is usually 1,500,000 units in 60 minutes. Intracoronary infusion is done with an initial 20,000-unit bolus and then 2000 units per minute for 60 minutes.
- **Tenecteplase** (TNKase®) is used to treat acute MI with large ST elevation. It is administered in a onetime bolus over 5 seconds and should be administered within 30 minutes of event.
- **Urokinase** (Abbokinase®) is used for DVT and pulmonary embolism. Dose is calculated according to patient's weight. Urokinase is given in an initial loading dose of 15 mL over 10 minutes and then with an infusion pump, 15 mL/hr over 12 hours.

Gastrointestinal

Acute abdominal trauma

Acute abdominal trauma may be blunt or penetrating:
- **Blunt injuries** from motor vehicle accidents (MVA), sports injuries, falls, and assaults are common causes of abdominal injury and comprise crush (compression), shear (tearing), and burst (sudden increased pressure). MVA often results in liver injury in the passenger with impact on that side and spleen injury in the driver with impact on the driver's side. Other injuries from blunt trauma include damage to the diaphragm, retroperitoneal hematomas, and intestinal injuries, including perforation.
- **Penetrating wounds**, on the other hand, are almost always related to gunshot wounds (high energy) or knife assaults (low energy). Gunshot wounds tend to cause more extensive damage than stab wounds, especially to the colon, liver, spleen and diaphragm. Interior injury may be extensive because the bullet damages tissue and may ricochet off of bone. Hemorrhage and peritonitis are common complications.

The spleen is the most frequently injured solid organ in blunt trauma. Injuries to the spleen are the most common because it's not well protected by the rib cage and is very vascular. Symptoms may be very non-specific. Kehr sign (radiating pain in left shoulder) indicates intra-abdominal bleeding and Cullen sign (ecchymosis around umbilicus) indicates hemorrhage from ruptured spleen. Some may have right upper abdominal pain although diffuse abdominal pain often occurs with blood loss, associated with hypotension. Splenic injuries are classified according to the degree of injury:
- Tear in splenic capsules or hematoma.
- Laceration of parenchyma (<3 cm).
- Laceration of parenchyma (>3 cm).
- Multiple lacerations of parenchyma or burst-type injury.

Treatment may be supportive if injury is not severe; otherwise, suturing of spleen may be needed. Because there is a risk of infection with splenectomy, every effort (bed rest, transfusion, reduced activity for at least 8 weeks) is done to avoid surgery because the spleen will often heal spontaneously.

Hepatic injury is the most common cause of death (mortality rates of 8-25%) from abdominal trauma and is often associated with multiple organ damage, so symptoms may be non-specific. Automobile accidents cause most blunt trauma. Elevation in liver transaminase levels indicates damage that may require CT examination with double contrast. Liver injuries are classified according to the degree of injury:
I. Tears in capsule with hematoma.
II. Laceration(s) of parenchyma (<3 cm).
III. Laceration(s) of parenchyma (<3 cm).
IV. Destruction of 25-75% of lobe from burst injury.
V. Destruction of >75% of lobe from burst injury.
VI. Avulsion [tearing away].

Hemodynamically stable patients are managed medically, but surgical repair may be necessary if the patient is unstable or bleeding. Hemorrhage is common complication of hepatic injury and may require ligation of hepatic arteries or veins. Treatment often includes intravenous fluids for fluid volume deficit as well as blood products (plasma, platelets) for coagulopathies.

Gastric injuries may result in perforation, primarily at the greater curvature. The risk increases if the person is injured with a full stomach after eating a meal and suffers blunt or penetrating force to the abdomen. Perforation results in severe pain, rigid abdomen, and bloody nasogastric drainage with peritonitis developing within hours, so early diagnosis and surgical repair must be done.

Intestinal injuries may occur from blunt or penetrating trauma. Indications of rupture often appear 24-48 hours when the person presents with symptoms of peritonitis resulting from leakage of intestinal contents into the peritoneum. Symptoms may include distention, abdominal pain, absent bowel sounds, leukocytosis, fever, dyspnea, nausea and vomiting. Sepsis and abscess or fistula formation can occur. Treatment includes prompt antibiotic therapy, and surgical repair with peritoneal lavage. The abdominal wound may be left open to heal by secondary intention.

Abdominal trauma with pronounced shock increases risk of compartment syndrome for a number of reasons:
- Edema of the intestines because of trauma and surgical manipulation.
- Capillary leakage.
- Hemorrhage (retroperitoneal).
- Abdominal packing left in place to control bleeding.
- IV crystalloid administration.

Pressure within the abdomen may begin to rise rapidly if the abdomen is closed, resulting in decreased cardiac output from pressure on the vena cava, increased airway pressures and acute respiratory distress syndrome, decreased urinary output with decrease in renal blood flow and glomerular filtration, increased central venous pressure resulting in increased intracranial pressure and cerebral edema. Diagnosis is by measurement of intra-abdominal pressure (>25 cm H_2O) by Foley catheter or NG tube with pressure transducer or water-column manometry. If risk for compartment syndrome exists, the wound should not be closed. Sudden release of pressure and reperfusion may cause acidosis, vasodilation, and cardiac arrest, so the patient should be given crystalloid solutions before decompression.

Peritonitis

Peritonitis (inflammation of the peritoneum) may be primary (from infection of blood or lymph) or, more commonly, secondary, related to perforation or trauma of the gastrointestinal tract, Common causes include perforated bowel, ruptured appendix, abdominal trauma, abdominal surgery, peritoneal dialysis or chemotherapy, or leakage of sterile fluids, such as blood, into the peritoneum. Diagnosis is made according to clinical presentation, abdominal x-rays, which may show distention of the intestines or air in the peritoneum, and laboratory findings, such as leukocytosis. Blood cultures may indicate sepsis.

Symptoms
- Diffuse abdominal pain with rebound tenderness (Blumberg's sign).
- Abdominal rigidity.
- Paralytic ileus.

- Fever (with infection).
- Nausea and vomiting.
- Sinus tachycardia.

Treatment
- Intravenous fluids and electrolytes.
- Broad-spectrum antibiotics.
- Laparoscopy as indicated to determine cause of peritonitis and effect repair.

Acute gastrointestinal hemorrhage

Gastrointestinal (GI) hemorrhage may occur in the upper or lower gastrointestinal track. The primary cause (50-70%) of GI hemorrhage is peptic ulcer disease (gastric and duodenal ulcers), which results in deterioration of the gastromucosal lining, compromising the glycoprotein mucous barrier and the gastroduodenal epithelial cells that provide protection from gastric secretions. The secretions literally digest the mucosal and submucosal layers, damaging blood vessels and causing hemorrhage. The primary causes are NSAIDs and infection with *Helicobacter pylori.*

Symptoms
- Abdominal pain and distention.
- Hematemesis.
- Bloody or tarry stools.
- Hypotension with tachycardia.

Treatment
- Fluid replacement with transfusions if necessary.
- Antibiotic therapy for *Helicobacter pylori.*
- Endoscopic thermal therapy to cauterize or injection therapy (hypertonic saline, epinephrine, ethanol) to cause vasoconstriction.
- Arteriography with intraarterial infusion of vasopressin and/or embolizing agents, such as stainless steel coils, platinum microcoils, or Gelfoam pledgets.
- Vagotomy and pyloroplasty if bleeding persists.

Stress-related erosive syndrome (SRES) (stress ulcers) occurs most frequently in those who are critically ill, such as those with severe or multi-organ trauma, mechanical ventilation, sepsis, severe burns, and head injury with increased intracranial pressure. Stress induces changes in the gastric mucosal lining and decreased perfusion of the mucosa, causing ischemia. SRES involves hemorrhage in ≥30% with mortality rates of 30-80% so prompt identification and treatment is critical. The lesions tend to be diffuse, so they are more difficult to treat than peptic ulcers.

Symptoms
- Coffee ground emesis.
- Hematemesis
- Abdominal discomfort.

<u>Treatment</u>
Prophylaxis in those at risk:
- Sucralfate (Carafate®) protects mucosa against pepsin.
- Famotidine (Pepcid®), nizatidine (Axid®), ranitidine (Zantac®) or cimetidine (Tagamet®) reduces gastric secretions.

Treatment for active bleeding includes:
- Intraarterial infusion of vasopressin.
- Intraarterial embolization.
- Oversewing of ulcers or total gastrectomy if bleeding persists.

Bowel obstruction and infraction

Bowel obstruction occurs when there is a mechanical obstruction of the passage of intestinal contents because of constriction of the lumen, occlusion of the lumen, or lack of muscular contractions (paralytic ileus). Obstruction may be caused by congenital or acquired abnormalities/disorders. Symptoms include:
- Abdominal pain and distention.
- Abdominal rigidity.
- Vomiting and dehydration.
- Diminished or no bowel sounds.
- Severe constipation (obstipation).
- Respiratory distress from diaphragm pushing against pleural cavity.
- Shock as plasma volume diminishes and electrolytes enter intestines from bloodstream.
- Sepsis as bacteria proliferates in bowel and invade bloodstream.

Bowel infarction is ischemia of the intestines related to severely restricted blood supply. It can be the result of a number of different conditions, such as strangulated bowel or occlusion of arteries of the mesentery, and may follow untreated bowel obstruction. People present with acute abdomen and shock, and mortality rates are very high even with resection of infarcted bowel.

Intestinal perforation

Intestinal perforation is a complete rupture or penetration of the intestinal wall. There are a number of causes:
- Traumatic injuries, such as gunshot or knife wounds.
- NSAIDs and/or aspirin, especially in elderly with diverticulitis.
- Acute appendicitis.
- Peptic ulcer disease.
- Iatrogenic causes: laparoscopy, endoscopy, colonoscopy, radiotherapy
- Bacterial infections.
- Inflammatory bowel diseases, such as Crohn's disease or ulcerative colitis.
- Ingestion of toxic substances (acids) or foreign bodies (toothpicks).

The danger posed by infection after perforation varies depending upon the site. The stomach and proximal portions of the small intestine have little bacteria, but the distal portion of the small intestine contains aerobic bacteria, such as *E. coli,* as well as anaerobic bacteria.

Symptoms include abdominal pain and distention and rigidity, fever, guarding and rebound tenderness, tachycardia and paralytic ileus with nausea and vomiting. Treatment is as for peritonitis, with antibiotics and surgical repair.

Gastrointestinal surgery

The Whipple (pancreaticoduodenectomy) procedure is used to surgically remove the head of the pancreas the gallbladder, part of the bile duct, the duodenum, and sometimes the distal portion of the stomach. After excision, the remaining pancreas, bile duct and intestinal stump are sutured to the intestine so that secretions empty into the intestine. The Whipple procedure may be done as an open procedure or laparoscopically. This procedure is used primarily for malignant or benign tumors of the head of the pancreas but can also be used for chronic pancreatitis, duodenal cancer, cancer of the ampulla, and cholangiocarcinoma. Whipple is recommended only if the cancer has not spread beyond the pancreas and has not invaded major vessels. Usually, the pancreas is still able to produce adequate insulin, but production of pancreatic enzymes may be impaired. A pylorus-preserving variation preserves the stomach and part of the pylorus to decrease nutritional deficiencies and weight loss associated with the standard Whipple.

Gastrointestinal surgery for esophageal cancer

Esophageal cancer starts in the inner layer of the esophagus and spreads. It may develop after long-term reflux because of cell changes brought about by gastric acid. Symptoms of esophageal cancer may include throat or epigastric discomfort, increasing dysphagia and inability to swallow solids, unexplained weight loss, hoarseness, hiccups, hematemesis, and the feeling of something in the throat.

Treatment for esophageal cancer involves surgical removal of the affected portion of the esophagus. Two common procedures include:
- **Esophagectomy,** which is removal of all or part of the esophagus with the distal end resutured to the stomach or an intestinal graft used to replace the excised portion of the esophagus.
- **Esophago-gastrectomy** is removal of the distal portion of the esophagus, lymph nodes, and the upper portion of the stomach, after which the remaining esophagus and stomach are reattached.

Postoperative management for esophagectomy and esophago-gastrectomy

Postoperative management for esophagectomy and esophago-gastrectomy includes monitoring intubation and ventilation while in place, ensuring NG tube is patent (but do not replace if pulled out as it passes through anastomosis), maintaining NPO for 5 to 7 days, providing nutrition per jejunostomy tube (if in place), monitoring IV fluids (usually 100-200 mL/hr), encouraging pulmonary toilet and observing for respiratory distress syndrome, monitoring chest tubes (if in place) and drains (Penrose, Jackson-Pratt), providing anticoagulants (heparin) BID and compression stockings to prevent emboli, observing for signs of delirium tremens or delirium if patient has history of alcohol abuse (common with this type of surgery), , monitoring cardiovascular and neurological status, and managing pain, which is often severe. Prior to initiating oral intake, a fluoroscopic examination with water-soluble contrast will be done to check for leaks. If no leaks, patients begin with clear liquids and progress to 6 to 8 small meals per day, avoiding excessively cold, hot, or spicy foods.

Gastrointestinal surgery

Bariatric surgery is used to promote weight loss in the morbidly obese (100 pounds over normal weight or BMI of 35-40). Surgery is done to restrict intake and/or prevent absorption of calories. Procedures are open surgical or laparoscopic and include:

- **Banding** places a band around the upper portion of the stomach, creating a small pouch with a small distal opening to slow emptying.
- **Sleeve gastrectomy** removes about 2/3s of stomach, and a distal part of the small intestine is attached directly to the remaining stomach, bypassing part of the small intestine to reduce absorption.
- **Roux-en-Y** uses staples and a vertical band to decrease the size of the stomach, creating a small pouch. Then a section of the small intestine is attached to the pouch, bypassing the first and second segments of the intestine to reduce absorption.
- **Gastric ballooning,** placing a balloon in the stomach and filling it with liquid to decrease stomach capacity is used primarily in Europe.

Esophagogastroduodenoscopy

Esophagogastroduodenoscopy (EGD) with a flexible fiberscope equipped with a lighted fiberoptic lens allows direct inspection of the mucosa of the esophagus, stomach, and duodenum. The scope has a still or video camera attached to a monitor for viewing during the procedure. The scope may be used for biopsies or therapeutically to dilate strictures or treat gastric or esophageal bleeding. The patient is positioned on the left side (head supported) to allow saliva drainage. Conscious sedation (midazolam, propofol) is commonly used along with a topical anesthetic spray or gargle to facilitate placing the lubricated tube through the mouth into the esophagus. Atropine reduces secretions. A bite guard in the mouth prevents the patient from biting the scope. The airway must be carefully monitored through the procedure (which usually takes about 30 minutes), including oximeter to measure oxygen saturation. While perforation, bleeding, or infection may occur, most complications are cardiopulmonary in nature and relate to drugs (conscious sedation) used during the procedure, so reversal agents (flumazenil, naloxone) should be available.

Esophageal varices

Esophageal varices are torturous dilated veins in the submucosa of the esophagus (usually the distal portion), a complication of cirrhosis of the liver in which obstruction of the portal vein causes an increase in collateral vessels, a decrease in circulation to the liver, and an increase in pressure in the collateral vessels in the submucosa of the esophagus and stomach. This causes the vessels to dilate. Because they tend to be fragile and inelastic, they tear easily, causing sudden massive esophageal hemorrhage. Bleeding from varices occurs in 19-50% with associated mortality rates of 40-70%. Treatment may include:

- Fluid and blood replacement.
- Intravenous vasopressin, somatostatin, and octreotide to decreased portal venous pressure and provide vasoconstriction.
- Endoscopic injection with sclerosing agents.
- Endoscopic variceal band ligation.
- Esophagogastric balloon tamponade to apply direct pressure.

Transjugular intrahepatic portosystemic shunting (TIPS) creates a channel between systemic and portal venous systems to reduce portal hypertension. A variety of other shunts may be done surgically if bleeding persists.

Portal hypertension

Portal hypertension, obstructed blood flow increasing blood pressure throughout the portal venous system, prevents the liver from filtering blood and causes the development of collateral blood vessels that return unfiltered blood to the systemic circulation. Increasing serum aldosterone levels cause sodium and fluid retention in the kidneys, resulting in hypervolemia, ascites and esophageal varices. Portal hypertension can be caused by any liver disease, especially cirrhosis and inherited or acquired coagulopathies that cause thrombosis of the portal vein.

Symptoms
- Ascites with distended abdomen.
- Esophageal varices with bleeding.
- Dyspnea.
- Abdominal discomfort.
- Fluid and electrolyte imbalances.

Treatment
- Restricted sodium intake.
- Diuretics.
- Intravenous fluid and replacement blood products.
- Balloon tamponade and vasopressin for bleeding varices.
- Endoscopic treatment of obstruction.
- Portal vein shunting redirecting blood from the portal vein to the vena cava.
- Liver transplant in severe cases.

Hepatic cirrhosis

Cirrhosis is a chronic hepatic disease in which normal liver tissue is replaced the fibrotic tissue that impairs liver function. There are 3 types:
- **Alcoholic** (from chronic alcoholism) is the most common type and results in fibrosis about the portal areas. The liver cells become necrotic, replaced by fibrotic tissue, with areas of normal tissue projecting in between, giving the liver a hobnail appearance.
- **Postnecrotic** with broad bands of fibrotic tissue is the result of acute viral hepatitis.
- **Biliary**, the least common type is caused by chronic biliary obstruction and cholangitis, with resulting fibrotic tissue about the bile ducts.

Cirrhosis may be either compensated or decompensated. Compensated cirrhosis usually involves non-specific symptoms, such as intermittent fever, epistaxis, ankle edema, indigestion, abdominal pain, and palmar erythema. Hepatomegaly and splenomegaly may also be present. Decompensated cirrhosis occurs when the liver can no longer adequately synthesize proteins, clotting factors, and other substances so that portal hypertension occurs.

Symptoms
- Hepatomegaly. Chronic elevated temperature. Clubbing of fingers.
- Purpura resulting from thrombocytopenia, with bruising and epistaxis.

- Portal obstruction resulting in jaundice and ascites. Bacterial peritonitis with ascites. Esophageal varices.
- Edema of extremities and presacral area resulting from reduced albumin in the plasma. Vitamin deficiency from interference with formation, use, and storage of vitamins, such as A, C, and K.
- Anemia from chronic gastritis and ↓dietary intake.
- Hepatic encephalopathy with alterations in mentation.
- Hypotension.
- Atrophy of gonads.

Treatment
- Treatment varies according to the symptoms and is supportive rather than curative as the fibrotic changes in the liver cannot be reversed:
- Dietary supplements and vitamins.
- Diuretics (potassium sparing), such as Aldactone® and Dyrenium®, to decrease ascites.
- Colchicine to reduce fibrotic changes.
- Liver transplant (the definitive treatment).

Malabsorption

Short gut (bowel) syndrome occurs when removal of part of the small intestine results in a malabsorptive condition. Symptoms relate to the amount of bowel removed and the area of resection:
- Resection of the terminal ileum interferes with absorption of bile salts and vitamin B12. If <100 cm removed, malabsorption of bile salts causes watery diarrhea. Treatment includes salt binding resins (cholestyramine 2 to 4 g three times daily). If >100 cm removed, steatorrhea with resultant malabsorption of fat-soluble vitamins occurs. Additional treatment includes low fat diet, vitamins, and calcium supplements to prevent oxalate kidney stone.
- Resection of >40-50% of small bowel results in weight loss, diarrhea, and electrolyte imbalance. If colon and 100cm of proximal jejunum are retained, a low fat, high complex carbohydrate diet, and electrolytes may maintain nutrition, but if the colon is removed, 200 cm of jejunum is required for adequate nutrition. Otherwise, parenteral nutrition is required, and this can lead to liver failure and death or liver/intestine transplantation

Crohn's disease manifests with inflammation of the GI system. Inflammation is transmural (often leading to intestinal stenosis and fistulas), focal and discontinuous with aphthous ulcerations progressing to linear and irregular shaped ulcerations. Granulomas may be present. Common sites of inflammation are the terminal ileum and cecum. Condition is usually chronic, but an acute flare-up may mimic appendicitis. Children may have delayed development and stunted growth, affecting adult stature. There is a genetic component to the disease.

Symptoms
- Perirectal abscess/fistula in advanced disease.
- Diarrhea usually present with colonic disease. May have nocturnal bowel movements, watery stools, and rectal hemorrh-age.
- Anemia may develop with chronic bleeding.
- Abdominal pain most common in lower right quad-rant, usually indicating trans-mural inflammation; may include post-prandial pain and cramping.

- Nausea and vomiting (usually related to strictures of small intestine).
- Malabsorption.
- Fever, night sweats.

Treatment
- Corticosteroids and antibiotics for acute exacerbations.
- Immunomodulatory agents (ciclo-sporine, methotrexate, azathioprine).
- Anti-diarrheals.
- Amino-salicylates (Sufasalazine).
- Antibiotics (Ciprofloxacin, metronidazole).
- Tumor necrosis factor antagonists (Infliximab).
- Enteral feedings or TPN.

Celiac disease
- Pathology: Autoimmune disorder with intolerance to gluten, which causes destruction of surface epithelium of the small intestine.
- Symptoms: Loss of weight. Diarrhea, bloat-ing, steatorrhea (fatty stools), azotorrhea (nitrogenous wastes in stool-urine). Anemia. Vitamin/Iron deficiency (folate, B12.
- Treatment: Gluten-free diet.

Lactose intolerance
- Pathology: Deficiency of intestina lactase causes increased lactose in intestine.
- Symptoms: Diarrhea, cramping.
- Treatment: Oral lactase (Lactaid®). Dairy-free diet.

Parasitic diseases (Giardiasis, strongyloidiasis, coccidiosis)
- Pathology: Parasites live & multiply within the intestines, causing damage to the intestinal mucosa.
- Symptoms: (Varies with parasitic agent). Loss of weight. Diarrhea, steatorrhea.
- Treatment: Antipara-sitic drugs as indicat-ed for the specific parasite.

Acute pancreatitis

Acute pancreatitis is related to chronic alcoholism or cholelithiasis in 90% of patients. Pancreatitis may be triggered by a variety of drugs (tetracycline,thiazides, acetaminophen, oral contraceptives). Pain is usually acute and may be in mid-epigastric, left upper abdominal, or more generalized. Nausea and vomiting as well as abdominal distention may be present. Complications may include shock, acute respiratory distress syndrome, and multi-organ failure. Diagnostic tests include:
- Serum lipase >2x normal value.
- Serum amylase (less accurate than lipase).
- CT with contrast to determine if there is pancreatic necrosis.
- Ultrasound to check bile duct for obstruction.
- MR cholangiopancreatography may be used in place of CT and ultrasound where available.

Treatment is usually supportive with oral intake NPO or restricted to clear liquids to help manage vomiting, ileus, and aspiration. Rehydration with intravenous fluids may be needed or TPN. Hemodynamic support as needed. Biliary obstruction needs to be removed with cholecystectomy. Antibiotics are given if necrosis is related to infection. Analgesia may be indicated, but avoid morphine as it may cause spasms in the sphincter of Oddi.

Gastrointestinal feeding tube placement

- **Surgical placement:** There are both open and laparoscopic surgical techniques for tubes to the stomach or jejunum. The three most common methods are the Janeway, the Stamm, and the Witzel techniques.
- **Endoscopic placement:** Percutaneous endoscopic gastrostomy (PEG) involves intubation of the esophagus with the endoscope and insertion of a sheathed needle with a guidewire through the abdomen and stomach wall so that a catheter can be fed down the esophagus, snared, and pulled out through the opening where the needle was inserted and secured. Similar endoscopic procedures can be done in the jejunum.
- **Radiologic placement:** Through fluoroscopy, ultrasound and/or CT, gastrostomy tube is inserted through the epigastrium and secured with a balloon and external bumper or disk. Insertion into the jejunum is done in a similar manner through the duodenum into the jejunum. A gastrojejunostomy tube, which both drains the stomach and feeds the jejunum, is another procedure.

Preventing displacement of enteral feeding tubes

The displacement of an enteral feeding tube is usually the result of inadequate stabilization. Foley catheters must be marked where they exit the stoma to check for migration. Gastrostomy tubes with an internal balloon or mushroom tip, measured markings, and an external disk are easier to stabilize, but internal device should be checked daily by gently pulling until resistance is felt. External stabilizing devices can be applied to the skin to hold the tube in place. The tube may also be taped to the abdomen or secured with a binder. Sometimes surgeons suture the tube in place, especially those with no balloon, such as jejunostomy tubes, which can become easily dislodged. A solid skin barrier with the tube fed through an anchored baby nipple is an inexpensive stabilizer. Position and length of tube should be carefully documented. Balloon volume should be checked weekly to insure there are no leaks. Skin beneath disks/ bumpers should be checked frequently.

Preventing and treating occlusion of enteral feeding tubes.

Prevention of occlusion involves proper administration of medications and feedings, and maintaining a regular schedule of flushing. Tubes should be flushed with 30 ml of water at least every 4 hours as well as before and after feedings and administration of medications. *Medications* should be in liquid form or crushed completely and enteric-coated or delayed release preparations should be avoided. Feeding solutions should be liquid consistency. Patient should be positioned with head elevated for feedings.

Flushing of occluded tube involves first checking for kinks or obvious problems, attaching a 30-60 ml syringe and aspirating fluid. Then, 5-10 ml of water can be slowly instilled (over about a minute) and aspirated a number of times to try to loosen occlusion. After clamping for 10-15 minutes, the flushing procedure can be repeated with warm water. If the water fails, a multi-enzyme cocktail or pancrease and sodium bicarbonate solution succeed. If all flushing fails, the physician should be notified.

Problems related to enteral feedings

Vomiting and/or aspiration

Causes:
- Tube incorrectly placed.

Solutions:
- Delayed gastric emptying.
- Contaminated formula.
- Increased residual volume.
- Check tube position.
- Delay feeding one hour and check residual volume before resuming.
- Elevate head of bed 30-45° or have patient sit in chair.
- Refrigerate formula, check dates and discard after 24 hours.

Diarrhea

Causes:
- Rapid feeding.
- Medications (such as antibiotics).
- Contaminated formula.
- Lactose intolerance.
- Low-fiber/hypertonic formula.
- Distal movement of tube.

Solutions:
- Slow rate of feeding or use continuous drip.
- Evaluate medications.
- Change tubing every 24 hours and avoid hanging feedings for more than 8 hours.
- Change formula (add fiber, decrease sodium).
- Check position of tube before feedings.

Constipation

Causes:
- Inadequate fluids.
- Fecal impaction.
- Medications.
- Formula.

Solutions:
- Increase fluids (30 mL/kg/body weight).
- Manual examination for fecal impaction.
- Evaluate medications.
- Consult dietician regarding formula.

<u>Dehydration</u>

Causes:
- Diarrhea/vomiting High protein formula.
- Poor fluid intake.
- Hyperosmotic diuresis.

Solutions:
- Treat as for diarrhea/vomiting (above).
- Consult dietician for change in formula. Increase fluids.
- Monitor blood glucose levels.

Total parenteral nutrition

Total parenteral nutrition (TPN) is an intravenous hypertonic solution containing glucose, fat emulsion, protein, minerals, and vitamins. Long (24 inch) PICCs may be inserted in the basilic or cephalic veins and advanced into central circulation for short-term TPN. Central venous catheters are usually inserted into the subclavian or jugular vein and advanced to the tip of the superior vena cava for long-term TPN. Central solutions are more hypertonic than peripheral. Risks include hypoglycemia, hyperglycemia, electrolyte imbalance, infection, air embolus, phlebitis, thrombosis, and nutritional deficiencies. Precautions:
- Use aseptic technique for feedings, dressing changes.
- Use micropore filter (solutions without fat emulsion).
- Use 1.2-micron filter (solutions with fat emulsion).
- Change filters and IV tubing every 24 hours.
- Monitor VS every 4 hours.
- Check daily weight.
- Laboratory tests 3 x weekly until stable and then weekly: Glucose, electrolytes, CBC, urea nitrogen, and hepatic enzymes.
- Check label and ingredients before administration.
- Discard cloudy solutions (contamination).
- Change solution at 24 hours.
- Check for infection.

Commercially-prepared TPN solutions contain dextrose and protein (amino acids), but electrolytes, vitamins, and trace elements are individualized. A total nutrient admixture that contains fat emulsion, dextrose, and amino acids is widely used although fat emulsion may be administered separately. Generally, fat emulsions should not provide >30% of total energy, with maximum dose of 2.5/g/kg per day over 12 to 24 hours. Protein levels of 1.5 to 2 g/kg/ per day are common. Vitamins and trace minerals are usually added to meet MDRs. TPN is initiated slowly with infusion rate gradually increasing over 24 to 48 hours. Because hyperglycemia is a common complication, blood glucose levels should be monitored every 4 to 6 hours at bedside. Insulin may be ordered (sliding scale) to maintain glucose level <150 mg/dL. Infusion rate should not be changed to manage hyperglycemia or hypoglycemia. TPN should be administered with an infusion pump so that rate of infusion can be precisely managed, and the rate of infusion and amount infused should be checked every 30 to 60 minutes.

Complications of TPN

Insertion trauma
- Signs/Symptoms: Pneumothorax, hemothorax: Dyspnea, diminished breath sounds, Dysrhythmia Air embolism, Brachial plexus injury: Numbness/weakness in arm
- Management: Emergency treatment as indicated, including removal/replacement of catheter.

Thrombus
- Signs/symptoms: Intraluminal blood clot. Occluded catheter.
- Management: Heparinization of PN solution

Phlebitis
- Signs/symptoms: Inflammation at insertion site (erythema, pain, edema) from infiltration into tissues.
- Management: Infusion of Intralipid solution.

Fluid imbalance
- Signs/symptoms: Overload or dehydration: Change in urinary output, increase or decrease of BUN, creatinine, hematocrit, serum sodium and serum osmolality
- Management: Recalculate fluid requirements. Evaluate for fluid loss, fever, renal insufficiency, cardiac insufficiency.

Hyperglycemia
- Signs/symptoms: Increase in serum glucose/urine glucose. Increased urinary output.
- Management: Decrease glucose concentration. Slow rate of infusion. Administer insulin.

Hypoglycemia
- Signs/symptoms: Decrease in serum glucose. Diaphoresis, pallor. Lethargy, confusion. Weakness, dizziness.
- Management: Stop insulin. Increase dextrose concentration. Slow rate of infusion. Evaluate for sepsis.

Electrolyte imbalance
- Signs/symptoms: Varies according to imbalance. Maintenance requirements:
  - Na: 2 to 4 mEq/kg/d.
  - K: 2 to 4 mEq/kg/d.
  - Mg: 0.25 to 1.0 mEq/kg/d.
  - Ca: 0.5 to 3 mEq/kg/d.
  - P: 0.5 to 2 mmol/kg/d.
- Management: Frequent laboratory monitoring and adjustment in electrolyte administration

Hyperammonemia
- Signs/symptoms: Lethargy, change in mental status. Asterixis (flapping, tremors of hands).
- Management: Evaluate for hepatic insufficiency. Decrease protein concentration in PN formula.

Azotemia
- Signs/symptoms: Evidence of dehydration: Dry mucous membranes, decreas-ed skin turgor Increas-ed BUN and urinary specific gravity.
- Management: Decrease amino acids in PN formula or change to NephrAmine

Deficiency of EFAs
- Signs/symptoms: Dry skin, flakiness. Thrombocytopenia
- Management: Increase lipid intake with lipids at least 2 x weekly as well as oral fats (if possible) and topical fats.

Hyperlipidemia
- Signs/symptoms: Triglyceride level increasing. Blood specimen cloudy.
- Management: Decrease lipid administration or stop if triglyceride $\geq$400 mg/dL. Monitor triglycerides every 4 hours initially and then daily.

Drains

- **Simple drains** are latex or vinyl tubes of varying sizes and lengths inserted into a wound to provide drainage of serous material, blood, pus, or other discharge. This type of drain is usually placed through a stab wound near the area of involvement.
- **Penrose drains** are soft rubber/latex tubes that are flat in appearance and are placed in surgical wounds to drain fluid by gravity and capillary action. They are available in various diameters and lengths.
- **Sump drains** are double-lumen or tri-lumen tubes (with a third lumen for infusions). A large outflow lumen and small inflow lumen produces venting when air enters the inflow lumen and forces drainage into the large lumen.
- **Percutaneous drainage catheter** is inserted into wound to provide continuous drainage for infection or symptoms from collection of drainage in the wound. Irrigation of the catheter may need to be done to maintain patency. Skin barriers and pouching systems may be necessary.

Closed drainage systems

Closed drainage systems use low-pressure suction to provide continuous gravity drainage of wounds. Drains are attached to collapsible suction reservoirs that provide negative pressure. *Management* includes daily dressing changes about tube insertion site, inspection of skin for inflammation or drainage, monitoring type and amount of drainage from drain, and emptying device by holding it lower than the wound, opening the plug, draining, squeezing all air out to reestablish suction and negative pressure, and reinserting plug. There are two closed drainage systems that are in frequent use:
- **Jackson-Pratt®** is a bulb-type drain that is about the size of a lemon. A thin plastic drain from the wound extends to a squeeze bulb that can hold about 100ml of drainage.
- **Hemovac®** is a round drain with coiled springs inside that are compressed after emptying to create suction. The device can hold up to 500 ml of drainage.

Liver function studies

- **Bilirubin** - Determines the ability of the liver to conjugate and excrete bilirubin: direct 0.0-0.3 mg/dL, total 0.0-0.9 mg/dL, and urine bilirubin should be 0.
- **Total protein** - Determines if the liver is producing protein in normal amounts: 7.0-7.5 g/dL: Albumin: 4.0-5.5 g/dL.
- **Globulin** - 1.7=3.3 g/dL. Serum protein electrophoresis is done to determine the ratio of proteins. Albumin/globulin (A/G) ratio: 1.5:1 to 2.5:1. (Albumin should be greater than globulin.)
- **Prothrombin time (PT)**- 100% or clot detection in 10 to 13 seconds. PT increased with liver disease. International normalized ratio (INR) (PT result/normal average): <2 for those not receiving anticoagulation and 2.0 to 3.0 those receiving anticoagulation. Critical value: >3 in patients receiving anticoagulation therapy.
- **Alkaline phosphatase** - 17-142 adults. (Normal values vary with method.) Indicates biliary tract obstruction if no bone disease
- **AST (SGOT)** - 10-40 units. (Increases in liver cell damage.)
- **ALT (SGPT)** - 5-35 units. (Increases in liver cell damage.)
- **GGT, GGTP** - 5-55 µ/L females, 5-85 µ/L males. (Increases with alcohol abuse.)
- **LDH** - 100-200 units. (Increases with alcohol abuse.)
- **Serum ammonia** - 150-250 mg/dL (Increases in liver failure.)
- **Cholesterol** - Increases with bile duct obstruction and decrease with parenchymal disease.

Malnutrition

The physical assessment is an important part of nutritional assessment to determine malnutrition or problems with self-feeding:

- **Hair** may be dry and brittle or thinning.
- **Skin** may show poor turgor, ecchymosis, tears, pressure areas, ulcerations, abrasions, or other compromises.
- **Mouth** may show dry mucous membranes. Lips may have cheilosis, cracking at the corners, and scaly lips (riboflavin deficiency). Gums may be swollen or bleeding, teeth loose or needing care, or dentures poorly-fitting. Tongue may be inflamed, dry, cracked, or have sores.
- **Nails** may become brittle.   Spoon shaped or pale nail bed indicates low iron.
- **Hands** may be crippled or arthritic, making eating difficult.
- **Vision** may be compromised so that people can't see to prepare food or have difficulty feeding themselves.
- **Mental status** may be impaired to the point that people can't understand diet instructions or prepare or eat meals.
- **Motor skills** may decrease, including hand-mouth coordination or ability to hold utensils.

Protein malnutrition (kwashiorkor or hypoalbuminemia), inadequate protein but adequate fats and carbohydrates, can result from chronic diarrhea, renal disease, infection, hemorrhage, burns, traumatic injuries or other illnesses. Onset is usually rapid with loss of visceral protein while skeletal muscle mass is retained, so it may be difficult to detect on a physical exam. Symptoms include:

- Hypoalbuminemia and anemia
- Edema
- Delayed healing of wound, immuno-incompetence.

Protein-calorie malnutrition (marasmus), inadequate protein and calories, is usually more obvious. Visceral protein is usually intact as is immune function because weight loss is gradual. However, patients are often very thin or emaciated from loss of skeletal muscle mass. Many are elderly and have chronic illnesses. Symptoms include:

- Decreased basal metabolism, hypothermia
- Lack of subcutaneous fat, decreased tissue turgor
- Bradycardia

Mixed protein-calorie malnutrition (combination) is common in hospitalized patients and has an acute onset with low visceral protein as well as rapid loss of weight, skeletal muscle mass, and fat.

Nutritional lab monitoring

Total protein levels can be influenced by many factors, including stress and infection, but it may be monitored as part of an overall nutritional assessment. Protein is critical for general health and wound healing, and because metabolic rate increases in response to a wound, protein needs increase:

- Normal values: 5-9g/kL.
- Diet requirements for wound healing: 1.25-1.5 g/kg per day.

Albumin is a protein that is produced by the liver and is a necessary component for cells and tissues. Levels decrease with renal disease, malnutrition, and severe burns. Albumin levels are the most common screening to determine protein levels. Albumin has a half-life of 18-20 days, so it is sensitive to long-term protein deficiencies more than short-term.

- Normal values: 3.5-5.5 g/dL
- Mild deficiency: 3-3.5 g/dL
- Moderate deficiency: 2.5-3.0 g/dL
- Severe deficiency: <2.5 g/dL.

Levels below 3.2 correlate with increased morbidity and death. Dehydration (poor intake, diarrhea, or vomiting) elevates levels, so adequate hydration is important to ensure meaningful results.

Prealbumin (transthyretin) is most commonly monitored for acute changes in nutritional status because it has a half-life of only 2-3 days. Prealbumin is a protein produced in the liver, so it is often decreased with liver disease. Oral contraceptives and estrogen can also decrease levels. Levels may rise with Hodgkin's disease or the use of steroids or NSAIDs. Prealbumin is necessary for transportation of both thyroxine and vitamin A throughout the body, so if levels fall, both thyroxine and vitamin A utilization are also affected:

- Normal values: 16-40 mg/dL.
- Mild deficiency: 10-15mg/dL
- Moderate deficiency: 5-9 mg/dL.
- Severe deficiency: <5 mg/dL.

Prealbumin is a good measurement because it quickly decreases when nutrition is inadequate and rises quickly in response to increased protein intake. Protein intake must be adequate to maintain levels of prealbumin. Death rates increase with any decrease in prealbumin levels.

Transferrin, which transports about one-third of the body's iron, is a protein produced by the liver. It transports iron from the intestines to the bone marrow where it is used to produce hemoglobin. The half-life of transferrin is about 8-10 days. It is sometimes used as a measure of nutritional status; however, transferrin levels are sensitive to many different things. Levels rapidly decrease with protein malnutrition. Liver disease and anemia can also depress levels, but a decrease in iron, commonly found with inadequate protein, stimulates the liver to produce more transferrin, which increases levels but also decreases production of albumin and prealbumin. Levels may also increase with pregnancy, use of oral contraceptives, and polycythemia. Thus, transferrin levels alone are not always reliable measurements of nutritional status:

- Normal values: 200-400 mg/dL.
- Mild deficiency: 150-200 mg/dL.
- Moderate deficiency: 100-150 mg/dL.
- Severe deficiency: <100 mg/dL.

Histamine receptor antagonists

Histamine (H) receptor antagonists (actually reverse agonists) are used to treat conditions in which excessive stomach acid causes heartburn and GERD. They block histamine 2 (H_2) (parietal) cell receptors in the stomach, thereby decreasing acid production. These drugs are used less commonly now than proton-pump inhibitors. Common H_2 antagonists include:

- **Cimetidine (Tagamet®):** The first H_2 antagonist, it is used less frequently than others because of inhibition of enzymes that results in drug interactions, especially with contraceptive agents and estrogen.
- **Ranitidine (Zantac®):** This was developed to decrease drug interactions and improve patient tolerance. Its activity is about 10 times that of cimetidine. It may be used in combination with other drugs to treat ulcers.
- **Famotidine (Pepcid®):** This may be combined with an antacid to increase the speed of effects as it has a slow onset. It may be used pre-surgically to reduce post-operative nausea.
- **Nizatidine (Axid®):** The last H_2 antagonist developed, it is about equal in potency and action to ranitidine.

Serotonin antagonists

Serotonin antagonists block $5\text{-}HT_2$ receptors of serotonin in the central and peripheral nervous systems and gastrointestinal system. An open channel can result in agitation, nausea, and vomiting, but antagonists close the channel and reduce these symptoms. Serotonin antagonists are frequently used to treat to prevent/treat nausea associated with chemotherapy and anesthesia. Medications include:

- **Metoclopramide** (Reglan®) is used to reduce nausea and vomiting from a wide range of causes. It is also a prokinetic drug that increases gastrointestinal contractions and promotes faster gastric emptying, so it is used for heartburn, GERD, and diabetic gastroparesis.
- **Ondansetron** (Zofran®) reduces vagal stimulation of medulla oblongata (vomiting center) and is used for nausea related to chemotherapy.
- **Tropisetron** (Navoban®) is used to reduce nausea related to chemotherapy.
- **Granisetron** (Kytril®) is used to reduce nausea related to chemotherapy, surgery, and radiation.

Serotonin antagonists have fewer side effects than other antiemetics, but may cause muscle cramping, agitation, diarrhea/constipation, dizziness, and headache.

Antacids

Antacids are medications used to reduce stomach acids by raising the pH and neutralizing the acids present. They are commonly used to treat heartburn or indigestion. Adverse reactions are relatively rare unless taken to excess or with renal impairment. Drugs include:

- **Aluminum hydroxide** (Amphojel®) may cause constipation and with renal impairment, hypophosphatemia and osteomalacia.
- **Magnesium hydroxide** (Milk of Magnesia®) may cause diarrhea and with renal impairment can cause hypermagnesemia.
- **Aluminum hydroxide with magnesium hydroxide** (Maalox®, Mylanta®).
- **Calcium carbonate** (TUMS®, Rolaids®, Titralac®) may cause gastric distention. Excess calcium intake may cause toxic reactions, including kidney stones and renal failure; so excess intake should be avoided.
- **Alka-Seltzer®** combines sodium bicarbonate with aspirin and citric acid so this compound may cause gastric irritation, nausea and vomiting, and tarry stools.
- **Bismuth subsalicylate** (Pepto-Bismol®). Pepto-Bismol® may react with sulfur in the body to create a black tongue and black stools, but this is temporary. Pepto-Bismol® has been associated with Reye's syndrome in children with influenza or chickenpox.

Proton pump inhibitors

Proton pump inhibitors (PPIs) are now used more frequently than histamine receptor antagonists. PPIs interfere with an acid-producing enzyme in the stomach wall, reducing stomach acid. PPIs are used to treat GERD, stomach ulcers, and *H. pylori* (with antibiotics). PPIs are similar in action and include:

- Esomeprazole (Nexium®)
- Lansoprazole (Prevacid®)
- Omeprazole (Prilosec®)
- Pantoprazole (Protonix®)
- Rabeprazole (Aciphex®)
- Omeprazole/sodium bicarbonate (Zegerid®) (Long-acting form of omeprazole.

Common side effects include gastrointestinal upset (nausea, diarrhea, and constipation), headache, and rash. In rare instances, PPIs may cause severe muscle pain; however, they are usually well-tolerated with few adverse effects. PPIs may interfere with the absorption of some drugs, such as those that are affected by stomach acid. Absorption of ketoconazole is impaired, and absorption of digoxin is increased, sometimes leading to toxicity. Omeprazole impacts the hepatic breakdown of drugs more than other PPIs and may cause increased levels of diazepam, phenytoin, and warfarin.

Renal

Acute renal failure

Acute renal failure is abrupt and almost complete failure of kidney function with decreased glomerular filtration rate (GFR), occurring over a period of hours/days. It most commonly occurs in hospitalized patients but may occur in others as well. The BUN increases and nitrogenous wastes are retained (azotemia). There are 3 primary categories, related to cause:

- **Prerenal disorders,** such as myocardial infraction, heart failure, sepsis, anaphylaxis, and hemorrhage result in hypoperfusion of the kidney and decreased GFR.
- **Intrarenal disorders** include burns, trauma, infection, transfusion reactions, and nephrotoxic agents that cause damage to glomeruli or kidney tubules, such as acute tubular necrosis. Burns and crush trauma injuries release myoglobin and hemoglobin from tissues, causing renal toxicity and/or ischemia. With transfusion reactions, hemolysis occurs, and the broken down hemoglobin concentrates and precipitates in tubules. Medications, such as NSAIDs and ACE inhibitors may interfere with kidney function and cause hypoperfusion and ischemia.
- **Post renal disorders** involve distal obstruction that increases pressure in tubules and decreased GFR.

Treatment includes discovering cause, renal diet, fluid restriction and dialysis.

Acute tubular necrosis

Acute tubular necrosis (ATN) occurs when a hypoxic condition causes renal ischemia that damages tubular cells of the glomeruli so they are unable to adequately filter the urine, leading to acute renal failure. Causes include hypotension, hyperbilirubinemia, sepsis, surgery (especially cardiac or vascular), and birth complications. ATN may result from nephrotoxic injury related to obstruction or drugs, such as chemotherapy, acyclovir, and antibiotics, such as sulfonamides and streptomycin. Symptoms may be non-specific initially and can include life-threatening complications.

Symptoms
- Lethargy.
- Nausea and vomiting.
- Hypovolemia with low cardiac output and generalized vasodilation.
- Fluid and electrolyte imbalance leading to hypertension, CNS abnormalities, metabolic acidosis, arrhythmias, edema, and congestive heart failure.
- Uremia leading to destruction of platelets and bleeding, neurological deficits, and disseminated intravascular coagulopathy (DIC).
- Infections can include pericarditis and sepsis.

Treatment
- Identifying and treating underlying cause, discontinuing nephrotoxic agents.
- Supportive care.
- Loop diuretics (in some cases), such as Lasix®.
- Antibiotics for infection (can include pericarditis and sepsis).
- Kidney dialysis.

Loop diuretics

Diuretics increase renal perfusion and filtration, thereby reducing preload and decreasing peripheral and pulmonary edema, hypertension, CHF, diabetes insipidus, and osteoporosis. There are different types of diuretics: loop, thiazide, and potassium sparing.

Loop diuretics inhibit the reabsorption of sodium and chloride (primarily) in the ascending loop of Henle. They also cause increased secretion of other electrolytes, such as calcium, magnesium, and potassium, and this can result in imbalances that cause dysrhythmias. Other side effects include frequent urination, postural hypotension, and increased blood sugar and uric acid levels. They are short-acting so are less effective than other diuretics for control of hypertension:

- **Bumetanide** (Bumex®) is given intravenously after surgery to reduce preload or orally to treat heart failure.
- **Ethacrynic acid** (Edecrin®) is given intravenously after surgery to reduce preload.
- **Furosemide** (Lasix®) is used for the control of congestive heart failure as well as renal insufficiency. It is used after surgery to decrease preload and to reduce the inflammatory response caused by cardiopulmonary bypass (post-perfusion syndrome).

Thiazide diuretics

Thiazide diuretics inhibit the reabsorption of sodium and chloride primarily in the early distal tubules, forcing more sodium and water to be excreted. Thiazide diuretics increase secretion of potassium and bicarbonate, so they are often given with supplementary potassium or in combination with potassium-sparing diuretics. Thiazide diuretics are the first line of drugs for treatment of hypertension. They have a long duration of action (12-72 hours, depending on the drug) so they are able to maintain control of hypertension better than short-acting drugs. They may be given daily or 3-5 days per week. There are numerous thiazide diuretics, including:

- **Chlorothiazide** (Diuril®)
- **Bendroflumethiazide** (Naturetin®)
- **Chlorthalidone** (Hygroton)
- **Trichlormethiazide** (Naqua®)

Side effects include, dizziness, lightheadedness, postural hypotension, headache, blurred vision, and itching, especially during initial treatment. Thiazide diuretics cause sensitivity to sun exposure, so people should be counseled to use sunscreen.

Potassium-sparing diuretics

Potassium-sparing diuretics inhibit the reabsorption of sodium in the late distal tubule and collecting duct. They are weaker than thiazide or loop diuretics, but do not cause a reduction in potassium level; however, if used alone, they may cause an increase in potassium, which can cause weakness, irregular pulse, and cardiac arrest. Because potassium-sparing diuretics are less effective alone, they are often given in a combined form with a thiazide diuretic (usually chlorothiazide), which mitigates the potassium imbalance. Typical side effects include dehydration, blurred vision, nausea insomnia, and nasal congestion, especially in the first few days of treatment:

- **Spironolactone** (Aldactone®) is a synthetic steroid diuretic that increases the secretion of both water and sodium and is used to treat congestive heart failure. It may be given orally or intravenously.

- **Eplerenone** is similar to spironolactone but has fewer side effects so it may be used with patients who can't tolerate the other drug.

Chronic renal failure

Chronic renal failure (resulting in end-stage renal disease) occurs when the kidneys are unable to filter and excrete wastes, concen-trate urine, and maintain electrolyte balance because of hypoxic conditions, kidney disease, or obstruction in the urinary tract. It results first in azotemia (increase in nitrogenous waste in the blood) and then in uremia (nitrogenous wastes cause toxic symptoms.) When >50% of the functional renal capacity is destroyed, the kidneys can no longer carry out necessary functions and progressive deterioration begins over months or years. Symptoms are often non-specific in the beginning with loss of appetite and energy.

Symptoms and complications
- Weight loss. Headaches, muscle cramping, general malaise.
- Increased bruising and dry or itching skin.
- Increased BUN and creatinine.
- Sodium and fluid retention with edema.
- Hyperkalemia. Metabolic acidosis.
- Calcium and phosphorus depletion, resulting in altered bone metabolism, pain, and retarded growth.
- Anemia with decreased production on RBCs. Increased risk of infection.
- Uremic syndrome.

Treatment
- Supportive symptomatic therapy.
- Dialysis and transplantation.
- Diet control: Low protein, salt, potassium, and phosphorus.
- Fluid limitations.
- Calcium and vitamin supplementation
- Phosphate binders.

IVP and radionucleotide renal scan

Intravenous pyelogram (IVP) is done to identify structural defects and tumors and to observe urinary structures. The patient is administered an IV contrast medium and may be administered antihistamine or corticosteroid before test to minimize allergic response. Serum creatinine and BUN are done prior to the IVP to ensure that the contrast medium can be excreted. During the procedure, radiographs are taken every minute x 5 and then after 15 minutes (giving the contrast medium time to pass into the bladder). A post-voiding radiograph shows how efficient the bladder is in emptying. Fluid intake should be increased post-procedure to flush contrast.

Radionucleotide renal scan with dimercaptosuccinic acid (DMSA) requires IV administration of a radioactive element followed by a series of CT scans taken over 20 minutes to 4 hours. The scan is used to assess function and perfusion of the kidney and can detect lesions, atrophy and scars and differentiate among different causes for hydronephrosis. The patient must be well-hydrated and may need to be catheterized to measure output of urine.

End-stage renal disease

Uremic syndrome is a number of disorders that can occur with end-stage renal disease and renal failure, usually after multiple metabolic failures and decrease in creatinine clearance to <10mL/min. There is compromise of all normal functions of the kidney: fluid balance, electrolyte balance, acid-base homeostasis, hormone production, and elimination of wastes. Metabolic abnormalities related to uremia include:

- **Decreased RBC production:** The kidney is unable to produce adequate erythropoietin in the peritubular cells, resulting in anemia, which is usually normocytic and normochromic. Parathyroid hormone levels may increase, causing calcification of the bone marrow, causing hypoproliferative anemia as RBC production is suppressed.
- **Platelet abnormalities:** Decreased Platelet count, increased turnover, and reduced adhesion leads to bleeding disorders.
- **Metabolic acidosis:** The tubular cells are unable to regulate acid-base metabolism, and phosphate, sulfuric, hippuric, and lactic acids increase, leading to congestive heart failure and weakness.
- **Hyperkalemia:** The nephrons cannot excrete adequate amounts of potassium. Some drugs, such as diuretics that spare potassium may aggravate the condition.
- **Renal bone disease:** decreased Calcium, increased phosphate, increased parathyroid hormone, decreased utilization of vitamin D lead to demineralization. In some cases, calcium and phosphate are deposited in other tissues (metastatic calcification).
- **Multiple endocrine disorders:** Thyroid hormone production is decreased and reproductive hormones abnormalities may result in infertility/impotence. Males have decreased testosterone but increased estrogen and LH. Females experience irregular cycles, lack of ovulation and menses. Insulin production may increase but with decreased clearance, resulting in episodes of hypoglycemia or decreased hyperglycemia in those who are diabetic.
- **Cardiovascular disorders:** Left ventricular hypertrophy is most common, but fluid retention may cause congestive heart failure and electrolyte imbalances, dysrhythmias. Pericarditis, exacerbation of valvular disorders, and pericardial effusions may occur.
- **Anorexia and malnutrition:** Nausea and poor appetite contribute to hypoalbuminemia, sometimes exacerbated by restrictive diets.

Renal dialysis

Renal dialysis is used primarily for those who have progressed from renal insufficiency to uremia with end stage renal disease (ESRD). It may also be temporarily for acute conditions. People can be maintained on dialysis, but there are many complications associated with dialysis so many people are considered for renal transplantation. There are a number of different approaches to dialysis:

- **Peritoneal dialysis:** An indwelling catheter is inserted surgically into the peritoneal cavity with a subcutaneous tunnel and a Dacron cuff to prevent infection. Sterile dialysate solution is slowly instilled through gravity, remains for a prescribed length of time, and is then drained and discarded. Peritoneal dialysis may be used for those who want to be more independent, don't live near a dialysis center, or want fewer dietary restrictions.
- **Continuous ambulatory peritoneal dialysis:** A series of exchange cycles are repeated 24 hours a day.
- **Continuous cyclic peritoneal dialysis:** A prolonged period of retaining fluid occurs during the day with drainage at night.

- **Hemodialysis**, the most common type of dialysis, is used for both short-term dialysis and long-term for those with ESRD. Treatments are usually done 3 times weekly for 3-4 hours or short daily dialysis with treatment either during the night or in short daily periods. Hemodialysis is often done for those who can't manage peritoneal dialysis or who live near a dialysis center, but it does interfere with work or school attendance and requires strict dietary and fluid restrictions between treatments. Short daily dialysis allows more independence, and increased costs may be offset by lower morbidity. A vascular access device, such as a catheter, fistula, or graft must be established for hemodialysis, and heparin is used to prevent clotting. With hemodialysis, blood is circulated outside of the body through a dialyzer (a synthetic semipermeable membrane), which filters the blood. There are many different types of dialyzers. High flux dialyzers use a highly permeable membrane that shortens the duration of treatment and decreases the need for heparin.
- **Continuous renal replacement therapy** (**CCRT**) circulates the blood by hydrostatic pressure through a semipermeable membrane. It is used in critical care and can be instituted quickly:
  - **Continuous arteriovenous hemofiltration** (CAVH) circulates blood from an artery (usually the femoral) to a hemofilter using only arterial pressure and not a blood pump. The filtered blood is then returned to the patients venous system, often with added fluids to offset those lost. Only the fluid in filtered.
  - **Continuous arteriovenous hemodialysis** (CAVHD) is similar to CAVH except that dialysate circulates on one side of the semipermeable membrane to increase clearance of urea.
  - **Continuous venovenous hemofiltration** (CVVH) pumps blood through a double-lumen venous catheter to a hemofilter, which returns the blood to the patient in the same catheter. It provides continuous slow removal of fluid, is better tolerated with unstable patients, and doesn't require arterial access.
  - **Continuous venovenous hemodialysis** is similar to CVVH but uses a dialysate to increase clearance of uremic toxins.

Dialysis complications

There are many **complications** associated with dialysis, especially when used for long-term treatment:
- **Hemodialysis***:* Long-term use promotes atherosclerosis and cardiovascular disease. Anemia and fatigue are common as are infections related to access devices or contamination of equipment. Some experience hypotension and muscle cramping during treatment. Dysrhythmias may occur. Some may exhibit dialysis disequilibrium from cerebral fluid shifts, causing headaches, nausea and vomiting, and alterations of consciousness.
- **Peritoneal dialysis:** Most complications are minor, but it can lead to peritonitis, which requires removal of the catheter if antibiotic therapy is not successful in clearing the infection within 4 days. There may be leakage of the dialysate around the catheter. Bleeding may occur, especially in females who are menstruating as blood is pulled from the uterus through the fallopian tubes. Abdominal hernias may occur with long use. Some may have anorexia from feeling of fullness or sweet taste in mouth from absorption of glucose.

Fluid balance/fluid deficit

Body fluid is primarily intracellular fluid (ICF) or extracellular space (ECF). By 3 years of age, the fluid balance has stabilized and remains throughout adulthood:
- ECF: 20-30% (intrastitial fluid, plasma, transcellular fluid).
- ICF: 40-50% (fluid within the cells)

The fluid compartments are separated by semipermeable membranes that allow fluid and solutes (electrolytes and other substances) to move by osmosis. Fluid also moves through diffusion, filtration, and active transport. In fluid volume deficit, fluid is out of balance and ECF is depleted; an overload occurs with increased concentration of sodium and retention of fluid. Signs of fluid deficit include:
- Thirsty, restless to lethargic.
- Increasing pulse rate, tachycardia.
- Fontanels depressed (infants).
- Decreased urinary output.
- Normal BP progressing hypotension.
- Dry mucous membranes
- 3-10% decrease in body weight.

Electrolyte imbalances

Sodium (Na) regulates fluid volume, osmolality, acid-base balance, and activity in the muscles, nerves and myocardium. It is the primary cation (positive ion) in ECF, necessary to maintain ECF levels that are needed for tissue perfusion:
- Normal value: 135-145 mEq/L.
- Hyponatremia: <135 mEq/L.
- Hypernatremia: >145 mEq/L.

Hyponatremia
May result from inadequate sodium intake or excess loss, through diarrhea, vomiting, NG suctioning. It can occur as the result of illness, such as severe burns, fever, SIADH, and ketoacidosis.

- Symptoms vary: Irritability to lethargy to lethargy and alterations in consciousness. Cerebral edema with seizures and coma. Dyspnea to respiratory failure.
- Treatment: Identify and treat underlying cause and provide Na replacement.

Hypernatremia
May result from renal disease, diabetes insipidus, and fluid depletion.

- Symptoms include irritability to lethargy to confusion to coma, seizures, flushing, muscle weakness and spasms, and thirst.
- Treatment includes identifying and treating underlying cause, monitoring Na levels carefully, and IV fluid replacement.

Potassium (K) is the primary electrolyte in ICF with about 98% inside cells and only 2% in ECF, although this small amount is important for neuromuscular activity. K influences activity of the skeletal and cardiac muscles. K level is dependent upon adequate renal functioning because 80% is excreted through the kidneys and 20% through the bowels and sweat:

- Normal values: 3.5-5.5 mEq/L.
- Hypokalemia: <3.5 mEq/L.
- Critical value: <2.5 mEq/L.
- A healthy NPO patient will need about 40 mEq of K per day to maintain serum K levels. (expect alterations in renal disease and other disease processes)

Hypokalemia
Note: K levels have a reciprocal change with serum pH.

Caused by loss of K through diarrhea, vomiting, gastric suction, and diuresis, alkalosis, decreased K intake with starvation, and nephritis. Symptoms include:

- Lethargy and weakness.
- Nausea and vomiting.
- Paresthesias and tetany.
- Dysrhythmias with EKG abnormalities: PVCs, flattened T waves.
- Muscle cramps with hyporeflexia.
- Hypotension.

Treatment: Identify and treat underlying cause and replace K. When possible, oral replacement is preferable to IV, as it allows slower adjustment of K levels. When given IV, K should be given no faster than 20 mEq/hour.

Hyperkalemia
>5.5 mEq/L.   Critical value: >6.5 mEq/L
Note: When a tourniquet is on, if a patient is opening and closing the hand, it can lead to falsely elevated K levels.

Caused by renal disease, adrenal insufficiency, metabolic acidosis, severe dehydration, burns, hemolysis, and trauma. It rarely occurs without renal disease but may be induced by treatment (such as NSAIDs and potassium-sparing diuretics). Untreated renal failure results in reduced excretion. Those with Addison's disease and deficient adrenal hormones suffer sodium loss that results in potassium retention. The primary symptoms relates to the effect on the cardiac muscle:

- Ventricular arrhythmias with increasing changes in EKC leading to cardiac and respiratory arrest.
- Weakness with ascending paralysis and hyperreflexia.
- Diarrhea.
- Increasing confusion.

Treatment includes identifying underlying cause and discontinuing sources of increased K:

- Calcium gluconate to decrease cardiac effects.
- Sodium bicarbonate shifts K into the cells temporarily. Insulin and hypertonic dextrose shift K into the cells temporarily. Cation exchange resin (Kayexalate®) to decrease K.
- Peritoneal dialysis or hemodialysis

More than 99% of **calcium (Ca)** is in the skeletal system with 1% in serum, but it is important for transmitting nerve impulses and regulating muscle contraction and relaxation, including the myocardium. Calcium activates enzymes that stimulate chemical reactions and has a role in coagulation of blood:
- Normal values: 8.2 to 10.2 mg/dL.
- Hypocalcemia: <8.2. Critical value: <7 mg/dL.
- Hypercalcemia: >10.2 mg/dL. Critical value: >12 mg/dL.

Hypocalcemia
May be caused by hypoparathyroidism and occurs after thyroid and parathyroid surgery, pancreatitis, renal failure, inadequate vitamin D, alkalosis, magnesium deficiency and low serum albumin.

Symptoms include: Tetany, tingling, seizures, altered mental status, ventricular tachycardia, positive Trousseau's sign, positive Chvostek's sign, and hypotension.

Treatment: Calcium replacement and vitamin D. It is preferable to give oral calcium, but if IV is given, carefully monitor EKG while giving 10% calcium gluconate 20 mL IV over 10 minutes.

Hypercalcemia
May be caused by acidosis, kidney disease, hyperparathyroidism, prolonged immobilization, and malignancies. Crisis carries a 50% mortality rate.

Symptoms include: Increasing muscle weakness with hypotonicity. Anorexia, nausea and vomiting. Constipation. Bradycardia and cardiac arrest.

Treatment: Identify and treat underlying cause, loop diuretics, and IV fluids.

Calcium levels should be interpreted with albumin levels. Calcium is inversely proportional to the pH of blood.

Phosphorus, or phosphate, (PO_4) is necessary for neuromuscular and red blood cell function, the maintenance of acid-base balance, and provides structure for teeth and bones. About 85% is in the bones, 14% in soft tissue, and <1% in ECF.
- Normal values: 2.4 – 4.5 mEq/L Hypophosphatemia: <2.4mEq/L.
- Hyperphosphatemia; > 4.5 mEq/L.

Hypophosphatemia
Occurs with severe protein-calorie malnutrition, excess antacids with magnesium, calcium or albumin, hyperventilation, severe burns, and diabetic ketoacidosis.

Symptoms include: Irritability, tremors, seizures to coma. Hemolytic anemia. Decreased myocardial function. Respiratory failure.

Treatment: Identify and treat underlying cause and replace phosphorus.

Hyperphosphatemia

Occurs with renal failure, hypoparathyroidism, excessive intake, and neoplastic disease, diabetic ketoacidosis, muscle necrosis, and chemotherapy.

Symptoms include: Tachy-cardia. Muscle cramping, hyperreflexia, and tetany. Nausea and diarrhea.

Treatment: Identify and treat underlying cause, correct hypocalcemia, and provide antacids and dialysis.

Magnesium (Mg) is the second most common intracellular electrolyte (after potassium) and activates many intracellular enzyme systems. Mg is important for carbohydrate and protein metabolism, neuromuscular function, and cardiovascular function, producing vasodilation and directly affecting the peripheral arterial system:
- Normal values: 1.6 to 2.6 mEq/L. Hypomagnesemia: <1.6 mEq/L. Critical value: <1.2 mg/dL.
- Hypermagnesemia: >2.6 mEq/L. Critical value: >4.9 mg/dL.

Hypomagnesemia

Occurs with chronic diarrhea, chronic renal disease, chronic pancreatitis, excess diuretic or laxative use, hyperthyroidism, hypoparathyroid-ism, severe burns, and diaphoresis.

Symptoms include: Neuro-muscular excitability/ tetany. Confusion, headaches and dizziness, seizure and coma. Tachycardia with ventricular arrhythmias. Respiratory depression.

Treatment: Identify and treat underlying cause, provide magnesium replacement.

Hypermagnesemia

Occurs with renal failure or inadequate renal function, diabetic ketoacidosis, hypothyroidism, and Addison's disease.

Symptoms include muscle weak-ness, seizures, and dysphagia with decreased gag reflex, tachycardia with hypotension.

Treatment: Identify and treat underlying cause, IV hydration with calcium, and dialysis.

Metabolic vs. respiratory acidosis

Pathophysiology
- Metabolic: Increase in fixed acid and inability to excrete acid or loss of base, with compensatory increase of CO_2 excretion by lungs
- Respiratory: Hypoventilation and CO_2 retention, with renal compensatory retention of bicarbonate (HCO_3-) and increased excretion of hydrogen.

Laboratory
- Metabolic: Decreased Serum pH and PCO_2 normal if uncompensated, and decreased if compensated. Decreased HCO_3-. Urine pH <6 if compensated.
- Respiratory: Increased serum pH and increased PCO_2. Increased HCO_3- if compensated and normal if uncompensated. Urine pH >6 if compensated.

<u>Causes</u>
- Metabolic: DKA, lactic acidosis, diarrhea, starvation, renal failure, shock, renal tubular acidosis, starvation
- Respiratory: COPD, overdose of sedative or barbiturate, obesity, severe pneumonia/atelectasis, muscle weakness (Guillain-Barré), mechanical hypoventilation.

<u>Symptoms</u>
- Metabolic: Neuro/muscular: drowsiness, confusion headache, coma. Cardiac: Decreased BP, arrhythmias, flushed skin. GI: nausea, vomiting, abdominal pain, diarrhea. Respiratory: Deep inspired tachypnea
- Respiratory: Neuro/muscular: drowsiness, dizziness, headache, coma, disorientation, seizures. Cardiac: Flushed skin, VF, decreased BP. GI: absent. Respiratory: Hypoventilation with hypoxia.

Metabolic vs. respiratory alkalosis

<u>Pathophysiology</u>
- Metabolic: Decreased strong acid or increased base, with compensatory CO_2 retention by lungs Respiratory: Hyperventilation and increased excretion of CO_2, with compensatory HCO_3- excretion by kidneys.

<u>Laboratory</u>
- Metabolic: Increased serum pH. PCO_2 normal if uncompensated and increased if compensated. Increased HCO_3- Urine pH >6 if compensated
- Respiratory: Increased serum pH. Decreased PCO_2 HCO_3- normal if uncompensated and decreased if compensated. Urine pH >6 if compensated.

<u>Causes</u>
- Metabolic: Excessive vomiting, gastric suctioning, diuretics, potassium deficit, excessive mineralocorticoids and $NaHCO_3$- intake.
- Respiratory: Encephalopathy, septicemia, brain injury, salicylate overdose, mechanical hyperventilation.

<u>Symptoms</u>
- Metabolic: Neuro/muscular: dizziness, confusion, nervousness, anxiety, tremors, muscle cramping, tetany, tingling, seizures. Cardiac: Tachycardia and arrhythmias. GI: Nausea, vomiting, anorexia. Respiratory: Compensatory hypoventilation.
- Respiratory: Neuro/muscular: Light-headed, confused, lethargic. Cardiac: Tachycardia and arrhythmias.GI: Epigastric pain, nausea and vomiting. Respiratory: Hyperventilation.

Hydronephrosis

Hydronephrosis is a symptom of a disease involving swelling of the kidney pelvises and calyces because of an obstruction that causes urine to be retained in the kidney. In chronic conditions, symptoms may be delayed until severe kidney damage has occurred. Over time, the kidney begins to atrophy. The primary conditions that predispose to hydronephrosis include:
- Vesicoureteral reflux.
- Obstruction at the ureteropelvic junction.

- Renal edema (non-obstructive)
- Any condition that impairs drainage of the ureters can cause backup of the urine.

<u>Symptoms</u>
- Symptoms vary widely depending upon cause and whether the condition is acute or chronic.
- Acute episodes are usually characterized by flank pain, abnormal creatinine and electrolyte levels, and increased pH.
- The enlarged kidney may be palpable as a soft mass

<u>Treatment</u>
- Treatment requires identifying the cause of obstruction and correcting it to ensure adequate drainage.
- A nephrostomy tube, ureteral stent or pyeloplasty may be done surgically in some cases.
- A urinary catheter may be inserted if there is outflow obstruction from the bladder.

Renal and ureteral calculi

Renal and urinary calculi occur frequently, more commonly in males, and can relate to diseases (hyperparathyroidism, renal tubular acidosis, gout) and lifestyle factors, such as sedentary work. Additionally, some medications can precipitate calculi. Calculi can form at any age, most composed of calcium, and can range in size from very tiny to >6mm. Those <4mm can usually pass in the urine easily. *Diagnostic* studies include clinical findings, UA, pregnancy test to rule out ectopic pregnancy, BUN and creatinine if indicated, ultrasound (for pregnant women and children, IV urography. Helical CT (non-contrast) is diagnostic.

<u>Symptoms</u>
- Symptoms occur with obstruction and are usually of sudden onset and acute:
- Severe flank pain radiating to abdomen and ipsilateral testicle or labium majorum, abdominal or pelvic pain (young children).
- Nausea and vomiting.
- Diaphoresis.
- Hematuria.

<u>Treatment</u>
- Analgesia: opiates and NSAIDs.
- Instructions and equipment for straining urine.
- Antibiotics if concurrent infection.
- Extracorporeal shock-wave lithotripsy.
- Surgical removal: Percutaneous/standard nephrolithotomy.

Urinary tract infections

Pyelonephritis is a potentially organ-damaging bacterial infection of the parenchyma of the kidney. Pyelonephritis can result in abscess formation, sepsis, and kidney failure. Pyelonephritis is especially dangerous for those who are immunocompromised, pregnant, or diabetic. Most infections are caused by *Escherichia coli. Diagnostic* studies include urinalysis, blood and urine cultures. Patients may require hospitalization or careful follow-up.

<u>Symptoms</u>

Symptoms vary widely but can include:

- Dysuria and frequency, hematuria, flank and/or low back pain.
- Fever and chills.
- Costovertebral angle tenderness.
- Change in feeding habits (infants).
- Change in mental status (geriatric)

Young women often exhibit symptoms more associated with lower urinary infection, so the condition may be overlooked.

<u>Treatment</u>

- Analgesia.
- Antipyretics.
- Intravenous fluids
- Antibiotics: started initially but may be changed based on cultures.
  - IV ceftriaxone with fluoroquinolone orally for 14 days.
  - Monitor BUN. Normal 7-8 mg/dL (8-20 mg/dL >age 60). Increase indicates impaired renal function, as urea is end product of protein metabolism.

Renal function studies

- **Specific gravity** 1.015-1.025. Determines kidney's ability to concentrate urinary solutes.
- **Osmolality (urine)** 350-900 mOsm/kg/24 hours. Shows early defects if kidney's ability to concentrate urine is impaired.
- **Osmolality (serum)** 275-295 mOsm/kg. Gives a picture of the amount of soultes in blood.
- **Uric acid** Male 4.4-7.6, Female 2.3-6.6. Levels increase with renal failure.
- **Creatinine clearance (24-hour)** Male 85 to 125 mL/min/1.73 m², Female 75 to 115 mL/min/1.73 m². Evaluates the amount of blood cleared of creatinine in 1 minute. Approximates the glomerular filtration rate.
- **Serum creatinine** 0.6-1.2mg/dL. Increases with impaired renal function, urinary tract obstruction, and nephritis. Level should remain stable with normal functioning.
- **Urine creatinine** Male 14 to 26 mg/kg/24 hr, Female 11 to 20 mg/kg/24 hr. Product of muscle breakdown that should be cleared by the kidneys. Increases with decreased renal function.
- **Blood urea nitrogen (BUN)** 7-8 mg/dL (8-20 mg/dL >age 60). Increase indicates impaired renal function, as urea is end product of protein metabolism.
- **BUN/creatinine ratio** 10:1. Increases with hypovolemia. With intrinsic kidney disease, the ratio is normal, but the BUN and creatinine are increased.

Urinalysis

- Color: Pale yellow/ amber and darkens when urine is concentrated or other substances (such as blood or bile) or present.
- Appearance: Clear but may be slightly cloudy.
- Odor: Slight. Bacteria may give urine a foul smell, depending upon the organism. Some foods, such as asparagus, change odor.
- pH: Usually ranges between 4.5 to 8 with average of 5 to 6.

- Sediment: Red cell casts from acute infections, broad casts from kidney disorders, and white cell casts from pyelonephritis. Leukocytes > 10 per ml^3 are present with urinary tract infections.
- Glucose, ketones, protein, blood, bilirubin, & nitrate: Negative. Urine glucose may increase with infection (with normal blood glucose). Frank blood may be caused by some parasites and diseases but also by drugs, smoking, excessive exercise, and menstrual fluids. Increased red blood cells may result from lower urinary tract infections.
- Uro-bilinogen: 0.1-1.0 units.

Kidney regulatory functions

Kidney regulatory functions include maintaining fluid balance. Fluid excretion balances intake with output so increased intake results in a large output and vice versa:
- **Osmolality** (the number of electrolytes and other molecules per kg/urine) measures the concentration or dilution. With dehydration, osmolality increases; with fluid retention, osmolality decreases. With kidney disease, urine is dilute and the osmolality is fixed.
- **Specific gravity** compares the weight of urine (weight of particles) to distilled water (1.000). Normal urine is 1.010-1.025 with normal intake. High intake lowers the specific gravity and low intake raises it. In kidney disease, it often does not vary.
- **Antidiuretic hormone** (ADH/vasopressin) regulates the excretion of water and urine concentration in the renal tubule by varying water reabsorption. When fluid intake decreases, blood osmolality rises and this stimulates release of ADH, which increases reabsorption of fluid to return osmolality to normal levels. ADH is suppressed with increased fluid intake, so less fluid is reabsorbed.

Radical nephrectomy

Radical nephrectomy is done for adenocarcinoma of the kidney, which may be associated with paraneoplastic syndromes, and, because this type of cancer is associated with smoking, patients may have underlying coronary artery or respiratory disease. Some patients have erythrocytosis, but many are anemic and may require transfusions in preparation for surgery to increase hemoglobin to >10 g/dL. Surgery is done under endotracheal general anesthesia with an anterior subcostal, flank, or thoracoabdominal (preferred for large tumors) incision. The kidney and its adrenal gland with surrounding fat and fascia are removed together. Blood loss may be extensive because the tumors tend to be vascular and large, requiring multiple transfusions. However, controlled hypotension should be limited to brief periods because it may impair renal function. Mannitol is given prior to dissection. Continual direct arterial pressure monitoring and central venous cannulation must be done. Nephron-sparing surgery (partial nephrectomy), often by laparoscopy, may be done if the renal cell carcinoma is <4 cm diameter. Postoperative analgesia and pulmonary hygiene are essential.

Renal biopsy

Renal biopsy to remove a small segment of cortical tissue helps to identify the extent of kidney disease with acute renal failure, transplant rejection, glomerulopathies, and persistent hematuria or proteinuria. Preoperative coagulation studies determine risk of bleeding. Biopsy is done percutaneously per needle biopsy (guided by fluoroscopy or ultrasound) or surgically through a small flank incision. A urine specimen must be obtained so it can be compared with a post-procedure specimen. Post-procedure:

- Maintain patient in supine position immediately after procedure for 4-6 hours and on bedrest overnight. Monitor urine for hematuria and compare with preop specimen.
- Monitor VS every 5 to 15 minutes for first hour and then less frequently. To minimize bleeding maintain bp <140/90.
- Note anorexia, vomiting, abdominal discomfort that suggest bleeding.
- Note pain: Severe colicky pain may indicate clot in the ureter.
- Monitor urinalysis and CBC post procedure.
- Maintain fluid intake at 3000 mL/day in absence of renal insufficiency.

Provide blood component therapy and surgical repair if bleeding occurs.

Renal ultrasound

Renal ultrasound is a non-invasive method of viewing the urinary structures. Most patients that present with with kidney disease of unknown origin should undergo renal ultrasound to assess for possible obstruction. Ultrasound uses ultrasonic sound waves transmitted by a transducer, which picks up reflected sound waves that a computer converts to electronic images. Ultrasound can show fluid accumulation, the movement of blood through the kidney, masses, malformations (congenital abnormalities), change in size of the kidney or other structures, and obstructions, such as renal calculi. Ultrasound is usually done before a renal biopsy, and may be done with a needle biopsy to guide placement of needle. Patient preparation includes drinking two 8-ounce glasses of water one hour before the examination to ensure that the bladder is full. The patient should be reminded not to urinate before the ultrasound. The patient usually remains in supine position throughout the procedure but may be asked to turn to the side. No special precautions are necessary post-procedure.

Multisystem

Management of near-drowning asphyxia

Submersion asphyxiation can cause profound damage to the central nervous system, pulmonary dysfunction related to aspiration, cardiac hypoxia with life-threatening arrhythmias, fluid and electrolyte imbalances, and multi-organ damage, so treatment can be complex. Hypothermia related to near drowning has some protective affect because blood is shunted to the brain and heart. Treatment includes:

- Immediate establishment of airway, breathing and circulation (ABCs).
- NG tube and decompression to reduce risk of aspiration.
- Neurological evaluation.
- Pulmonary management includes monitoring for ≥ 72 hours for respiratory deterioration. Ventilation may need positive-end expiratory pressure (PEEP), but this poses danger to cardiac output and can cause barotrauma, so use should be limited.
- In patients that are symptomatic but do not yet need intubation, use supplemental oxygen to keep $SpO_2 > 94\%$.
- Monitoring of cardiac output and function.
- Neurological care to reduce cerebral edema and increased intracranial pressure, and prevent secondary injury.
- Rewarming if necessary (0.5 to $1°C/hr$).

Traumatic asphyxia

Asphyxia may relate to a number of different injuries:

- **Traumatic asphyxia** most commonly involves a crush injury of the thorax, and traumatic injuries to multiple organs may be present. Crush injuries are characterized by petechiae in the area of compression although tight-fitting clothing, such as a woman's bra, may prevent petechiae from forming.
- **Manual strangulation** may involve crush injuries to the throat, such as hyoid fracture. Often the face appears cyanotic while the rest of the body does not. Petechiae may be present on the face as well. Bruising may be noted about the throat.
- **Ligature strangulation** is similar to manual although throat markings are different, with an indented area surrounding the neck.
- **Hanging** produces a V-shaped marking on the throat and does not encircle the neck.
- **Choking** obstructs the airway. (May require bronchoscopy to remove foreign object).

In all cases, immediate establishment of airway, breathing, and circulation (ABCs) takes precedence. Surgical intervention may be needed for traumatic crush injuries.

Shock

There are a number of different types of shock, but there are general characteristics that they have in common. In all types of shock, there is a marked decrease in tissue perfusion related to hypotension, so that there is insufficient oxygen delivered to the tissues and, in turn, inadequate removal of cellular waste products, causing injury to tissue:

- Hypotension (systolic below 90 mm Hg). This may be somewhat higher (110 mm Hg) in those who are initially hypertensive.
- Decreased urinary output (<0.5 mL/kg/hr), especially marked in hypovolemic shock
- Metabolic acidosis.
- Hypoxemia <90 mm Hg for children and adults birth-50; < 80mm Hg for those 51 to 70 and <70 for those over 70.
- Peripheral/cutaneous vasoconstriction/vasodilation resulting in cool, clammy skin.
- Alterations in level of consciousness.

Types of Shock

Distributive
Preload: decrease(sometimes stays same)
Cardiac Output: increase
SVR: decrease

Cardiogenic
Preload: increase
Cardiac Output: decrease
SVR: increase

Hypovolemic
Preload: decrease
Cardiac Output: decrease
SVR: increase

Neurogenic shock is a type of distributive shock that occurs when injury to the CNS (from trauma resulting in acute spinal cord injury (from both blunt and penetrating injuries), neurological diseases, drugs, or anesthesia, impairs the autonomic nervous system that controls the cardiovascular system. The degree of symptoms relates to the level of injury with injuries above T1 capable of causing disruption of the entire sympathetic nervous system and lower injuries causing various degrees of disruption. Even incomplete spinal cord injury can cause neurogenic shock.

Symptoms
- Hypotension and warm dry skin related to lack of vascular tone that results in hypothermia from loss of cutaneous heat.
- Bradycardia is a common but not universal symptom.

Treatment
- ABCDE (airway, breathing, circulation, disability evaluation, exposure)
- Rapid fluid administration with crystalloid to keep mean arterial pressure at 85-90 mm Hg.
- Placement of pulmonary artery catheter to monitor fluid overload.

- Inotropic agents (dopamine, dobutamine) if fluids don't correct hypotension.
- Atropine for persistent bradycardia.

Distributive shock occurs with adequate blood volume but inade-quate intravascular volume because of arterial/venous dilation that results in decreased vascular tone and hypoperfusion of internal or-gans. Cardiac output may be normal or blood may pool, decreasing cardiac output. Distributive shock may result from anaphylactic shock, septic shock, neurogenic shock, and drug ingestions.

Symptoms
- Hypotension (systolic <90mm Hg or <40mm Hg from nor-mal), tachypnea, tachycardia (>90) (may be lower if patient receiving β-blockers.
- Skin initially warm, later hypoperfused.
- Hyper- or hypothermia (>38°C or <36°C).
- Hypoxemia.
- Alterations in mentation.
- Decreased Urinary output.
- Symptoms related to underlying cause.

Treatment
- Treating underlying cause and stabilizing hemodynamics:
  o Septic shock or anaphylactic therapy and monitoring as indicated.
  o Oxygen with endotracheal intubation if necessary.
  o Rapid fluid administration at 0.25-0.5L NS or isotonic crystalloid every 5-10 minutes as needed to 2-3 L.
  o Inotropic agents (dopamine, dobutamine, norepinephrine) if necessary, for patients with profound hypotension

Anaphylaxis syndrome

Anaphylaxis syndrome is a sudden acute systemic immunoglobulin E (IgE) or non-immunoglobulin E (non-IgE) inflammatory response affecting the cardiopulmonary and other systems.
- **IgE-mediated response** (anaphylactic shock) is an antibody-antigen reaction against an allergen, such as milk, peanuts, latex, insect bites, or fish. This is the most common type.
- **Non IgE-mediated response** (anaphylactoid reaction) is a systemic reaction to infection, exercise, radio contrast material or other triggers. While the response is almost identical to the other type, it does not involve IgE.

Typically, with IgE-mediated response, an antigen triggers release of substances, such as histamine and prostaglandins, which affect the skin, cardiopulmonary, and GI systems. Histamine causes initial erythema and edema by inducing vasodilation. Each time the person has contact with the antigen, more antibodies form in response, so allergic reactions worsen with each contact. In some cases, initial reactions may be mild, but subsequent contact can cause severe life-threatening response.

Symptoms
Symptoms may recur after the initial treatment (biphasic anaphylaxis), so careful monitoring is essential:
- Sudden onset of weakness, dizziness, confusion.
- Severe generalized edema and angioedema. Lips and tongue may swell.
- Urticaria
- Increased permeability of vascular system and loss of vascular tone.
- Severe hypotension leading to shock.
- Laryngospasm/bronchospasm with obstruction of airway causing dyspnea and wheezing.
- Nausea, vomiting, and diarrhea.
- Seizures, coma and death.

Treatment
- Establish patent airway and intubate if necessary for ventilation.
- Provide oxygen at 100% high flow.
- Monitor VS.
- Administer epinephrine (Epi-pen® or solution).
- Albuterol per nebulizer for bronchospasm.
- Intravenous fluids to provide bolus of fluids for hypotension.
- Diphenhydramine if shock persists.
- Methylprednisolone is no response to other drugs.

Primary and secondary multi-organ dysfunction syndrome

Multi-organ dysfunction syndrome (MODS) is progressive deterioration and failure of 2 or more organ systems with mortality rates of 45-50% with 2 organ systems involved and up to 80-100% if there are ≥3 systems failing. Trauma patients and those with severe conditions, such as shock, burns, and sepsis, are particularly vulnerable, especially in those >65. MODS may be primary or secondary:
- **Primary** MODS relates to direct injury/disorder of the organ systems, resulting in dysfunction, such as with thermal injuries, traumatic pulmonary injuries, and invasive infections.
- **Secondary** MODS relates to dysfunction of organ systems not directly involved in injury/disorder but developing as the result of a systemic inflammatory response syndrome (SIRS) as the patient's immune and inflammatory responses become dysregulated. In some patients, failure of organ systems is sequential, usually progressing from the lungs, the liver, the gastrointestinal system, and the kidneys to the heart. However, in other cases, various organ systems may fail at the same time.

Multisystem complications of burn injuries

Burn injuries begin with the skin but can affect all organs and body systems, especially with a major burn:
- **Cardiovascular**: Cardiac output may fall by 50% as capillary permeability increases with vasodilation and fluid leaks from the tissues.
- **Urinary**: Decreased blood flow causes kidneys to increase ADH, which increases oliguria. BUN and creatinine levels increase. Cell destruction may block tubules, and hematuria may result from hemolysis.

- 150 -

- **Pulmonary**: Injury may result from smoke inhalation or (rarely) aspiration of hot liquid. Pulmonary injury is a leading cause of death from burns and is classified according to degree of damage:
    - First: Singed eyebrows and nasal hairs with possible soot in airways and slight edema.
    - Second: (At 24 hours) Stridor, dyspnea, and tachypnea with edema and erythema of upper airway, including area of vocal chords and epiglottis.
    - Third: (At 72 hours) worsening symptoms if not intubated and if intubated, bronchorrhea and tachypnea with edematous, secreting tissue.
- **Neurological**: Encephalopathy may develop from lack of oxygen, decreased blood volume and sepsis. Hallucinations, alterations in consciousness, seizures and coma may result for recovery is usual.
- **Gastrointestinal**: Ileus and ulcerations of mucosa often result from poor circulation. Ileus usually clears within 48-72 hours, but if it returns it is often indicative of sepsis.
- **Endocrine/Metabolic:** The sympathetic nervous system stimulates the adrenals to release epinephrine and norepinephrine to increase cardiac output and cortisol for wound healing. The metabolic rate increases markedly. Electrolyte loss occurs with fluid loss from exposed tissue, especially phosphorus, calcium and sodium, with an increase in potassium levels. Electrolyte imbalance can be life-threatening if burns cover >20% of BSA. Glycogen depletion occurs within 12-24 hours and protein breakdown and muscle wasting occurs without sufficient intake of protein.

Management of burn injuries

Management of burn injuries must include both wound care and systemic care to avoid complications that can be life threatening. Treatment includes:
- Establishment of airway and treatment for inhalation injury as indicated:
    - Supplemental oxygen, incentive spirometry, nasotracheal suctioning.
    - Humidification.
    - Bronchoscopy as needed to evaluate bronchospasm and edema.
    - β-Agonists for bronchospasm, followed by aminophylline if ineffective.
    - Intubation and ventilation if there are indications of respiratory failure. This should be done prior to failure. Tracheostomy may be done if ventilation >14 days.
- Intravenous fluids and electrolytes, based on weight and extent of burn. Parkland formula: 4 ml/kg/wt x BSA per 24 hours.
- Enteral feedings, usually with small lumen feeding tube into the duodenum.
- NG tube for gastric decompression to prevent aspiration.
- Indwelling catheter to monitor urinary output. Urinary output should be 0.5-2 ml/kg/hr.
- Analgesia for reduction of pain and anxiety.
- Topical and systemic antibiotics.
- Wound care with removal of eschar and dressings as indicated.

Severe infections

There are a number of terms used to refer to severe infections and often used interchangeably, but they are part of a continuum:
- **Bacteremia** is the presence of bacteria in the blood but without systemic infection.
- **Septicemia** is a systemic infection caused by pathogens (usually bacteria or fungi) present in the blood.

- **Systemic inflammatory response syndrome** (SIRS), a generalized inflammatory response affecting may organ systems, may be caused by infectious or non-infectious agents, such as trauma, burns, adrenal insufficiency, pulmonary embolism, and drug overdose. If an infectious agent is identified or suspected, SIRS is an aspect of sepsis. Infective agents include a wide range of bacteria and fungi, including *Streptococcus pneumoniae* and *Staphylococcus aureus*. SIRS includes 2 of the following:
  - Elevated (>38°C) or subnormal rectal temperature (<36°C).
  - Tachypnea or $PaCO_2$ <32 mm Hg.
  - Tachycardia.
  - Leukocytosis (>12,000) or leukopenia (<4000).

Infections can progress from bacteremia, septicemia, and SIRS to the following:
- **Sepsis** is presence of infection either locally or systemically in which there is a generalized life-threatening inflammatory response (SIRS). It includes all the indications for SIRS as well as one of the following:
  - Changes in mental status.
  - Hypoxemia (<72 mm Hg) without pulmonary disease.
  - Elevation in plasma lactate.
  - Decreased urinary output <5 mL/kg/wt for ≥1 hour.
- **Severe sepsis** includes both indications of SIRS and sepsis as well as indications of increasing organ dysfunction with inadequate perfusion and/or hypotension.
- **Septic shock** is a progression from severe sepsis in which refractory hypotension occurs despite treatment. There may be indications of lactic acidosis.
- **Multi-organ dysfunction syndrome** *(MODS)* is the most common cause of sepsis-related death. Cardiac function becomes depressed, acute respiratory distress syndrome (ARDS) may develop, and renal failure may follow acute tubular necrosis or cortical necrosis. Thrombocytopenia appears in about 30% of those affected and may result in disseminated intravascular coagulation (DIC). Liver damage and bowel necrosis may occur.

Septic shock

Septic shock is caused by toxins produced by bacteria and cytokines that the body produces in response to severe infection, resulting in a complex syndrome of disorders. Symptoms are wide-ranging:
- Initial: Hyper- or hypothermia, increased temperature (above 38°C) with chills, tachycardia with increased pulse pressure, tachypnea, alterations in mental status (dullness), hypotension, hyperventilation with respiratory alkalosis ($PaCO_2$ ≤30 mm Hg), increased lactic acid, and unstable BP, and dehydration with increased urinary output.
- Cardiovascular: Myocardial depression and dysrhythmias.
- Respiratory: Adults respiratory distress syndrome (ARDS).
- Renal: acute renal failure (ARF) with decreased urinary output and increased BUN.
- Hepatic: Jaundice and liver dysfunction with an increase in transaminase, alkaline phosphatase and bilirubin.
- Hematologic: Mild or severe blood loss (from mucosal ulcerations), neutropenia or neutrophilia, decreased platelets, and DIC.
- Endocrine: Hyperglycemia, hypoglycemia (rare).
- Skin: cellulitis, erysipelas, and fascitis, acrocyanotic and necrotic peripheral lesions.
- Septic shock is most common in newborns, those >50, and those who are immunocompromised. There is no specific test to confirm a diagnosis of septic shock, so

diagnosis is based on clinical findings and tests that evaluate hematologic, infectious, and metabolic states: CBC, DIC panel, electrolytes, liver function tests, BUN, creatinine, blood glucose, ABGs, urinalysis, ECG, radiographs, blood and urine cultures.

Treatment must be aggressive and includes:
- Oxygen and endotracheal intubation as necessary.
- IV access with 2-large bore catheters and central venous line.
- Rapid fluid administration at 0.5L NS or isotonic crystalloid every 5-10 minutes as needed (to 4-6 L).
- Monitoring urinary output to optimal >30mL/hr.
- Inotropic agents (dopamine, dobutamine, norepinephrine) if no response to fluids or fluid overload.
- Empiric IV antibiotic therapy (usually with 2 broad spectrum antibiotics for both gram-positive and gram-negative bacteria) until cultures return and antibiotics may be changed.
- Hemodynamic and laboratory monitoring.
- Removing source of infection (abscess, catheter).

Toxic ingestions

Treatment for toxic ingestions is related to the type of toxin and whether or not it is identified:
- **Administration of reversal agent** if substance is known and an antidote exists. Antidotes for common toxins include:
  o Opiates: Naloxone (Narcan®).
  o Toxic alcohols: Ethanol infusion and/or dialysis.
  o Acetaminophen: N-acetylcysteine.
  o Calcium channel blockers, beta-blockers: Calcium chloride, Glucagon.
  o Tricyclic antidepressants: Sodium bicarbonate.
  o Ethylene glycol: fomepizole.
  o Iron: deferoxamine
- **GI decontamination** at one time was standard procedures (Ipecac® and gastric lavage followed by activated charcoal). It is no longer advised for routine use although selective gastric lavage may be appropriate if done within 1 hour of ingestion.
- **Activated charcoal** (1 g/kg/wt) orally or per NG tube binds to many toxins if given within one hour of ingestion. It may also be used in multiple doses (q 4-6 hrs) to enhance elimination
- **Forced diuresis** with alkalinization of urine (>7.5) may prevent absorption of drugs that are weak bases or acids.

Acetaminophen toxicity

Acetaminophen toxicity from accidental or intentional overdose has high rates of morbidity and mortality unless promptly treated. Diagnosis is by history and acetaminophen level, which should be completed within 8 hours of ingestion if possible. Toxicity occurs with dosage >140 mg/kg in one dose or >7.5g in 24 hours.

<u>Symptoms</u>
Symptoms occur in stages:
- (Initial) Minor gastrointestinal upset.
- (Days 2-3) Hepatotoxicity with RUQ pain and increased AST, ALT, and bilirubin.
- (Days 3-4) Hepatic failure with metabolic acidosis, coagulopathy, renal failure, encephalopathy, nausea, vomiting, and possible death.
- (Days 5-12) Recovery period for survivors.

<u>Treatment</u>
- GI decontamination with activated charcoal (orally or NG) <24 hours.
- Toxicity is plotted on the Rumack-Matthew nomogram with serum levels >150 requiring antidote. The antidote is most effective ≤8 hours of ingestion but decreases hepatotoxicity even >24 hours.
- Antidote: 72-hour N-acetylcysteine (NAC) protocol includes 140 mg/kg initially and 70 mg/kg every 4 hours for 17 more doses (orally or IV).
- Supportive therapy.

Caustic ingestions

Caustic ingestions of acids (pH <7) such as sulfuric, acetic, hydrochloric, and hydrofluoric found in many cleaning agents and alkalis (pH >7) such as sodium hydroxide, potassium hydroxide, sodium tripolyphosphate (in detergents) and sodium hypochlorite (bleach) can result in severe injury and death. Acids cause coagulation necrosis in the esophagus and stomach and may result in metabolic acidosis, hemolysis, and renal failure if systemically absorbed. Alkali injuries cause liquefaction necrosis, resulting in deeper ulcerations, often of the esophagus, but may involve perforation and abdominal necrosis with multi-organ damage. Diagnosis is by detailed history, airway examination (oral intubation if possible), arterial blood gas, electrolytes, CBC, hepatic and coagulation tests, radiograph, and CT for perforations.

<u>Symptoms</u>
Symptoms may vary but can include:
- Pain.
- Dyspnea.
- Oral burns.
- Dysphonia.
- Vomiting.

<u>Treatment</u>
- Supportive and symptomatic therapy.
- NO ipecac, charcoal, neutralization, or dilution.
- NG tube for acids only to aspirate residual.
- Endoscopy in first few hours to evaluate injury/perforations.
- Sodium bicarbonate for pH <7.10.
- Prednisolone (alkali injuries).

Amphetamine and cocaine toxicity

Amphetamine toxicity may be caused by IV, inhalation, or insufflation of various substances that include methamphetamine (MDA or "ecstasy"), methylphenidate (Ritalin®),

- 154 -

methylenedioxymethamphetamine (MDMA), and ephedrine and phenylpropanolamine. Cocaine may be ingested orally, IV or by insufflation while crack cocaine may be smoked. Amphetamines and cocaine are CNS stimulants that can cause multi-system abnormalities.

Symptoms may include chest pain, dysrhythmias, myocardial ischemia, MI, seizures, intracranial infarctions, hypertension, dystonia, repetitive movements, unilateral blindness, lethargy, rhabdomyolysis with acute kidney failure, perforated nasal septum (cocaine) and paranoid psychosis (amphetamines). Crack cocaine may cause pulmonary hemorrhage, asthma, pulmonary edema, barotrauma, and pneumothorax. Swallowing packs of cocaine can cause intestinal ischemia, colitis, necrosis, and perforation. Diagnosis includes clinical findings, CBC, chemistry panel, toxicology screening, ECG, and radiography.

Treatment includes:
- Gastric emptying (≤1 hour). Charcoal administration.
- IV access. Supplemental oxygen.
- Sedation for seizures: Lorazepam 2m, diazepam 5mg IV titrated in repeated doses. Agitation: Haloperidol.
- Hypertension: Nitroprusside, phentolamine 2.5-5mg IV.
- Cocaine quinidine-like effects: Sodium bicarbonate.

Gastric emptying for toxic substance ingestion

Gastric emptying for toxic substance ingestion should be done ≤60 minutes of ingestion for large life-threatening amounts of poison. The patient requires IV access, oximetry, and cardiac monitoring. Sedation (1-2 mg IV midazolam) or RSI and endotracheal intubation may be necessary. Patients should be positioned in left lateral decubitus position with head down at 20° to prevent passage of stomach contents into duodenum although intubated patients may be lavaged in the supine position. With a bite block in place, an orogastric Y-tube (36-40 Fr. for adults) should be inserted after estimating length. Placement should be confirmed with injection of 50 mL of air confirmed under auscultation and aspiration of gastric contents. Irrigation is done by gravity instillation of about 200-300 mL warmed (45° C) tap water or NS. The instillation side is clamped and drainage side opened. This is repeated until fluid returns clear. A slurry of charcoal is then instilled, and tube clamped and removed when procedures completed.

Carbon monoxide poisoning

Carbon monoxide (CO) poisoning occurs with inhalation of fossil fuel exhausts from engines, emission of gas or coal heaters, indoor use of charcoal, and smoke and fumes. The CO binds with hemoglobin, preventing oxygen carriage and impairing oxygen delivery to tissue. Diagnosis includes history, on-site oximetry reports, neurological examination, and CO neuropsychological screening battery (CONSB) done with patient breathing room air, CBC, electrolytes, ABGs, ECG, chest radiograph (for dyspnea).

Symptoms
- Cardiac: chest pain, palpitations, decreased capillary refill, hypotension, cardiac arrest.
- CNS: malaise, nausea, vomiting, lethargy, stroke, coma, seizure.
- Secondary injuries: rhabdomyolysis with renal failure
- Non-cardiogenic pulmonary edema
- Multiple organs failure (MOF).

- DIC.
- Encephalopathy.

Treatment
- Immediate support of airway, breathing, and circulation.
- Non-barometric oxygen (100%) by non-breathing mask with reservoir or ETT if necessary.
- Mild: Continue oxygen for 4 hours with reassessment.
- Severe: hyperbaric oxygen therapy (usually 3 treatments) to improve oxygen delivery.

Cyanide poisoning

Cyanide poisoning, from hydrogen cyanide (HCN) or cyanide salts, can result from inhalation of burning plastics, intentional or accidental ingestion or dermal exposure, occupation exposure, ingestion of some plant products, manufacture of PCP, and sodium nitroprusside infusions. Inhalation of HCN causes immediate symptoms; and ingestion of cyanide salts, within minutes. Diagnosis is by history, clinical examination, and normal PaO_2 and metabolic acidosis.

Symptoms
Symptoms increase in severity and alter with the amount of exposure:
- **Cardiovascular**: Tachycardia, hypertension, bradycardia, hypotension, and cardiac arrest.
- **Skin**: May appear pink or cherry-colored because of oxygen remaining in the blood.
- **CNS**: Headaches, lethargy, seizures, coma.
- **Respiratory**: Dyspnea, tachypnea, and respiratory arrest.

Treatment
- Supportive care as indicated.
- Removal of contaminated clothes.
- Gastric decontamination.
- Copious irrigation for topical exposure.
- Antidotes:
  - Amyl nitrate ampule cracked and inhaled 30 seconds.
  - Sodium nitrite (3%) 10 mL IV.
  - Sodium thiosulfate (25%) 50 mL IV.

Salicylate toxicity

Salicylate toxicity may be acute or chronic and is caused by ingestion of OTC drugs containing salicylates, such as ASA, Pepto-Bismol®, and products used in hot inhalers. Diagnosis is by ferric chloride or Ames Phenistix tests. Symptoms vary according to age and amount of ingestion. Co-ingestion of sedatives may alter symptoms.

Symptoms
- <150 mg/kg: Nausea and vomiting.
- 150-300 mg/kg: Vomiting, hyperpnea, diaphoresis, tinnitus, alterations in acid-base balance.
- >300 mg/kg (usually intentional overdose): Nausea, vomiting, diaphoresis, tinnitus, hyperventilation, respiratory alkalosis and metabolic acidosis. Chronic toxicity results in hyperventilation, tremor, papilledema, alterations in mental status, pulmonary edema, seizures, and coma.

- 156 -

<u>Treatment</u>
- Gastric decontamination with lavage (≤1 hour) and charcoal.
- Volume replacement (D5W).
- Sodium bicarbonate 1-2mEq/kg.
- Monitoring of salicylate concentration, acid-base, electrolytes every hour.
- Whole-bowel irrigation (sustained release tablets).

Benzodiazepine toxicity

Benzodiazepine toxicity may result from accidental or intentional overdose with such drugs as Xanax®, Librium®, Valium®, Ativan®, Serax®, Versed®, and Restoril®. Mortality is usually the result of co-ingestion of other drugs. Diagnosis is based on history and clinical exam, as benzodiazepine level does not correlate well with toxicity.

<u>Symptoms</u>
- Non-specific neurological changes: lethargy, dizziness, alterations in consciousness, ataxia.
- Respiratory depression and hypotension are rare complications.
- Coma and severe central nervous depression are usually caused by co-ingestions.

<u>Treatment</u>
- Gastric emptying (<1 hour).
- Charcoal.
- Concentrated dextrose, thiamine and naloxone if co-ingestions suspected, especially with altered mental status.
- Monitoring for CNS/respiratory depression.
- Supportive care.
- Flumazenil (antagonist) 0.2mg each minute to total 3mg may be used in some cases but not routinely advised because of complications related to benzodiazepine dependency or co-ingestion of cyclic antidepressants. Flumazenil is contraindicated in the presence of increased intracranial pressure.

Ethanol overdose

Ethanol overdose affects the central nervous system as well as other organs in the body. Ethanol is absorbed through the mucosa of the mouth, stomach, and intestines, with concentrations peaking about 30-60 minutes after ingestion. If people are easily aroused, they can usually safely sleep off the effects of ingesting too much alcohol, but if the person is semi-conscious or unconscious, emergency medical treatment should be initiated.

<u>Symptoms</u>
- Altered mental status with slurred speech and stupor.
- Nausea and vomiting.
- Hypotension.
- Bradycardia with arrhythmias
- Respiratory depression and hypoxia.
- Cold, clammy skin or flushed skin (from vasodilation).
- Acute pancreatitis with abdominal pain.

- Lack of consciousness
- Circulatory collapse leading to death.

Treatment
- Careful monitoring of arterial blood gases and oxygen saturation.
- Ensure patent airway with intubation and ventilation if necessary.
- Intravenous fluids.
- Dextrose to correct hypoglycemia if indicated.
- Maintain body temperature (warming blanket).
- Dialysis may be necessary in severe cases.

Pain assessment

Pain is subjective and may be influenced by the individual's pain threshold (the smallest stimulus that produces the sensation of pain) and pain tolerance (the maximum degree of pain that a person can tolerate). The most common current pain assessment tool for adults and pre-teens/adolescents is the 1-10 scale:
- = no pain.
- 1-2 = mild pain.
- 3-5 = moderate pain.
- 6-7 = severe pain.
- 8-9 = very severe pain.
- 10 = excruciating pain.

However, there is more to pain assessment than a number on a scale. Assessment includes information about onset, duration, and intensity. Identifying what triggers pain and what relieves it can be very useful when developing a plan for pain management. Patients may show very different behavior when they are in pain: Some may cry and moan with minor pain, and others may exhibit little difference in behavior when truly suffering. Thus, judging pain by behavior can lead to the wrong conclusions.

Patients with cognitive impairment or inability to verbalize pain may not be able to indicate the degree of pain, even by using a face scale with pictures of smiling to crying faces. The Pain Assessment in Advanced Dementia (PAINAD) scale may be helpful, especially for those with Alzheimer's disease. Careful observation of non-verbal behavior can indicate that the patient is in pain:
- **Respirations**: Patients often have more rapid and labored breathing as pain increases with short periods of hyperventilation or Cheyne-Stokes respirations.
- **Vocalization**: Patients may remain negative in speech or speak quietly and reluctantly. They may moan or groan. As pain increases, they may call out, moan or groan loudly, or cry.
- **Facial expression:** Patients may appear sad or frightened, may frown or grimace, especially on activities that increase pain.
- **Body language:** Patients may be tense, fidgeting, pacing and as pain increases may become rigid, clench fists, or lie in fetal position. They may become increasingly combative.
- **Consolability**: Patients are less distractible or consolable with increased pain.

Adverse systemic effect of pain

Acute pain causes adverse systemic affects that can negatively affect many body systems.

- **Cardiovascular**: Tachycardia and increased BP is a common response to pain, causing increased cardiac output and systemic vascular resistance. In those with pre-existing cardiovascular disease, such as compromised ventricular function, cardiac output may decrease. The increased myocardial need for oxygen may cause or worsen myocardial ischemia.
- **Respiratory**: Increased need for oxygen causes an increase in minute ventilation at the same time that and splinting because of pain may compromise pulmonary function. If the chest wall movement is constrained, tidal volume falls, impairing the ability to cough and clear secretions. Bed rest further compromises ventilation.
- **Gastrointestinal**: Sphincter tone increases and motility decreases, sometimes resulting in ileus. There may be increased secretion of gastric acids, which irritate the gastric lining and can cause ulcerations. Nausea, vomiting, and constipation may occur. Reflux may result in aspiration pneumonia. Abdominal distention may occur.
- **Urinary**: Increased sphincter tone and decreased motility result in urinary retention.
- **Endocrine**: Hormone levels are affected by pain. Catabolic hormones, such as catecholamine, cortisol and glucagon increase and anabolic hormones, such as insulin and testosterone decrease. Lipolysis increases along with carbohydrate intolerance. Sodium retention can occur because of increased ADH, aldosterone, angiotensin, and cortisol. This in turn causes fluid retention and a shift to extracellular space.
- **Hematologic**: There may be reduced fibrinolysis, increased adhesiveness of platelets, and increased coagulation.
- **Immune**: Leukocytosis and lymphopenia may occur, increasing risk of infection.
- **Emotional**: Patients may become depressed, anxious, angry, depressed appetite, and sleep-deprived. This type of response is most common in those with chronic pain, who usually don't have typical systemic responses of those with acute pain.

Pain management

Patient-controlled analgesia (PCA) allows the patient to control administration of pain medication by pressing a button on an intravenous delivery system with a computerized pump. The device is filled with opioid (as prescribed) and must be programmed correctly and checked regularly to ensure that it is functioning properly and that controls are set. Current recommendations are that most patients that have an open (and some laparoscopic) surgical procedure use a PCA pump for pain control post operatively until they are tolerating fluids well orally. They may then be switched to oral pain medications.

The most-commonly administered medications include morphine, meperidine, fentanyl, and sufentanil. Most devices can be set to deliver continuous infusion of opioid as well as patient-controlled bolus. Each element must be set:

- **Bolus**: Determines the amount of medication received when the patient delivers a dose.
- **Lockout interval:** Time required between administrations of boluses.
- **Continuous infusion:** Rate at which opioid is delivered per hour for continuous analgesia.
- **Limit** (usually set at 4 hours): Total amount of opioid that can be delivered in the preset time limit.

With Authorized Agent Controlled Analgesia (AACA), people who are trained and authorized (such as nurse, family member, and caregiver) may administer the medication as well as the patient.

Therapeutic hypothermia

Therapeutic hypothermia is used to reduce ischemic tissue damage associated with cardiac arrest, ischemic stroke, traumatic brain/spinal cord injury, neurogenic fever, and related coma (3 on Glasgow scale). Hypothermia has a neuroprotective effect by making cell membranes less permeable. Hypothermia should be initiated immediately after an ischemic event if possible but some benefit remains up to 6 hours. Desflurane or meperidine is given to reduce the shivering response. Hypothermia to 33°C may be induced by cooled saline through a femoral catheter, reducing temperature 1.5 to 2° C per hour, with by an electronic control unit. Hypothermic water blankets covering ≥80% of body the body surface can also lower body temperature. In some cases, both a femoral cooling catheter and water blanket are used for rapid reduction of temperature. Rectal probes measure core temperature. Hypothermia increases risk of bleeding (decreased clotting time), infection (due to impairing leukocyte function and introducing catheters), arrhythmias, hyperglycemia, and DVT. Rewarming is done slowly at 0.5 to 1° C/hr. through warmed intravenous fluids, warm humidified air, and/or warming blanket. The warming process is a critical time as it causes potassium to be moved from extracellular to intracellular spaces and the patient's electrolyte levels must be monitored regularly.

Delayed emergence

Delayed emergence (failure to emerge for 30-60 minutes after anesthesia ends) is more common in the elderly because of slowed metabolism of anesthetic agents but may have a variety of causes, such as drug overdose during surgery, overdose related to preinduction use of drugs or alcohol that potentiates intraoperative drugs. In this case, naloxone or flumazenil may be indicated if opioids or benzodiazepines are implicated. Physostigmine may also be used to reverse effects of some anesthetic agents. Hypothermia may also cause delay in emergence, especially core temperatures <33°C, and may require forced-air warming blankets to increase the temperature. Other metabolic conditions, such as hypoglycemia or hyperglycemia may also affect emergence. Patients suffering from delayed emergence must be evaluated for perioperative stroke, especially after neurological, cardiovascular, or cerebrovascular surgery. Metabolic disturbance may also delay emergence.

Postoperative nausea and vomiting

Post-operative nausea and vomiting (PONV) varies with the type of anesthetic agent used. It occurs in about 20-30% of post-anesthesia patients and may be delayed up to 24 hours. Inhalational agents have a higher incidence of PONV than intravenous, and the incidence is lower with epidural or subarachnoid administration although it may indicate the onset of hypotension. PONV correlates with the duration of surgery, with longer surgeries causing increased PONV. If high doses of narcotics, propofol, or nitrous oxide are used, PONV is often a problem. PONV is most common in young women and also relates to menstruation. It is also increased in those with a history of smoking or motion sickness. Some surgical procedures correlate with PONV: strabismus repair, ear surgery, laparoscopy, tonsillectomy, orchiopexy, and gynecological procedures to retrieve ova. PONV may be associated with post-operative pain, so managing pain is an important factor in preventing PONV.

Post-anesthetic respiratory complications

Respiratory complications are most common in the postanesthesia period, so monitoring of oxygen levels is critical to preventing hypoxemia:

- **Airway obstruction** may be partial or total. Partial obstruction is indicated by sonorous or wheezing respirations, and total by absence of breath sounds. Treatment includes supplemental oxygen, airway insertion, repositioning (jaw thrust), or succinylcholine and positive-pressure ventilation for laryngospasm. If edema of the glottis is causing obstruction, IV corticosteroids may be used.
- **Hypoventilation** ($PaCO_2$ >45 mm Hg) is often mild but may cause respiratory acidosis. It is usually related to depression caused by anesthetic agents. A number of factors may slow emergence (hypothermia, overdose, metabolism) and cause hypoventilation. It may also be related to splinting because of pain, requiring additional pain management.
- **Hypoxemia** (mild is PaO_2 500-60 mm Hg) is usually related to hypoventilation and/or increased right to left shunting and is usually treated with supplementary oxygen (30-60%) with or without positive airway pressure.

Post-anesthetic cardiovascular complications

Cardiovascular complications are sometimes related to respiratory complications, which may need to be addressed as well. Complications include:

- **Hypotension** is most often mild and requires no specific treatment. It is most commonly caused by hypovolemia and is significant if BP falls 20-30% below normal baseline. A bolus (100-250 mL IV colloid) is used to confirm hypovolemia. If severe, then medications, such as epinephrine, may be indicated. Hypotension may occur with pneumothorax so careful respiratory assessment must be done.
- **Hypertension** usually occurs ≤ 30 minutes after surgery and is common in those with history of hypertension. It may be secondary to hypoxemia or metabolic acidosis. Mild increases usually don't require treatment but medications may be used for moderate (β-adrenergic blockers) or severe (nitroprusside).
- **Arrhythmias** usually relate to respiratory complications or effects of anesthetic agents. Bradycardia may relate to cholinesterase inhibitors, opioids, or propranolol. Tachycardia may relate to anticholinergics, β-agonists, and vagolytic drugs. Hypokalemia and hypomagnesemia may cause premature atrial and ventricular beats.

Behavioral/Psychosocial

Injuries consistent with domestic violence

Characteristic injuries
- Ruptured eardrum.
- Rectal/genital injury—burns, bites, trauma.
- Scrapes and bruises about the neck, face, head, trunk, arms.
- Cuts, bruises, and fractures of the face.

Patterns of injuries
- Bathing suit pattern—injuries on parts of body that are usually covered with clothing as the perpetrator abuses but hides evidence of abuse.
- Head and neck injuries (50%).

Abusive injuries (rarely attributable to accidents)
- Bites, bruises, rope and cigarette burns, welts in the outline of weapons (belt marks).
- Bilateral injuries of arms/legs.

Defensive injuries
- Back of the body injury from being attacked while crouched on the floor face down.
- Soles of the feet from kicking at perpetrator.
- Ulnar aspect of hand or palm from blocking blows.

Elder abuse

Age and disability increase risks of elder abuse with people >80 more than twice as likely to suffer abuse than younger adults. Patients with dementia, such as Alzheimer's disease, are at risk of abuse in both the home environment, where they are often cared for by adult children, and in institutions. Caregivers often lose patience and become frustrated, especially if the patient's behavior is belligerent, combative, or disruptive. About 5-14% of those with dementia are victims of elder abuse compared to 1-3% of the general population. This type of abuse can be very difficult to diagnose, as the patient is usually unable to corroborate abuse. In fact, even older adults who are not cognitively impaired may be afraid to report abuse because they depend on the abusers to care for them. Older and/or disabled adults who are dependent on others for assistance with ADLs, such as dressing, bathing, and food preparation are also particularly at risk for outright abuse and neglect. Abusers often suffer from depression and or substance abuse and may be financially dependent on the victim. Indications of abuse include unexplained or multiple bruises consistent with abuse and fearful demeanor.

Sexual abuse

Rape and sexual abuse victims (both male and female) should be treated sensitively and questioned privately.

Examination
Should include:
- Assault history that includes what happened, when, where, and by whom.
- Medical history to determine if there is a risk of pregnancy and when and if the last consensual sex occurred that might interfere with laboratory findings.
- Physical examination should include examination of the genitals, rectum, and mouth. The body should be examined for bruising or other injuries. Toluidine dye should be applied to the perineum before insertion of a speculum into the vagina to detect small vulvar lacerations.

Treatment
- Pelvic examination.
- Rape kit (within 72 hours of assault).
- STD screening.
- Prophylactic antibiotics.
- HIV testing and follow up.
- Suturing/repair of open wounds.
- Emergency contraception.
- Victims may be severely traumatized and require psychological and emotional support. All victims of sexual abuse should be referred for psychological counseling. Cognitive behavioral therapy has proven effective in helping victims cope more effectively.

Violence and aggression

Violence and aggression is sometimes seen in the critical care setting. The nurse must be aware of signs of impending violence or aggression in order to intervene:
- **Violence** is a physical act perpetrated against an inanimate object, animal, or other person with the intent to cause harm. Violence often results from anger, frustration, or fear and occurs because the perpetrators believe that they are threatened or that their opinion is right and the victim is wrong. Violence may occur suddenly without warning or following aggressive behavior. Violence can result in death or severe injury if the individual attacks a fellow individual or staff member.
- **Aggression** is the communication of a threat or intended act of violence and will often occur before an act of violence. This communication can occur verbally or nonverbally. Gestures, shouting, speaking increasingly loudly, invasion of personal space, or prolonged eye contact are examples of aggression requiring the individual be redirected or removed from the situation.

Use of restraints

Restraints are used to restrict movement, activity, and access. There are two primary types of restraints used with individuals: behavioral and clinical. Behavioral restraints are more commonly used in the psychiatric unit or when individuals are at risk of hurting themselves or others. More commonly, clinical restraints are used to ensure that the individual does not interfere with safe care. The federal government and the Joint Commission have issued strict guidelines for temporary restraints or those not part of standard care (such as post-surgical restraint):

- There must be a written policy.
- An assessment must be completed.
- An alternative method should be tried before applying a restraint.
- An order must be written.
- The least restrictive effective restraint should be used.
- A nurse must remove the restraint, assess, and document findings at least every 2 hours.
- Physical restraints may involve the use of a person physically restraining an individual or the use of a mechanical device to restrict movement.

Chemical restraints

Chemical restraints involve the use of medications, such as lorazepam or haloperidol, to manage an individual's behavior problems. This type of restraint is indicated when individuals are extremely agitated or violent in order to prevent injury to themselves or others. Chemical restraints inhibit individuals' physical movements and make their behavior more manageable. Medication used on an ongoing basis as part of treatment is not legally considered a chemical restraint, which is used only in emergent situations, even though the medications may be the same. There is little consensus about the use of chemical restraints although benzodiazepines and/or antipsychotics are frequently used to control severe agitation. Oral medications should be tried first before injections, as oral medication is less coercive. The trend in psychiatric medicine is to target medications to treat particular symptoms, such as severe agitation, rather than simply to chemically restrain the individual.

Delirium

Delirium is an acute sudden change in consciousness, characterized by reduced ability to focus or sustain attention, language and memory disturbance, disorientation, confusion, audiovisual hallucinations, sleep disturbance, and psychomotor activity disorder. Delirium differs from disorders with similar symptoms in that delirium is fluctuating. Delirium occurs in 10-40% of hospitalized older adults and about 80% of patients who are terminally ill. Delirium may result from drugs, such as anticholinergics, and numerous conditions, including infection, hypoxia, trauma, dementia, depression, vision and hearing loss, surgery, alcoholism, untreated pain, fluid/electrolyte imbalance, and malnutrition. Delirium increases risks of morbidity and death, especially if untreated. Diagnosis includes interview to identify triggers and history and chart review. Asking patient to count backward from 20 to 1 and spell first name backward can identify attention deficit. Treatment includes providing sitter to ensure safety and decreasing dosage of hypnotics and psychotropics. Medications to reduce symptoms include trazodone, lorazepam, and haloperidol.

The **Confusion Assessment Method** is used to assess the development of delirium and is intended for those without psychiatric training. The tool covers 9 factors. Some factors have a range of possibilities and others are rated only as to whether the characteristic is present, not present, uncertain, or not applicable. The tool provides room to describe abnormal behavior. Factors indicative of delirium include:

- **Onset**: Acute change in mental status.
- **Attention**: Inattentive, stable or fluctuating.
- **Thinking**: Disorganized, rambling conversation, switching topics, illogical,

- **Level of consciousness:** Altered, ranging from alert to coma.
- **Orientation**: Disoriented (person, place, time)
- **Memory**: Impaired.
- **Perceptual disturbances:** Hallucinations, illusions.
- **Psychomotor abnormalities:** Agitation (tapping, picking, moving) or retardation (staring, not moving).
- **Sleep-wake cycle:** Awake at night and sleepy in the daytime.

Alzheimer's disease

There are a number of methods for staging Alzheimer's disease. Staging is done by a combination of physical exam, history (often provided by family or caregivers), and mental assessment, as there is no definitive test for Alzheimer's.

The 7-stage classification system (developed by Gary Reisberg, MD) is used by the Alzheimer's Association:

Stage 1: Pre-clinical with no evident impairment although slight changes may be occurring within the brain.

Stage 2: Very mild cognitive decline with some misplacing of items and forgetting things or words, but impairment is not usually noticeable to others or found on medical examination.

Stage 3: Mild, early-stage cognitive decline with short-term memory loss, problems with reading retention, remembering names, handling money, planning, and organizing. May misplace items of value.

Stage 4: Moderate cognitive decline with decreased knowledge of current affairs or family history, difficulty doing complex tasks, and social withdrawal. This stage is more easily recognized on exam and may persist for 2-10 years, during which the patients may be able to manage most activities of daily living and hygiene.

Stage 5: Moderately-severe cognitive decline as the cerebral cortex and hippocampus shrink and the ventricles enlarge. Patients are obviously confused and disoriented to date, time, and place. Patients may have difficulty using/understanding speech and managing activities of daily living. They may forget address and telephone number. They may dress inappropriately, forget to eat and lose weight, or eat a poor diet. They may be unable to do simple math, such as counting backward by 2s.

Stage 6: Moderately severe cognitive decline as the brain continues to shrink and neurons die. Patients are profoundly confused and unable to care for themselves and may undergo profound personality changes. They may confuse fiction and reality. They may fail to recognize family members, experience difficulty toileting, and begin to pace obsessively or wander away. Sundowner's syndrome, in which the person has disruption of waking/sleeping cycles and tends to get restless and wander about at night, is common. Patients may develop obsessive behaviors, such as tearing items, pulling at the hair, or wringing hands. This stage (with stage 7) may be prolonged, lasting 1-5 years.

Stage 7: Very severe cognitive decline during which most patients are wheelchair bound or bedbound and lose most ability to speak beyond a few words. They are incontinent of urine and feces; may be unable to sit unsupported or hold head up; choke easily and have increased weakness and muscle rigidity.

Alzheimer's disease drugs

Treatment for Alzheimer's disease is aimed at slowing the progression of the disease and ensuring patient safety. Two types of drugs are FDA approved, but many clinical trials are taking place. In some cases 2 drugs (such as Aricept® and Namenda®) may be given. Patients must take medication daily and be monitored care-fully as some drugs may worsen symptoms in some patients, so different drugs may need to be tried.

Cholin-esterase inhibitors (Prevents breakdown of acetylcholine, needed for learning and memory)
Type of drug and indication
- Donepezil (Aricept®): All stages of Alzheimer's.
- Rivastigmine (Exelon®): Mild to moderate disease.
- Galantamine (Razadyne): Mild to moderate disease.
  - *Adverse effects*
    - Nausea, vomiting, loss of appetite, and frequent bowel movements
- Tacrine (Cognex®): Mild to moderate disease
  - *Adverse effects*
    - Nausea, vomiting, and possible damage to the liver

Memantine (Targets glutamate, involved in learning and memory)
Type of drug and indication
- Namenda®: Moderate to severe
  - *Adverse effects*
    - Headache, confusion, dizziness, and constipation

Non-Alzheimer's dementias

Non-Alzheimer's dementia includes:
- **Creutzfeld-Jakob disease** - This causes rapidly progressive dementia with impaired memory, behavioral changes, and incoordination.
- **Dementia with Lewy Bodies** - Cognitive and physical decline is similar to Alzheimer's, but symptoms may fluctuate frequently. This form of dementia may include visual hallucinations, muscle rigidity, and tremors.
- **Fronto-temporal dementia** - This may cause marked changes in personality and behavior and is characterized by difficulty using and understanding language.
- **Mixed dementia** - Dementia mirrors Alzheimer's and another type because of two different causes of dementia.
- **Normal pressure hydrocephalus** - This is characterized by ataxia, memory loss, and urinary incontinence.
- **Parkinson's dementia** - This form of dementia may involve impaired decision making, and difficulty concentrating, learning new material, understanding complex language, and sequencing. Inflexibility. Short or long-term memory loss may occur.
- **Vascular dementia** - Memory loss may be less pronounced than that common to Alzheimer's, but symptoms are similar.

Cognitive assessment

Individuals with evidence of dementia or short-term memory loss, often associated with Alzheimer's disease, should have cognition assessed. The Mini-mental state exam (MMSE) or the Mini-cog test is commonly used. Both require the individual to carry out specified tasks.

MMSE:
- Remembering and later repeating the names of 3 common objects.
- Counting backward from 100 by 7s or spelling "world" backward.
- Naming items as the examiner points to them.
- Providing the location of the examiner's office, including city, state, and street address.
- Repeating common phrases.
- Copying a picture of interlocking shapes.
- Following simple 3-part instructions, such a picking up a piece of paper, folding it in half, and placing it on the floor.
- A score of ≥24/30 is considered a normal functioning level.

Mini-cog:
- Remembering and later repeating the names of 3 common objects.
- Drawing the face of a clock with all 12 numbers and the hands indicating the time specified by the examiner.

Developmental delays

Intellectual disability is usually diagnosed <18. Individuals may have difficulty adapting to changing environments, need guidance in decision-making, and have self-care or communication deficits. Behaviors range from shy and passive to hyperactive or aggressive. Those with associated physical characteristics (Down syndrome) or problems are often diagnosed early. Intellectual disability may be inherited (Tay-Sachs), toxin-related (maternal alcohol consumption), perinatal (hypoxia), environmental (lack of stimulation/neglect), or acquired (encephalitis, brain injury). Diagnosis involves performance results from standardized tests along with behavior analysis. Intellectual disability classifications are based on IQ:

55 to 69 – mild (85%): Educable to about 6th grade level. May not be diagnosed until adolescence. Usually able to learn skills and be self-supporting but may need assistance and supervision.

40 to 54 – moderate (10%): Trainable and may be able to work and live in sheltered environments or with supervision.

25 to 39 – severe (3-4%): Language usually delayed and can learn only basic academic skills and perform simple tasks.

≤25 profound (1-2%): Usually associated with neurological disorder with sensorimotor dysfunction. Require constant care and supervision.

Autism spectrum disorders (ASD), pervasive developmental disorders (PDD), present with a wide range of symptoms. These patients are often isolated with an inability to socialize. Their communication abilities are limited. Autism is characterized by delay in social interactions with others, social use of language, or exercise of imagination. Symptoms range from mild (Asperger's) to severe. Diagnostic criteria include at least 6 of the following:

- **Impairment of social interactions** (in at least 2 areas): Inability to use/understand non-verbal communication, inability to establish peer relationships, lack of socialization skills, and inability to express emotions.
- **Impairment of communication** (In at least one area): Delay or lack of spoken language without attempt to compensate, such as through gestures, inability to carry out a conversation with others, repetitive use of language (echolalia), and inability to carry out make-believe play or imitation appropriate to developmental level.
- **Restrictive repetitive or stereotyped behavior** (in at least one area): Preoccupation with some behavior patterns (head banging, rituals), inflexibility, and/or preoccupation with objects.

Failure to thrive

Failure to thrive is used in older adults as a descriptive term for those who show general decline, with evidence of malaise and loss of appetite and weight. Failure to thrive is often associated with cognitive impairment, depression, decreased motor activity/function, and malnutrition. Failure to thrive may result from chronic illness, medications, or socioeconomic factors, such as homelessness, poverty, and/or isolation. In some cases, especially with cognitive or physical impairment, failure to thrive may stem from neglect by caregivers. A complete physical assessment and laboratory studies and assessment of nutrition can help to identify underlying medical causes. Medications that may contribute to failure to thrive include anticonvulsants, antidepressants, opioids, SSRIs, neuroleptics, diuretics, β-blockers, anticholinergics, α-antagonists, and benzodiazepines. Functional assessment should review the patient's ability to carry out activities of daily living and a cognitive assessment should assess the patient's ability to reason. The geriatric depression scale helps to assess the degree of depression, which is often a contributing factor.

Functional assessment

Part of nutritional/functional assessment includes functional impairment and dentition. Dentition relates directly to the ability to chew food and eat, so ill-fitting dentures, caries, or edentulous condition may require intervention or adjustment of diet. Functional impairment may affect the ability to prepare and receive adequate fluids and nutrition. **Functional assessment** includes:

- **Activities of daily living** (ADL): This is the ability to care for oneself, including dressing, bathing, and preparing food. Inability to carry out ADL may relate to physical impairment (paralysis, paresis, frailty), or cognitive impairment (dementia, confusion).
- **Instrumental activities of daily living** (IADL): This includes managing affairs (including finances), arranging transportation, using prosthetic devices, shopping, telephoning. Inability to carry out IADL may relate to cognitive impairment, poverty, or inaccessibility and can prevent people from shopping for or ordering food.

Each individual is different, so once an assessment is completed, then an individualized plan for assisting the older adult can be developed.

Geriatric Depression Scale

The Geriatric Depression Scale (GDS) is a self-assessment tool to identify older adults with depression. The test can be used with those with normal cognition and those with mild to moderate impairment. The test poses 15 questions to which patients answer "yes" or "no." A score of >5 "yes" answers is indicative of depression:

1. Are you basically satisfied with your life?
2. Have you dropped many of your activities and interests?
3. Do you feel your life is empty?
4. Do you often get bored?
5. Are you in good spirits most of the time?
6. Are you afraid that something bad is going to happen to you?
7. Do you feel happy most of the time?
8. Do you often feel helpless?
9. Do you prefer to stay at home rather than going out and doing new things?
10. Do you feel you have more problems with memory than most?
11. Do you think it is wonderful to be alive now?
12. Do you feel pretty worthless the way you are now?
13. Do you feel full of energy?
14. Do you feel that your situation is hopeless?
15. Do you think that most people are better off than you are?

Bipolar disorders

Bipolar disorder is a mood disorder characterized by mania, depression, or both. Subtypes include:

- **Bipolar I:** Characterized by at least one manic episode, sometime following an episode of depression. This form of bipolar usually includes cycling between mania and depression with episodes of psychosis that include paranoia and hallucinations.
- **Bipolar II:** Characterized by at least one episode of depression and at least one episode of hypomania (shorter lasting and less severe than mania) with the depressive periods of longer duration than hypomanic periods.
- **Cyclothymia (Bipolar III):** Characterized by milder mood swings.
- **Bipolar NOS:** Mood disorder without clear pattern.

Some people with bipolar disorder may experience rapid cycling between depression and mania, often more than 4 times in a year with mood changes occurring rapidly, such as within a few hours. Additionally, some people may experience a mixed type of bipolar disorder in which depression and mania both occur at the same time.

Bipolar disorder is characterized by manic episodes alternating with depressive episodes that occur in varying patterns interspersed with periods of normal mood (euthymia). A **manic episode** is a distinct period characterized by extremely elevated mood, energy, and unusual thought patterns, causing impairment in occupational functioning and social activities for at least one week. Criteria include presence of at least three of the following during the same period:

- Unrealistic, grandiose beliefs about one's abilities or powers.
- Rapid and pressured speech.
- Racing thoughts, jumping quickly from one idea to the next.
- Looseness of thought patterns.
- Easily distracted and unable to concentrate.
- Feeling unusually "high" and optimistic.
- Increased interest in goal-directed activity.
- Acting recklessly without thinking about the consequences:
  o Questionable business transactions.

- o Wasteful expenditures of money.
  - o Unsafe sexual activity.
  - o Unusual social interactions.
  - o Highly vocal arguments uncharacteristic of previous behaviors.
- Decreased need for sleep, but feeling extremely energetic.
- Delusions and hallucinations (in severe cases).

The symptoms of the depressive phase of bipolar disorder are the opposite of those symptoms that occur during the manic phase; additionally, suicide is a constant concern for those suffering through the depressive phase. Depressive episodes include:
- Feelings of hopelessness or helplessness.
- Putting affairs in order as if leaving somewhere.
- Acting recklessly as if not caring about one's life.
- Suicidal ideation: Seeking out weapons or pills that could be used to commit suicide.
- Loss of interest in enjoyable pastimes.
- Physical and mental sluggishness.
- Appetite or weight changes.
- Sleeping too much.
- Concentration and memory problems.
- Feelings of self-loathing, shame, or guilt.
- Ruminating about death, self-harm, or suicide.

Lithium

Lithium, used for bipolar disorder, has a very narrow therapeutic window, and toxicity is a medical emergency that can lead to death. Lithium is cleared from the body by the kidneys and can negatively affect thyroid function. An initial assessment should include an evaluation of kidney function. Tests include a urinalysis (UA), BUN and creatinine levels, an electrolyte panel, 24-hour urine for creatinine clearance, screening for diabetes, hypertension and any history of diuretic medications or over use of analgesics. NSAIDs, SSRIs, phenothiazines, and diuretics may cause drug interactions. Thyroid function must also be evaluated. A TSH, T3, T4 and free thyroxine index should be drawn. About 1 individual in 25 develops goiter from lithium-induced hypothyroidism. A complete physical exam along with a complete family and individual history should be obtained. Other tests should include a 12-lead ECG, fasting blood glucose, and CBC. A complete initial assessment, ongoing assessments, frequent evaluations of lithium levels and individual education are all an essential part of the treatment plan.

Plasma levels of lithium must be frequently monitored for lithium toxicity, which can lead to death. The normal therapeutic range is 0.6 and 1.4 mEq/L for adults. Plasma levels will usually decrease to an acceptable level within 48 hours after discontinuation of the medication; however, in severe cases involving acute renal failure, dialysis may be necessary. An individual must be able to tell the difference between side effects and symptoms of toxicity. Side effects include hand tremors, twitching, nausea, diarrhea, seizures, confusion, and increase in urinary output. Symptoms of mild toxicity associated with blood levels between 1.5 – 2.5 mEq/L can include severe vomiting and diarrhea, increased muscle tremors and twitching, lethargy, body aches, ataxia, ringing in the ears, blurry vision, vertigo or hyperactive deep tendon reflexes. More severe symptoms associated with blood levels greater than 2.5 mEq/L can include elevated temperature, low urine output, hypotension, ECG abnormalities, decreased level of consciousness, seizures, coma or death.

Major depressive episode

A major depressive episode is a depressed mood, profound and constant sense of hopelessness and despair, or loss of interest in all or almost all activities for a period of at least two weeks. Family history of depression is a major risk factor. Developmental hormone changes at puberty or hormone disruption from disease can also contribute to depression. Depression is associated with neurotransmitter dysregulation, especially serotonin and norepinephrine. Major depression can be mild, moderate, or severe, and is characterized by a combination of symptoms that interfere with the ability to work, study, sleep, eat and enjoy once pleasurable activities. Criteria include at least five of the following (including the first two):
- Depressed mood most of the day.
- Diminished interest in most or all activities previously found enjoyable.
- Significant weight gain or loss without dieting.
- Insomnia or hypersomnia.
- Persistent pessimism.
- Constant fatigue.
- Feelings of worthlessness.
- Reduced ability to focus on tasks.
- Recurring thoughts of death or suicide.

Selective serotonin reuptake inhibitors

Selective serotonin reuptake inhibitors (SSRIs) are antidepressant medications that block reuptake of serotonin (neurotransmitter) in the brain, increasing the extracellular level of the neurotransmitter and improving transmission. Neurotransmitters allow neurons to communicate with "messages" passed from a presynaptic cell (sender) in one neuron to a post-synaptic receptor (receiver) in the other. The exact means by which SSRIs relieve depression is not clear. All SSRIs have similar action but may have different chemical properties that cause various side effects, so some people tolerate one better than others. Side effects include nausea, weight gain, sexual dysfunction, excitation and agitation, and insomnia, drowsiness, increased perspiration, headache, and diarrhea. In rare cases, serotonin syndrome may occur from high levels of serotonin from overdose or combination with MAO inhibitors, so SSRIs must not be taken within 2 weeks of each other. Symptoms include severe anxiety and agitation, hallucinations, confusion, blood pressure swings, fever, tachycardia, seizures, and coma. SSRIs are not addictive but abrupt cessation may trigger discontinuation syndrome (flu-like symptoms).

Tricyclic/cyclic antidepressants

Tricyclic antidepressants (named for the 3-ring chemical structure of the first of this group) inhibit the uptake of neurotransmitters, primarily norepinephrine and serotonin, and serve as antagonists to dopamine and histamine. Tricyclic antidepressants usually target 2 or 3 of these neurotransmitters while newer antidepressants, such as SSRIs, target only one. Tricyclic antidepressants treat depression, ADHD, nocturnal enuresis, and pain (migraine). They are sometimes referred to as cyclic antidepressants because newer drugs have a 4-ring structure. Tricyclic antidepressants are lipophilic and highly protein-bound, so they absorb rapidly. They affect the limbic system, decreasing β-receptors, which are stimulated by increased levels of norepinephrine, which interferes with receptor function. They have long half-lives, which increases toxic affects with overdose, and anticholinergic (primarily muscarinic) effects. Because of this, cyclic antidepressants tend to have more side effects than newer antidepressants: dry mouth, blurring vision, cardiac abnormalities, constipation, urinary retention, and hyperthermia. Alterations in memory and cognition, drowsiness, anxiety, muscle twitches, gynecomastia, and breast enlargement may occur. They are contraindicated with MAO inhibitors and cimetidine.

Extrapyramidal system

The extrapyramidal system is a group of neural connections outside of the medulla that control movement. Extrapyramidal effects are the result of drug influence on the extrapyramidal system and include:
- Akinesia (inability to start movement).
- Akathisia (inability to stop movement).
- Dystonia (extreme and uncontrolled muscle contraction, torticollis, flexing, and twisting).

The most common extrapyramidal symptom caused by antipsychotic agents is tardive dyskinesia, in which individuals are unable to control their movements, such as tics, lip smacking, and eye blinking. The term tardive refers to the delayed onset of the symptoms. Even after the discontinuation of a drug, extrapyramidal side effects may still be present. Oculogyric crisis is common in children, and features restlessness, staring, painful deviation or crossing of the eyes, jaw spasm and protruding tongue. Antipsychotics also cause Parkinsonian symptoms like lead-pipe muscle rigidity, but these symptoms occur most often in elderly adults.

Treatment for extrapyramidal effects

Extrapyramidal effects drastically alter an individual's quality of life by making him/her conspicuous in public. The individual can also develop frightening dysphagia (difficulty swallowing), uncontrollable tics and motor activity. All of these symptoms contribute to a worsening of depression. One must treat the symptoms in order to maintain an effective psychopharmacological therapy or risk the individual's discontinuation of the drugs due to their motor side effects. In some cases, discontinuing the causative medication is the only solution, but symptoms may persist. Symptom control agents of choice include:
- Anticholinergics, such as benztropine or biperiden.
- Antiviral amantadine hydrochloride, which mediate symptoms by increasing dopamine active in the brain.
- Bromocriptine.
- Pergolide.

Adult studies have shown that vitamin E may mediate extrapyramidal symptoms.

Second-generation antipsychotics

Second-generation antipsychotics (SGAs), also called atypical antipsychotics, are used for bipolar disorders, schizophrenia, and psychosis and include aripiprazole (Abilify®), clozapine (Clozaril®), olanzapine (Zyprexa®), quetiapine (Seroquel®), risperidone (Risperdal®), and ziprasidone (Geodon®). Females report more side effects than males, but the recommended doses for males and females are identical. Women were underrepresented when SGAs were clinically tested because researchers feared teratogenic effects on fetuses. Side-effects include constipation, increased appetite, weight gain, urinary retention, various sexual side effects, increased prolactin, menstrual irregularities, increased risk of diabetes mellitus, decreased blood pressure, dizziness, agranulocytosis, and leucopenia. Atypical antipsychotics may interact with fluvoxamine, phenytoin,

- 172 -

carbamazepine, barbiturates, nicotine, ketoconazole, phenytoin, rifampin, and glucocorticoids. The use of atypical antipsychotic agents correlates with significant weight gain. Overweight and obese individuals are likely to develop insulin resistance and glucose intolerance, which may lead to diabetes mellitus. Data show clozapine and olanzapine as the greatest offenders. Ziprasidone seems to present the lowest risk.

Alcohol withdrawal

Chronic abuse of ethanol (alcoholism) is associated with alcohol withdrawal syndrome *(delirium tremens)* with abrupt cessation of alcohol intake, resulting in hallucinations, tachycardia, diaphoresis, and sometimes-psychotic behavior. It may be precipitated by trauma or infection and has a high mortality rate, 5-15% with treatment and 35% without treatment. Management includes:

- Monitor vital signs and blood gases.
- Use the Clinical Instrument for Withdrawal for Alcohol (CIWA) to measure symptoms of withdrawal.
- Assess and monitor level of consciousness, orientation, alterations in sensory impressions, agitation, and anxiety.
- Provide an environment with minimal sensory stimulus (lower lights, close blinds).
- Implement fall and seizure precautions.
- Provide nutritional support and monitor intake and output.
- Implement measures to assure proper sleep and stress management.
- Express acceptance and reassurance.
- Maintain body temperature.

People easily aroused can usually safely sleep off the effects of ingesting too much alcohol but if semi-conscious or unconscious, emergency medical treatment (such as IV fluids and medications, intubation, and/or dialysis) may be necessary.

Alcohol use assessment (CAGE)

The CAGE tool is used as a quick assessment tool to determine if people are drinking excessively or are problem drinkers. Moderate drinking, (1-2 drinks daily or one drink a day for older adults), unless contraindicated by health concerns, is usually not harmful to people, but drinking more than that can lead to serious psychosocial and physical problems. One drink is defined as 12 ounces of beer/wine cooler, 5 ounces of wine, or 1.5 ounces of liquor.

C: Cutting down	Do you think about trying to cut down on drinking?
A: Annoyed at criticism	Are people starting to criticize your drinking?
G: Guilty feelings	Do you feel guilty or try to hide your drinking?
E: Eye opener	Do you increasingly need a drink earlier in the day?

"Yes" on one question suggests the possibility of a drinking problem while "yes" on ≥2 indicates a drinking problem, and the individual should be provided information about reducing drinking and appropriate referrals made.

Indicators of substance abuse

Many people with substance abuse (alcohol or drugs) are reluctant to disclose this information, but there are a number of indicators that are suggestive of substance abuse:

Physical signs
- Needle tracks on arms or legs.
- Burns on fingers or lips.
- Pupils abnormally dilated or constricted, eyes watery.
- Slurring of speech, slow speech.
- Lack of coordination, instability of gait.
- Tremors.
- Sniffing repeatedly, nasal irritation.
- Persistent cough.
- Weight loss.
- Dysrhythmias.
- Pallor, puffiness of face.

Other signs
- Odor of alcohol/marijuana on clothing or breath.
- Labile emotions, including mood swings, agitation, and anger.
- Inappropriate, impulsive, and/or risky behavior.
- Lying.
- Missing appointments.
- Difficulty concentrating/short term memory loss, disoriented/confused.
- Blackouts.
- Insomnia or excessive sleeping.
- Lack of personal hygiene.

Drug screening

A drug screen is used to determine use of illicit drugs. Testing varies according to the type of drug used, duration of use, and time of use. Different types of screens include:
- **Serum**: Most drugs can be detected within 24 hours and for up to 3-5 days, but this varies.
- **Saliva**: Similar to serum, drugs can usually be detected within 1 to 3 hours of use and for 2 or 3 days afterward.
- **Perspiration**: The person wears a special patch for up to 2 weeks to evaluate chronic drug use.
- **Urine**: Drugs show up in the urine in about 6 to 8 hours, but tests can be inaccurate if people dilute urine by drinking 1 to 2 liters of fluids or add adulterants that change the chemical makeup of the urine.
- **Hair**: Drugs and alcohol can usually be detected in hair within about two weeks of use and remain for about 90 days.

Cognitive-behavioral therapy

Cognitive-behavioral therapy (CBT) focuses on the impact that thoughts have on behavior and feelings and encourages the individual to use the power of rational thought to alter perceptions and behavior. This approach to counseling is usually short-term, about 12-20 sessions, with the first

- 174 -

sessions to obtain a history, middle sessions to focus on problems, and last sessions to review and reinforce. Individuals are assigned "homework" during the sessions to practice new ways of thinking and to develop new coping strategies. The therapist helps the individual identify goals and then find ways to achieve those goals. CBT acknowledges that all problems cannot be resolved, but one can deal differently with problems. The therapist asks many questions to determine the individual's areas of concern and encourages the individual to question his/her own motivations and needs. CBT is goal-centered so each counseling session is structured toward a particular goal, such as coping techniques. CBT centers on the concept of unlearning previous behaviors and learning new ones, questioning behaviors, and doing homework.

Management of suicidal patients

Patients may attempt suicide for many reasons, including severe depression, social isolation, situational crisis, bereavement, or psychotic disorder (schizophrenia). Suicidal patients should be referred for psychiatric evaluation. If a person attempts suicide, he/she should be hospitalized and assessed for continued risk after initial treatment, which depends upon the type of suicide attempt.

Suicidal indications
- Depression or dysphoria.
- Hostility to others.
- Problems with peer relationships, and lack of close friends.
- Post-crisis stress (divorce, death in family, graduation, college).
- Withdrawn personality,
- Quiet, lonely appearance, behavior.
- Change in behavior (drop in grades, wearing black clothes, unkempt appearance, sleeping excessively, or not sleeping).
- Co-morbid psychiatric problems (bipolar, schizophrenia).
- Drug abuse.

High risk for repeated suicide attempt
- Violent suicide attempt (knives, gunshots).
- Suicide attempt with low chance of rescue.
- Ongoing psychosis or disordered thinking.
- Ongoing severe depression and feeling of helplessness.
- History of previous suicide attempts.
- Lack of social support system.

Professional Caring and Ethical Practices

AACN Synergy model

The AACN Synergy model of nursing practice, developed by the AACN for nursing certification, places the needs of the patient as a central focus and defines the relationship between 8 patient characteristics and 8 nurse competencies. These competencies and characteristics are evaluated on a scale (1-5).

- **Patient characteristics** include resiliency, vulnerability, stability, complexity, resource availability, participation in care, participation in decision-making, and predictability.
- **Nurse competencies** include clinical judgment, advocacy, caring practices, collaboration, systems thinking, response to diversity, clinical inquiry, and facilitation of learning.
- **System or healthcare environment** is the third element of the model. It provides support for the needs of the patients and empowers and nurtures the practice of nursing, caring, and ethical practice.

All three of these systems are essential for Synergy. The needs of the patient are the driving force for nurse competencies and both are dependent on the healthcare system. When the needs, competencies, and system complement each other, Synergy is achieved, and outcomes for the nurse, the patient, and the system are optimized.

The AACN Synergy model is based on three levels of quality outcomes (patient, nurse, and system). Six general indicators of quality outcomes include:
- Satisfaction of patient and family.
- Adverse incidents rates.
- Rate of complications.
- Adherence to discharge plans.
- Mortality rate.
- Length of stay in hospital.

These general outcomes are based on outcomes derived from the patient, the nurse, and the system:
- **Patient outcomes** include functional change, behavioral change, trust, ratings, satisfaction, comfort, and quality of life.
- **Nurse outcomes** include physiological changes, presence or absence of complications, extent to which care of treatment objectives were attained.
- **System outcomes** include recidivism, costs, and resource utilization.

Advocacy/Moral Agency

Nurse competencies under the AACN Synergy model include **advocacy/moral agency**:
- **Advocacy** is working for the best interests of the patient despite personal values in conflict and assisting patients to have access to appropriate resources.
- **Agency** is openness and recognition of issues and a willingness to act.
- **Moral agency** is the ability to recognize needs and take action to influence the outcome of a conflict or decision.

The levels of advocacy/moral agency include:
- Level 1: This nurse works on behalf of the patient, assesses personal values, has awareness of patient's rights and ethical conflicts, and advocates for the patient when consistent with the nurse's personal values.
- Level 3: This nurse advocates for the patient/family, incorporates their values into the care plan even when they differ from the nurse's, and can utilize internal resources to assist patient/family with complex decisions.
- Level 5: This nurse advocates for patient/family despite differences in values and is able to utilize both internal and external resources to help to empower patient/family to make decisions.

Complementary therapies

Complementary therapies are used as well as conventional medical treatment and should be included if this is what the patient/family wants, empowering the family to take some control. Complementary therapies vary widely and most can easily be incorporated into the plan of care. The National Center for Complementary and Alternative Medicine recognizes the following:
- Whole medical systems include medical systems, such as homeopathic, naturopathic medicine, acupuncture, and Chinese herbal medications.
- Mind-body medicine can include support groups, medication, music, art, or dance therapy.
- Biologically-based practices include the use of food, vitamins, or nutrition for healing.
- Manipulative/body-based programs include massage or other types of manipulation, such as chiropractic treatment.
- Energy therapies may be biofield therapies intended to affect the aura (energy field) that some believe surrounds all living things. These therapies include therapeutic touch and Reiki. Bioelectromagnetic-based therapies use a variety of magnetic fields.

Ethical assessment

While the terms *ethics* and *morals* are sometimes used interchangeably, ethics is a study of morals and encompasses concepts of right and wrong. When making ethical assessments, one must consider not only what people should do but also what they actually do, as these two things are sometimes at odds. Ethical issues can be difficult to assess because of personal bias, and that is one of the reasons that sharing concerns with other internal sources and reaching consensus is so valuable. Issues of concern might include options for care, refusal of care, rights to privacy, adequate relief of suffering, and the right to self-determination. Internal sources might include the ethics committee, whose charge is to make decisions regarding ethical issues. Risk management can provide guidance related to personal and institutional liability. External agencies might include government agencies, such as the public health department.

Beneficence and nonmaleficence

Beneficence is an ethical principle that involves performing actions that are for the purpose of benefitting another person. In the care of a patient, any procedure or treatment should be done with the ultimate goal of benefitting the patient, and any actions that are not beneficial should be reconsidered. As conditions change, procedures need to be continually reevaluated to determine if they are still of benefit.

Nonmaleficence is an ethical principle that means healthcare workers should provide care in a manner that does not cause direct intentional harm to the patient:

- The actual act must be good or morally neutral.
- The intent must be only for a good effect.
- A bad effect cannot serve as the means to get to a good effect.
- A good effect must have more benefit than a bad effect has harm.

Autonomy and justice

Autonomy is the ethical principle that the individual has the right to make decisions about his/her own care. In the case of children or patients with dementia who cannot make autonomous decisions, parents or family members may serve as the legal decision maker. The nurse must keep the patient and/or family fully informed so that they can exercise their autonomy in informed decision-making.

Justice is the ethical principle that relates to the distribution of the limited resources of healthcare benefits to the members of society. These resources must be distributed fairly. This issue may arise if there is only one bed left and two sick patients. Justice comes into play in deciding which patient should stay and which should be transported or otherwise cared for. The decision should be made according to what is best or most just for the patients and not colored by personal bias.

Bioethics

Bioethics is a branch of ethics that involves making sure that the medical treatment given is the most morally correct choice given the different options that might be available and the differences inherent in the varied levels of treatment. In the acute/critical care unit, if the patients, parents, and the staff are in agreement when it comes to values and decision-making, then no ethical dilemma exists; however, when there is a difference in value beliefs between the patients/parents and the staff, there is a bioethical dilemma that must be resolved. Sometimes, discussion and explanation can resolve differences, but at times the institution's ethics committee must be brought in to resolve the conflict. The primary goal of bioethics is to determine the most morally correct action using the set of circumstances given.

Informed consent

Patients or guardians must provide informed consent for all treatment the patient receives. This includes a thorough explanation of all procedures and treatment and associated risks. Patients/guardians should be apprised of all options and allowed input on the type of treatments. Patients/guardians should be apprised of all reasonable risks and any complications that might be life threatening or increase morbidity. The American Medical Association has established guidelines for informed consent:

- Explanation of diagnosis.
- Nature and reason for treatment or procedure.
- Risks and benefits.
- Alternative options (regardless of cost or insurance coverage).
- Risks and benefits of alternative options.
- Risks and benefits of not having a treatment or procedure.
- Providing informed consent is a requirement of all states.

Patient/family rights

In order for patient/family rights to be incorporated into the plan of care, the care plan needs to be designed as a collaborative effort that encourages participation of patients and family members. There are a number of different programs that can be useful, such as including patients and families on advisory committees. Additionally, assessment tools, such as surveys for patients/families, can be utilized to gain insight in the issues that are important to them. While infants and small children and sometimes the elderly cannot speak for themselves, "patient" is generally understood to include not only the immediate family but also other groups or communities who have an interest in the care of an individual or individuals. Because many hospital stays are now short-term, programs that include follow-up interviews and assessments are especially valuable in determining if the needs of the patient/family were addressed in the care plan.

Confidentiality

Confidentiality is the obligation that is present in a professional-patient relationship. Nurses are under an obligation to protect the information they possess concerning the patient and family. Care should be taken to safeguard that information and provide the privacy that the family deserves. This is accomplished through the use of required passwords when family call for information about the patient and through the limitation of who is allowed to visit. There may be times when confidentiality must be broken to save the life of a patient, but those circumstances are rare. The nurse practitioner must make all efforts to safeguard patient records and identification. Computerized record keeping should be done in such a way that the screen is not visible to others, and paper records must be secured.

Ethical issues related to terminally ill patients

There are a number of ethical concerns that healthcare providers and families must face when determining the treatments that are necessary and appropriate for a terminally-ill patient. It is the nurse's responsibility to provide support and information to help parents/families make informed decisions:

Analgesia
- Advantages: Provide comfort. Ease the dying process.
- Disadvantages: Increase sedation and decrease cognition and interaction with family. Side effects. May hasten death.

Active treatments (such as antibiotics, chemotherapy)
- Advantages: Prolong life. Relieve symptoms. Reassure family.
- Disadvantages: Prolong the dying process. Side effects may be severe (as with chemotherapy).

Supplemental nutrition
- Advantages: Relieve family's anxiety that patient is hungry. Prolong life.
- Disadvantages: May cause nausea, vomiting. May increase tumor growth with cancer. May increase discomfort.

<u>IV fluids for hydration</u>
- Advantages: May cause nausea, vomiting. May increase tumor growth with cancer. May increase discomfort.
- Disadvantages: May result in congestive heart failure and pulmonary edema with increased dyspnea. Increased urinary output and incontinence may cause skin breakdown. Prolong dying process.

<u>Resuscitation efforts</u>
- Advantages: Allow family to deny death is imminent.
- Disadvantages: Cause unnecessary suffering and prolong dying process.

Rights and responsibilities

Empowering patients and families to act as their own advocates requires they have a clear understanding of their rights and responsibilities. These should be given (in print form) and/or presented (audio/video) to patients and families on admission or as soon as possible:
- **Rights** should include competent, non-discriminatory medical care that respects privacy and allows participation in decisions about care and the right to refuse care. They should have clear understandable explanations of treatments, options, and conditions, including outcomes. They should be apprised of transfers, changes in care plan, and advance directives. They should have access to medical records information about charges.
- **Responsibilities** should including providing honest and thorough information about health issues and medical history. They should ask for clarification if they don't understand information that is provided to them, and they should follow the plan of care that is outlined or explain why that is not possible. They should treat staff and other patients with respect.

Caring Practices

In the AACN Synergy model, caring practices encompass all nursing activities that respond to the individual patient's and family's needs in a caring, compassionate, and therapeutic environment to promote patient comfort and prevent unnecessary suffering. Caring practices recognize inner strength and its relation to healing and seeks to enhance the dignity of the individual through vigilance, nurturing, and skilled technical and basic nursing practices. Levels of caring practices include:
- Level 1: This nurse provides a safe environment and cares for the present basic needs of the patient without focus on future needs and considers death a potential outcome.
- Level 3: This nurse provides compassionate care, responding to changes in the patient and acts of kindness while accepting death as a possible outcome and providing measures to ensure good end-of-life care and a peaceful death.
- Level 5: This nurse is fully engaged in patient care and understands and interprets patient/family dynamics and needs, ensuring comfort, dignity, and safety while respecting the individual and family.

Problem solving

Problem solving to anticipate or prevent recurrences of patient/family dissatisfaction involves arriving at a hypothesis, testing, and assessing data to determine if the hypothesis holds true. If a problem has arisen, taking steps to resolve the immediate problem is only the first step if recurrence is to be avoided:

- **Define the issue:** Talk with the patient or family and staff to determine if the problem related to a failure of communication or other issues, such as culture or religion.
- **Collect data:** This may mean interviewing additional staff or reviewing documentation, gaining a variety of perspectives.
- **Identify important concepts:** Determine if there are issues related to values or beliefs.
- **Consider reasons for actions:** Distinguish between motivation and intention on the part of all parties to determine the reason for the problem.
- **Make a decision:** A decision on how to prevent a recurrence of a problem should be based on advocacy and moral agency, reaching the best solution possible for the patient and family.

Patients'/families' rights

Patients' (families') rights in relation to what they should expect from a healthcare organization are outlined in both standards of the Joint Commission and National Committee for Quality Assurance. Rights include:

- Respect for patient, including personal dignity and psychosocial, spiritual, and cultural considerations.
- Response to needs related to access and pain control.
- Ability to make decisions about care, including informed consent, advance directives, and end of life care.
- Procedure for registering complaints or grievances.
- Protection of confidentiality and privacy.
- Freedom from abuse or neglect.
- Protection during research and information related to ethical issues of research.
- Appraisal of outcomes, including unexpected outcomes.
- Information about organization, services, and practitioners.
- Appeal procedures for decisions regarding benefits and quality of care.
- Organizational code of ethical behavior.
- Procedures for donating and procuring organs/tissue.

Facilitating safe passage

Facilitating safe passage is part of caring practice that ensures patient safety, in a broad sense, from a variety of perspectives:

- Giving appropriate medications and treatment without errors that endanger the patient's health is essential.
- Providing information to the patient/family about treatments, changes, conditions, and other aspects related to care helps them to cope with the situations as they arise.
- Preventing infection is central to patient safety and includes staff using proper infection control methods, such as handwashing.
- Knowing the person requires the nurse to take the time and effort to understand the needs and wishes of the patient/family.

- Assisting with transitions involves not only helping the patient/family cope with moving from one form of treatment, or one unit to another but also with transitions in health, such as from illness to health or from illness to death.

Advance directives

In accordance to Federal and state laws, individuals have the right to self-determination in health care, including decisions about end of life care through advance directives such as living wills and the right to assign a surrogate person to make decisions through a durable power of attorney. Patients should routinely be questioned about an advanced directive as they may present at a healthcare provider without the document. Patients who have indicated they desire a do-not-resuscitate (DNR) order should not receive resuscitative treatments for terminal illness or conditions in which meaningful recovery cannot occur. Patients and families of those with terminal illnesses should be questioned as to whether the patients are Hospice patients. For those with DNR requests or those withdrawing life support, staff should provide the patient palliative rather than curative measures, such as pain control and/or oxygen, and emotional support to the patient and family. Religious traditions and beliefs about death should be treated with respect.

Pain management

Promoting a caring and supportive environment means ensuring that the patient is comfortable. According to Joint Commission guidelines and Federal law, all patients have to right to pain management, and this applies to all ages. It's not enough to recognize this; procedures must be in place to assure that all staff are committed to reducing pain and that patients/families be apprised of the right and benefits of pain management. There are steps that the institution can take in this process:
- Create an interdisciplinary team to research, provide guidelines, and communicate goals.
- Assess pain management procedures already in place to determine effectiveness or need for change.
- Establish a minimum standard that should be legally followed.
- Clarify responsibility for pain control and imbed this in the standards of practice.
- Provide information about pain control to all levels of care providers.
- Educate patients to understand they are entitled to rapid response.
- Educate staff to institutionalize pain management.

Supporting families of dying patients

Families of dying patients often do not receive adequate support from nursing staff that feel unprepared for dealing with families' grief and unsure of how to provide comfort, but families may be in desperate need of this support:

Before death
- Stay with the family and sit quietly, allowing them to talk, cry, or interact if they desire.
- Avoid platitudes, "His suffering will be over soon."
- Avoid judgmental reactions to what family members say or do and realize that anger, fear, guilt, and irrational behavior are normal responses to acute grief and stress.

- Show caring by touching the patient and encouraging family to do the same.
  - o Note: Touching hands, arms, or shoulders of family members can provide comfort, but follow clues of the family.
- Provide referrals to support groups if available.

Time of death
- Reassure family that all measures have been taken to ensure the patient's comfort.
- Express personal feeling of loss, "She was such a sweet woman, and I'll miss her" and allow family to express feelings and memories. Provide information about what is happening during the dying process, explaining death rales, Cheyne-Stokes respirations, etc.
- Alert family members to imminent death if they are not present. Assist to contact clergy/spiritual advisors.
- Respect feelings and needs of parents, siblings, and other family.

After death
- Encourage parents/family members to stay with the patient as long as they wish to say goodbye.
- Use the patient's name when talking to the family.
- Assist family to make arrangements, such as contacting funeral home.
- If an autopsy is required, discuss with the family and explain when it will take place.
- If organ donation is to occur, assist the family to make arrangements. Encourage family members to grieve and express emotions.
- Send card or condolence note.

Kübler-Ross's five stages of grief

Grief is a normal response to the death or severe illness/abnormality of a patient. How a person deals with grief is very personal, and each will grieve differently. Elisabeth Kübler-Ross identified five stages of grief in *On Death and Dying* (1969), which can apply to both patients and family members. A person may not go through each stage but usually goes through two of the five stages:

- **Denial**: Patients/families may be resistive to information and unable to accept that a person is dying/impaired. They may act stunned, immobile, or detached and may be unable to respond appropriately or remember what's said, often repeatedly asking the same questions.
- **Anger**: As reality becomes clear, patient/families may react with pronounced anger, directed inward or outward. Women, especially, may blame themselves and self-anger may lead to severe depression and guilt, assuming they are to blame because of some personal action. Outward anger, more common in men, may be expressed as overt hostility.
- **Bargaining**: This involves if-then thinking (often directed at a deity): "If I go to church every day, then God will prevent this." Patient/family may change doctors, trying to change the outcome.
- **Depression**: As the patient and family begin to accept the loss, they may become depressed, feeling no one understands and overwhelmed with sadness. They may be tearful or crying and may withdraw or ask to be left alone.
- **Acceptance**: This final stage represents a form of resolution and often occurs outside of the medical environment after months. Patients are able to accept death/dying/incapacity. Families are able to resume their normal activities and lose the constant preoccupation with their loved one. They are able to think of the person without severe pain.

Medication errors

There are about 7000 deaths yearly in the United States attributed to medication errors. Studies indicate that there are errors in 1 in 5 doses of medication given to patients in hospitals. A caring environment is one in which patient safety is ensured with proper handling and administering of medications:

- Avoid error-prone abbreviations or symbols. The Joint Commission has established a list of abbreviations to avoid, but mistakes are frequent with other abbreviations as well. In many cases, abbreviations and symbols should be avoided altogether or restricted to a limited approved list.
- Prevent errors from illegible handwriting. Handwritten orders should be block printed to reduce change of error.
- Institute bar coding and scanners that allow the patient's wristband and medications to be scanned for verification.
- Provide lists of similarly-named medications to educate staff.
- Establish an institutional policy for administering of medications that includes protocols for verification of drug, dosage, and patient as well as educating the patient about the medications.

Therapeutic communication

Therapeutic communication begins with respect for the patient/family and the assumption that all communication, verbal and non-verbal, has meaning. Listening must be done empathetically. Techniques that facilitate communication include:

Introduction
Make a personal introduction and use the patient's name: "Mrs. Brown, I am Susan Williams, your nurse."

Encouragement
Use an open-ended opening statement: "Is there anything you'd like to discuss?" Acknowledge comments: "Yes," and "I understand." Allow silence and observe non-verbal behavior rather than trying to force conversation. Ask for clarification if statements are unclear. Reflect statements back (use sparingly): Patient: "I hate this hospital." Nurse: "You hate this hospital?"

Empathy
Make observations: "You are shaking," and "You seem worried." Recognize feelings:
Patient: "I want to go home."
Nurse: "It must be hard to be away from your home and family."

Provide information as honestly and completely as possible about condition, treatment, and procedures and respond to patient's questions and concerns.

Exploration
Verbally express implied messages:
Patient: "This treatment is too much trouble."
Nurse: "You think the treatment isn't helping you?"

Explore a topic but allow the patient to terminate the discussion without further probing: "I'd like to hear how you feel about that.

<u>Orientation</u>
Indicate reality:
Patient: "Someone is screaming."
Nurse: "That sound was an ambulance siren."

Comment on distortions without directly agreeing or disagreeing:
Patient: "That nurse promised I didn't have to walk again."
Nurse: "Really? That's surprising because the doctor ordered physical therapy twice a day."

<u>Collaboration</u>
Work together to achieve better results: "Maybe if we talk about this, we can figure out a way to make the treatment easier for you."

<u>Validation</u>
Seek validation: "Do you feel better now?" or "Did the medication help you breathe better?"

Avoiding non-therapeutic communication

While using therapeutic communication is important, it is equally important to avoid interjecting non-therapeutic communication, which can effectively block effective communication. *Avoid the following:*

- Meaningless clichés: "Don't worry. Everything will be fine." "Isn't it a nice day?"
- Providing advice: "You should…" or "The best thing to do is…." It's better when patients ask for advice to provide facts and encourage the patient to reach a decision.
- Inappropriate approval that prevents the patient from expressing true feeling or concerns:
  o Patient: "I shouldn't cry about this."
  o Nurse: "That's right! You're an adult!"
- Asking for explanations of behavior that is not directly related to patient care and requires analysis and explanation of feelings: "Why are you upset?"
- Agreeing with rather than accepting and responding to patient's statements can make it difficult for the patient to change his/her statement or opinion later: "I agree with you," or "You are right."
- Negative judgments: "You should stop arguing with the nurses."
- Devaluing patient's feelings: "Everyone gets upset at times."
- Disagreeing directly: "That can't be true," or "I think you are wrong."
- Defending against criticism: "The doctor is not being rude; he's just very busy today."
- Subject change to avoid dealing with uncomfortable topics;
  o Patient: "I'm never going to get well."
  o Nurse: "Your family will be here in just a few minutes."
- Inappropriate literal responses, even as a joke, especially if the patient is at all confused or having difficulty expressing ideas:
  - Patient: "There are bugs crawling under my skin."
  - Nurse: "I'll get some buy spray,"
- Challenge to establish reality often just increases confusion and frustration:
  o "If you were dying, you wouldn't be able to yell and kick!"

Collaboration

In the AACN Synergy model, Collaboration is a team approach of working with a variety of others (physicians, nurses, dieticians, therapist, families, social workers, community leaders and members, clergy, intra- and inter-disciplinary teams) in a cooperative manner, using good therapeutic communication skills, to ensure that each person is contributing optimally toward reaching patient goals and positive outcomes. Collaboration requires mutual respect, professional maturity, common purpose, and a positive sense of self. Levels of collaboration include:

- Level 1: This nurse participates in collaborative activities, learns from others, including mentors, and respects the input of others.
- Level 3: This nurse not only participates in collaborative activities but also initiates them and actively seeks learning opportunities.
- Level 5: This nurse takes a leadership role in collaborative activities by mentoring and teaching others while still seeking learning opportunities and actively seeks additional resources as needed.

Communication skills

Collaboration requires a number of communication skills that differ from those involved in communication between nurse and patient. These skills include:

- **Using an assertive approach:** It's important for the nurse to honestly express opinions and to state them clearly and with confidence, but the nurse must do so in a calm non-threatening manner.
- **Making casual conversation:** It's easier to communicate with people with whom one has a personal connection. Asking open-ended questions, asking about other's work, or commenting on someone's contributions helps to establish a relationship. The time before meetings, during breaks, and after meetings presents an opportunity for this type of conversation.
- **Being competent in public speaking:** Collaboration requires that a nurse be comfortable speaking and presenting ideas to groups of people, and doing so helps the person to gain credibility. This is a skill that must be practiced.
- **Communicating in writing:** The written word remains a critical component of communication, and the nurse should be able to communicate clearly and grammatically.

Skills needed for collaboration

Nurses must learn the set of skills needed for collaboration in order to move nursing forward. Nurses must take an active role in gathering data for evidence-based practice to support nursing's role in health care and must share this information with other nurses and health professionals in order to plan staffing levels and to provide optimal care to patients.

Increased and adequate staffing has consistently been shown to reduce adverse outcomes, but there is a well-documented shortage of nurses in the United States, and more than half of current RNs work outside the hospital. Increased patient loads not only increase adverse outcomes but also increase job dissatisfaction and burnout. In order to manage the challenges facing nursing, nurses must develop skills needed for collaboration:

- Be willing to compromise.
- Communicate clearly.
- Identify specific challenges and problems.

- Focus on the task.
- Work with teams.

Delegation of tasks

The scope of nursing practice includes delegation of tasks to unlicensed assistive personnel, providing those personnel have adequate training and knowledge to carry out the tasks. Delegation should be used to manage the workload and to provide adequate and safe care. The nurse who delegates remains accountable for patient outcomes and for supervision of the person to whom the task was delegated, so the nurse must consider the following:
- Whether knowledge, skills, and training of the unlicensed assistive personnel provides the ability to perform the delegated task.
- Whether the patient's condition and needs have been properly evaluated and assessed.
- Whether the nurse is able to provide ongoing supervision.

Delegation should be done in a manner that reduces liability by providing adequate communication. This includes specific directions about the task, including what needs to be done, when, and for how long. Expectations related to consultation, reporting, and completion of tasks should be clearly defined. The nurse should be available to assist if necessary.

5 Rights of delegation

Prior to delegating tasks, the nurse should assess the needs of the patients and determine the task that needs to be completed, assure that he/she can remain accountable and can supervise the task appropriately and evaluate effective completion. The 5 rights of delegation include:
- **Right task:** The nurse should determine an appropriate task to delegate for a specific patient.
- **Right circumstance:** The nurse has considered the setting, resources, time factors, safety factors, and all other relevant information to determine the appropriateness of delegation.
- **Right person:** The nurse is in the right position to choose the right person (by virtue of education/skills) to perform a task for the right patient.
- **Right direction:** The nurse provides a clear description of the task, the purpose, any limits, and expected outcomes.
- **Right supervision:** The nurse is able to supervise, intervene as needed, and evaluate performance of the task.

Delegation of tasks in teams

On major responsibility of leadership and management in performance improvement teams is using delegation effectively. The purpose of having a team is so that the work is shared, and leaders can cripple themselves by taking on too much of the workload. Additionally, failure to delegate shows an inherent distrust in team members.

Delegation includes:
- Assessing the skills and available time of the team members, determining if a task is suitable for an individual.
- Assigning tasks, with clear instructions that include explanation of objectives and expectations, including a timeline.

- Ensuring that the tasks are completed properly and on time by monitoring progress but not micromanaging.
- Reviewing the final results and recording outcomes.

Because the leader is ultimately responsible for the delegated work, mentoring, monitoring, and providing feedback and intervention as necessary during this process is a necessary component of leadership. While delegated tasks may not always be completed successfully, they represent an opportunity for learning.

Creating a common vision of care

Facilitating the creation of a common vision for care within the healthcare system begins with the organization/facility, working collaboratively to create teams and an organization focused on serving the patient/family. A common vision should be the ideal in any organization, but achieving such a goal requires a true collaborative effort:
- Inclusion of all levels of staff across the organization/facility, both those in nursing and non-nursing positions.
- Consensus building through discussions, inservice, and team meetings to bring about convergence of diverse viewpoints.
- Facilitation that values creativity and provides encouragement during the process.
- Vision statement incorporating the common vision that accessible to all staff.

Recognition that a common vision is an organic concept that may evolve over time and should be reevaluated regularly and changed as needed to reflect the needs of the organization, patients, families, and staff.

Teambuilding

Leading, facilitating, and participating in performance improvement teams requires a thorough understanding of the dynamics of team building:
- **Initial interactions:** This is the time when members begin to define their roles and develop relationships, determining if they are comfortable in the group.
- **Power issues:** The members observe the leader and determine who controls the meeting and how control is exercised, beginning to form alliances.
- **Organizing:** Methods to achieve work are clarified and team members begin to work together, gaining respect for each other's contributions and working toward a common goal.
- **Team identification:** Interactions often become less formal as members develop rapport, and members are more willing to help and support each other to achieve goals.
- **Excellence:** This develops through a combination of good leadership, committed team members, clear goals, high standards, external recognition, spirit of collaboration, and a shared commitment to the process.

Effective team meetings

Leading and facilitating improvement teams requires utilizing good techniques for meetings. Considerations include:
- **Scheduling**: Both the time and the place must be convenient and conducive to working together, so the leader must review the work schedules of those involved, finding the most convenient time. Venues or meeting rooms should allow for sitting in a circle or around a

table to facilitate equal exchange of ideas. Any necessary technology, such as computers or overhead projectors, or other equipment, such as whiteboards, should be available.

- **Preparation**: The leader should prepare a detailed agenda that includes a list of items for discussion.
- **Conduction**: Each item of the agenda should be discussed, soliciting input from all group members. Tasks should be assigned to individual members based on their interest and part in the process in preparation for the next meeting. The leader should summarize input and begin a tentative future agenda.
- **Observation**: The leader should observe the interactions, including verbal and non-verbal communication, and respond to these.

Intra-and inter-disciplinary teams

There are a number of skills that are needed to lead and facilitate coordination of **intra-and inter-disciplinary teams:**

- Communicating openly is essential with all members encouraged to participate as valued members of a cooperative team.
- Avoiding interrupting or interpreting the point another is trying to make allows free flow of ideas.
- Avoiding jumping to conclusions, which can effectively shut off communication.
- Active listening requires paying attentions and asking questions for clarification rather than to challenge other's ideas.
- Respecting others opinions and ideas, even when opposed to one's own, is absolutely essential.
- Reacting and responding to facts rather than feelings allows one to avoid angry confrontations or diffuse anger.
- Clarifying information or opinions stated can help avoid misunderstandings.
- Keeping unsolicited advice out of the conversation shows respect for others and allows them to solicit advice without feeling pressured.

Leadership styles

Leadership styles often influence the perception of leadership values and commitment to collaboration. There are a number of different leadership styles:

Charismatic: Depends upon personal charisma to influence people, and may be very persuasive, but this type leader may engage "followers" and relate to one group rather than the organization at large, limiting effectiveness.

Bureaucratic: Follows organization rules exactly and expects everyone else to do so. This is most effective in handling cash flow or managing work in dangerous work environments. This type of leadership may engender respect but may not be conducive to change.

Autocratic: Makes decisions independently and strictly enforces rules, but team members often feel left out of process and may not be supportive. This type of leadership is most effective in crisis situations, but may have difficulty gaining commitment of staff

- 189 -

Consultative: Presents a decision and welcomes input and questions although decisions rarely change. This type of leadership is most effective when gaining the support of staff is critical to the success of proposed changes.

Participatory: Presents a potential decision and then makes final decision based on input from staff or teams. This type of leadership is time-consuming and may result in compromises that are not wholly satisfactory to management or staff, but this process is motivating to staff who feel their expertise is valued.

Democratic: Presents a problem and asks staff or teams to arrive at a solution although the leader usually makes the final decision. This type of leadership may delay decision-making, but staff and teams are often more committed to the solutions because of their input.

Laissez-faire (free rein): Exerts little direct control but allows employees/ teams to make decisions with little interference. This may be effective leadership if teams are highly skilled and motivated, but in many cases this type of leadership is the product of poor management skills and little is accomplished because of this lack of leadership.

Resistance to organizational change

Performance improvement processes cannot occur without organizational change, and resistance to change is common for many people, so coordinating collaborative processes requires anticipating resistance and taking steps to achieve cooperation. Resistance often relates to concerns about job loss, increased responsibilities, and general denial or lack of understanding and frustration. Leaders can prepare others involved in the process of change by taking these steps:
- Be honest, informative, and tactful, giving people thorough information about anticipated changes and how the changes will affect them, including positives.
- Be patient in allowing people the time they need to contemplate changes and express anger or disagreement.
- Be empathetic in listening carefully to the concerns of others.
- Encourage participation, allowing staff to propose methods of implementing change, so they feel some sense of ownership.
- Establish a climate in which all staff members are encouraged to identify the need for change on an ongoing basis.
- Present further ideas for change to management.

Conflict resolution

Conflict is an almost inevitable product of teamwork, and the leader must assume responsibility for conflict resolution. While conflicts can be disruptive, they can produce positive outcomes by forcing team members to listen to different perspectives and opening dialogue. The team should make a plan for dealing with conflict resolution. The best time for conflict resolution is when differences emerge but before open conflict and hardening of positions occur. The leader must pay close attention to the people and problems involved, listen carefully, and reassure those involved that their points of view are understood.

Steps to conflict resolution include:
- Allow both sides to present their side of conflict without bias, maintaining a focus on opinions rather than individuals.
- Encourage cooperation through negotiation and compromise.
- Maintain the focus, providing guidance to keep the discussions on track and avoid arguments.
- Evaluate the need for renegotiation, formal resolution process, or third party.
- Utilize humor and empathy to diffuse escalating tensions.
- Summarize the issues, outlining key arguments.
- Avoid forcing resolution if possible

Collaboration

One of the most important forms of collaboration is that between the nurse and the patient/family, but this type of collaboration is often overlooked. Nurses and others in the healthcare team must always remember that the point of collaborating is to improve patient care, and this means that the patient and patient's family must remain central to all planning. For example, including family in planning for a patient takes time initially, but sitting down and asking the patient and family, "What do you want?" and using the Synergy model to evaluate patient's (and family's) characteristics can provide valuable information that saves time in the long run and facilitates planning and expenditure of resources. Families, and even young children, often want to participate in care and planning and feel validated and more positive toward the medical system when they are included.

The critical care nurse must initiate and facilitate collaboration with external agencies because many have direct impacts on patient care and needs:
- Industry can include other facilities sharing interests in patient care or pharmaceutical companies. It's important for nursing to have a dialog with drug companies about their products and how they are used in specific populations because many medications are prescribed to women, children, or the aged without validating studies for dose or efficacy.
- Payors have a vested interest in containing health care costs, so providing information and representing the interests of the patient is important.
- Community groups may provide resources for patients and families, both in terms of information and financial or other assistance.
- Political agencies are increasingly important as new laws are considered about nurse-patient ratios and infection control in many states.
- Public health agencies are partners in health care with other facilities and must be included, especially in issues related to communicable disease.

Systems Thinking

In the AACN Synergy model, systems thinking is having the background knowledge and practical tools to manage both environmental and system resources, within and outside of the healthcare system, in order to solve problems for the patient/family and meet their needs. Solving problems requires a holistic view of the interrelationships and understanding of how structures, patterns, and events affect outcomes. Levels of systems thinking include:
- Level 1: This nurse views himself/herself as the primary resource to meet the needs of the patient within the confines of the unit and doesn't recognize the need to negotiate.

- Level 3: This nurse looks beyond the unit and personal contributions to care to view the patient's progress through the entire system and sees the need to negotiate with others to provide the best resources available although may lack the skills needed to do so,
- Level 5: This nurse is expert at understanding the organization holistically and uses a number of different strategies to negotiate with others and assist the patient with progress through the system.

Patient characteristics

The Synergy method for patient care recognizes that there are a number of patient characteristics that must be considered if a nurse's competencies are to match those of the patient/family:
- **Resiliency** is the ability to recover from a devastating illness and regain a sense of stability, both physically and emotionally. Things that often support resiliency are faith, a positive sense of hope, and a supportive network of friends and family.
- **Vulnerability** are those factors putting a person at increased risk and interfering with recovery and/or compliance, such as anxiety, fear, lack of support, chronic illness, prejudice, and lack of information.
- **Stability** allows a patient/family to maintain a state of equilibrium (physically and/or emotionally) despite illness and challenges. Important factors include relief from stress, conflicts, or emotional burdens, motivation, and values.
- **Complexity** occurs when more than one system is involved, and these can be internal (cardiac and renal systems) or external (addicted and homeless) or some combination (ill with poor family dynamics).

Barriers

Barriers to system thinking can arise with the individual, the department, or the administrative level:
- **Identification with role rather than purpose:** People see themselves from the perspective of their role in the system, as nurse or physician, and are not able to step outside their preconceived ideas to view situations holistically or to accept the roles of others. They may lack the ability to look at situations as human beings first, and professionals second.
- **Feelings of victimization:** People may blame the organization or the leadership for personal shortcomings or feel that there is nothing that they can do to improve or change situations. A feeling of victimization may permeate an institution to the point that meaningful communication cannot take place, and people are not open to change.
- **Relying on past experience:** New directions require new solutions, so being mired in the past or relying solely on past experience can prevent progress.
- **Autocratic views:** Some feel that their perceptions and practices are the only ones that are acceptable and often have a narrow focus so that they cannot view the system as a whole but focus on short-term outcomes. They fail to see that there are many aspects to a problem, affecting many parts of the system.
- **Failure to adapt:** Change is difficult for many individuals and institutions, but the medical world is changing rapidly, and this requires adaptability. Those who fail to adapt may feel threatened by changes and unsure of their ability to relearn new concepts, principles, and procedures.

- 192 -

- **Weak consensus**: Groups that arrive at easy or weak consensus without delving into important issues may delude themselves into believing that they have solved problems and remain fixed and often ignored rather than moving forward.

Delivery of care

The delivery of care is impacted by a numerous forces:
- **Social forces** are increasing demand for access to treatment and medical services, both traditional and complementary. As society views equitable medical care as a right, then delivery of care must be available to all.
- **Political forces** affect medical care as the Federal and state governments increasingly become purchasers of medical care, imposing their guidelines and limitations on the medical system.
- **Regulatory forces** may be local, state, or Federal and can have a profound effect of delivery of care and services, differing from one state or region to another.
- **Economic forces**, such as managed care or cost-containment committees, try to contain costs to insurers and facilities by controlling access to and duration of treatment, and limiting products. Economic pressure is working to prevent duplication of services in a geographical area, and providers are creating networks to purchase supplies and equipment directly.

Concepts of systems thinking

The promotion of organizational values and commitment requires that the organization embody systems thinking and the associated concepts. Systems thinking focuses on how systems interrelate, with each part affecting the entire system: Concepts include:
- **Individual responsibility**: Individuals are encouraged to establish their own goals within the organization and to work toward a purpose.
- **Learning process:** The internalized beliefs of the staff are respected while building upon these beliefs to establish a mindset based on continuous learning and improvement.
- **Vision**: A sharing of organizational vision helps staff to understand the purpose of change and builds commitment.
- **Team process:** Teams are assisted to develop good listening and collaborative skills so that there is an increase in dialogue and an ability to reach consensus.
- **Systems thinking:** Staff members are encouraged to understand the interrelationship of all members of the organization and to appreciate how any change affects the whole.

Steps to systems thinking

An approach to systems thinking is especially valuable in organizations in which there is lack of consensus, effective change is stalemated, and standards are inconsistent. Systems thinking is a critical thinking approach to problem solving that takes an organization-wide perspective. Steps include:
- **Define the issue:** Describe the problem in detail without judgment or solutions.
- **Describe behavior patterns:** This includes listing factors related to the problem, using graphs to outline possible trends.
- **Establish cause-effect relationships:** This may include using the Five Whys or other root cause analysis or feedback loops.

- **Define patterns of performance/behavior:** Determine how variables affect outcomes and the types of patterns of behavior currently taking place.
- **Find solutions:** Discuss possible solutions and outcomes.
- **Institute performance improvement activities:** Make changes and then monitor for changes in behavior.

Key concepts

There are a number of key concepts related to quality that must be communicated to all members of an organization through inservice, workshops, newsletters, fact sheets, and team meetings. Quality care/performance should be:
- **Appropriate** to needs and in keeping with best practices.
- **Accessible** to the individual despite financial, cultural, or other barriers.
- **Competent**, with practitioners well-trained and adhering to standards.
- **Coordinated** among all healthcare providers.
- **Effective** in achieving outcomes based on the current state of knowledge.
- **Efficient** in methods of achieving the desired outcomes.
- **Preventive**, allowing for early detection and prevention of problems.
- **Respectful** and caring with consideration of the individual needs given primary importance.
- **Safe** so that the organization is free of hazards or dangers that may put patients or others at risk.

Response to Diversity

In the AACN Synergy model, response to diversity is the ability to recognize a wide range of differences (social, cultural, ethnic, racial, economic, language, religious), to appreciate these differences and incorporate consideration for them into the plan of care. Diverse groups also include the disabled, gay and lesbians, and marginal groups, such as the homeless. Levels of response to diversity include:
- Level 1: This nurse can assess diversity with standardized questionnaires and provide care based on personal belief system and past experience, but doesn't seek assistance in dealing adequately with diversity.
- Level 3: This nurse takes a much more active role in asking about issues of diversity issues and incorporates needs into the plan of care, teaching the patient about the healthcare system.
- Level 5: This nurse considers issues of diversity in all aspects of care and presents patients with alternatives, responding to, anticipating, and integrating consideration of cultural and other differences.

Cultural competence

Different cultures view health and illness from very different perspectives, and patients often come from a mix of many cultures, so the acute care nurse must be not only accepting of cultural differences but must be sensitive and aware. There are a number of characteristics that are important for a nurse to have cultural competence:
- **Appreciating diversity:** This must be grounded in information about other cultures and understanding of their value system.

- **Assessing own cultural perspectives:** Self-awareness is essential to understanding potential biases.
- **Understanding intercultural dynamics:** This must include understanding ways in which cultures cooperate, differ, communicate, and reach understanding.
- **Recognizing institutional culture:** Each institutional unit (hospital, clinic, office) has an inherent set of values that may be unwritten but is accepted by the staff.
- **Adapting patient service to diversity:** This is the culmination of cultural competence as it is the point of contact between cultures.

Blood products and Jehovah Witnesses

Jehovah Witnesses have traditionally shunned transfusions and blood products as part of their religious belief. In 2004, the *Watchtower*, a Jehovah Witness publication presented a guide for members. When medical care indicates the need for blood transfusion or blood products and the patient and/or family members are practicing Jehovah Witnesses, this may present a conflict. It's important to approach the patient/family with full information and reasons for the transfusion or blood components without being judgmental, allowing them to express their feelings. In fact, studies show that while adults often refuse transfusions for themselves, they frequently allow their children to receive blood products, so one should never assume that an individual would refuse blood products based on the religion alone. Jehovah Witnesses can receive fractionated blood cells, thus allowing hemoglobin-based blood substitutes. The following guidelines are provided to church members:

Blood standards for Jehovah Witnesses
- Not acceptable: Whole blood: red cells, white cells, platelets, plasma
- Acceptable: Fractions from red cells, white cells, platelets, and plasma

Mexican patients

Many areas of the country have large populations of Mexican and Mexican-Americans. As always, it's important to recognize that cultural generalizations don't always apply to individuals. Recent immigrants, especially, have cultural needs that the nurse must understand:
- Many Mexicans are Catholic and may like the nurse to make arrangements for a priest to visit.
- Large extended families may come to visit to support the patient and family, so patients should receive clear explanations about how many visitors are allowed, but some flexibility may be required.
- Language barriers may exist as some may have limited or no English skills so translation services should be available around the clock.
- Mexican culture encourages outward expressions of emotions, so family may react strongly to news about a patient's condition, and people who are ill may expect some degree of pampering, so extra attention to the patient/family members may alleviate some of their anxiety.
- Some immigrant Mexicans have very little formal education, so medical information may seem very complex and confusing, and they may not understand the implications or need for follow-up care.
- Mexican culture perceives time with more flexibility than American, so if parents need to be present at a particular time, the nurse should specify the exact time (1:30 PM) and explain the reason rather than saying something more vague, such as "after lunch."

- People may appear to be unassertive or unable to make decisions when they are simply showing respect to the nurse by being deferent.
- In traditional families, the males make decisions, so a woman waits for the father or other males in the family to make decisions about treatment or care.
- Families may choose to use folk medicines instead of Western medical care or may combine the two.
- Children and young women are often sheltered and are taught to be respectful to adults, so they may not express their needs openly.

Middle Eastern patients

There are considerable cultural differences among Middle Easterners, but religious beliefs about the segregation of males and females are common. It's important to remember that segregating the female is meant to protect her virtue. Female nurses have low status in many countries because they violate this segregation by touching male bodies, so parents may not trust or show respect for the nurse who is caring for their family member. Additionally, male patients may not want to be cared for by female nurses or doctors, and families may be very upset at a female being cared for by a male nurse or physician. When possible, these cultural traditions should be accommodated:

- In Middle Eastern countries, males make decisions, so issues for discussion or decision should be directed to males, such as the father or spouse, and males may be direct in stating what they want, sometimes appearing demanding.
- If a male nurse must care for a female patient, then the family should be advised that *personal care* (such as bathing) will be done by a female while the medical treatments will be done by the male nurse.
- Families may practice strict dietary restrictions, such as avoiding pork and requiring that animals be killed in a ritual manner, so vegetarian or kosher meals may be required.
- People may have language difficulties requiring a translator, and same-sex translators should be used if at all possible.
- Families may be accompanied by large extended families that want to be kept informed and whom patients consult before decisions are made.
- Most medical care is provided by female relatives, so educating the family about patient care should be directed at females (with female translators if necessary).
- Outward expressions of grief are considered as showing respect for the dead.
- Middle Eastern families often offer gifts to caregivers. Small gifts (candy) that can be shared should be accepted graciously, but for other gifts, the families should be advised graciously that accepting gifts is against hospital policy.
- Middle Easterners often require less personal space and may stand very close.

Asian patients

There are considerable differences among different Asian populations, so cultural generalizations may not apply to all, but nurses caring for Asian patients should be aware of common cultural attitudes and behaviors:

- Nurses and doctors are viewed with respect, so traditional Asian families may expect the nurse to remain authoritative and to give directions and may not question, so the nurse should ensure that they understand by having them review material or give demonstrations and should provide explanations clearly, anticipating questions that the family might have but may not articulate.

- Disagreeing is considered impolite. "Yes" may only mean that the person is heard, not that they agree with the person. When asked if they understand, they may indicate that they do even when they clearly do not so as not to offend the nurse.
- Asians may avoid eye contact as an indication of respect. This is especially true of children in relation to adults and younger adults in relation to elders.
- Patients/families may not show outward expressions of feelings/grief, sometimes appearing passive. They also avoid public displays of affection. This does not mean that they don't feel, just that they don't show their feelings.
- Families often hide illness and disabilities from others and may feel ashamed about illness.
- Terminal illness is often hidden from the patient, so families may not want patients to know they are dying or seriously ill.
- Families may use cupping, pinching, or applying pressure to injured areas, and this can leave bruises that may appear as abuse, so when bruises are found, the family should be questioned about alternative therapy before assumptions are made.
- Patients may be treated with traditional herbs.
- Families may need translators because of poor or no English skills.
- In traditional Asian families, males are authoritative and make the decisions.

Clinical Inquiry

In the AACN Synergy model, clinical inquiry is a continual process of questioning and evaluating practice in order to provide innovative and outstanding care through application of the results of research and experience. Clinical inquiry requires a desire to acquire new knowledge, openness to accepting advice from mentors and other health and allied professionals, competency in identifying clinical problems, and the ability search the literature for research, critical skills to interpret research findings, and to willingness and ability to design and participate in research. Levels of clinical inquiry include:
- Level 1: This nurse recognizes problems and seeks advice, follows industry standards and guidelines, and seeks further knowledge.
- Level 3: This nurse questions industry standards and guidelines as well as current practice and utilizes research and education to improve patient care.
- Level 5: This nurse is able to deviate from industry standards and guidelines when necessary for the individual patients and utilizes literature review and clinical research to gain knowledge, establish new practices, and improve patient care.

Evidence-based guidelines

Steps to evidence-based practice guidelines include:
- **Focus on the topic/methodology:** This includes outlining possible interventions/treatments for review, choosing patient populations and settings and determining significant outcomes. Search boundaries (such as types of journals, types of studies, dates of studies) should be determined.
- **Evidence review:** This includes review of literature, critical analysis of studies, and summarizing of results, including pooled meta-analysis.
- **Expert judgment:** Recommendations based on personal experience from a number of experts may be utilized, especially if there is inadequate evidence based on review, but this subjective evidence should be explicated acknowledged.
- **Policy considerations:** This includes cost-effectiveness, access to care, insurance coverage, availability of qualified staff, and legal implications.

- **Policy:** A written policy must be completed with recommendations. Common practice is to utilize letter guidelines, with "A" the most highly recommended, usually based the quality of supporting evidence.
- **Review:** The completed policy should be submitted to peers for review and comments before instituting the policy.

Clinical/critical pathways

Clinical/critical pathway development is done by those involved in direct patient care. The pathway should require no additional staffing and cover the entire scope of an illness. Steps include:
- Selection of patient group and diagnosis, procedures, or conditions, based on analysis of data and observations of wide variance in approach to treatment and prioritizing organization and patient needs.
- Creation of interdisciplinary team of those involved in the process of care, including physicians to develop pathway.
- Analysis of data includes literature review and study of best practices to identify opportunities for quality improvement.
- Identification of all categories of care, such as nutrition, medications, nursing.
- Discussion, reaching consensus.
- Identifying the levels of care and number of days to be covered by the pathway.
- Pilot testing and redesigning steps as indicated.
- Educating staff about standards.
- Monitoring and tracking variances in order to improve pathways.

Basic research concepts

The nurse must be taught and understand the process of critical analysis and know how to conduct a survey of the literature. Basic research concepts include:
- **Survey of valid sources:** Information from a juried journal and an anonymous website or personal website are very different sources, and evaluating what constitutes a valid source of data is critical.
- **Evaluation of internal and external validity:** Internal validity shows a cause and effect relationship between two variables, with the cause occurring before the effect and no intervening variable. External validity occurs when results hold true in different environments and circumstances with different populations.
- **Sample selection and sample size:** Selection and size can have a huge impact on the results, but a sample that is too small may lack both internal and external validity. Selection may be so narrowly focused that the results can't be generalized to others groups.

Critical reading

There are a number of steps to critical reading to evaluate research:
- **Consider the source** of the material. If it is in the popular press, it may have little validity compared to something published in a juried journal.
- **Review the author's credentials** to determine if a person is an expert in the field of study.
- **Determine thesis**, or the central claim of the research. It should be clearly stated.
- **Examine the organization** of the article, whether it is based on a particular theory, and the type of methodology used.

- **Review the evidence** to determine how it is used to support the main points. Look for statistical evidence and sample size to determine if the findings have wide applicability.
- **Evaluate** the overall article to determine if the information seems credible and useful and should be communicated to administration and/or staff.

Internal and external validity, generalizability, and replication

Many research studies are most concerned with internal validity, adequate unbiased data properly collected and analyzed within the population studied, but studies that determine the efficacy of procedures or treatments, for example, should have external validity as well; that is, the results should be generalizable (true) for similar populations. Replication of the study with different subjects, researchers, and under different circumstances should produce similar results. For various reasons, some people may be excluded from a study so that instead of randomized subjects, the subjects may be highly selected so when data is compared with another population in which there is less or more selection, results may be different. The selection of subjects, in this case, would interfere with external validity. Part of the design of a study should include considerations of whether or not it should have external validity or whether there is value for the institution based solely on internal validation.

Selection and information bias

Selection bias occurs when the method of selecting subjects results in a cohort that is not representative of the target population because of inherent error in design. For example, if all patients who develop urinary infections are evaluated per urine culture and sensitivities for microbial resistance, but only those patients with clinically-evident infections are included, a number of patients with sub-clinical infections may be missed, skewing the results. Selection bias is only a concern when participants in studies are specifically chosen. Many surveillance studies do not involve selection of subjects.

Information bias occurs when there are errors in classification, so an estimate of association is incorrect. Non-differential misclassification occurs when there is similar misclassification of disease or exposure among both those who are diseased/exposed and those who are not. Differential misclassification occurs when there is a differing misclassification of disease or exposure among both those who are diseased/exposed and those who are not.

Qualitative and quantitative data

Both qualitative and quantitative data are used for analysis, but the focus is quite different:
- **Qualitative data**: Data are described verbally or graphically, and the results are subjective, depending upon observers to provide information. Interviews may be used as a tool to gather information, and the researcher's interpretation of data is important. Gathering this type of data can be time-intensive, and it can usually not be generalized to a larger population. This type of information gathering is often useful at the beginning of the design process for data collection.
- **Quantitative data**: Data are described in terms of numbers within a statistical format. This type of information gathering is done after the design of data collection is outlined, usually in later stages. Tools may include surveys, questionnaires, or other methods of obtaining numerical data. The researcher's role is objective.

Hypothesis and hypothesis testing

A hypothesis should be generated about the probable cause of the disease/infection based on the information available in laboratory and medical records, epidemiologic study, literature review, and expert opinion. A hypothesis, for example, should include the infective agent, the likely source, and the mode of transmission: "Wound infections with *Staphylococcus aureus* were caused by reuse and inadequate sterilization of single-use irrigation syringes used during wound care in the ICU." Hypothesis testing includes data analysis, laboratory findings, and outcomes of environmental testing. It usually includes case control studies, with 2-4 controls picked for each case of infection. They may be matched according to age, sex, or other characteristics, but they are not infected at the time they are picked for the study. Cohort studies, whose controls are picked based on having or lacking exposure, may also be instituted. If the hypothesis cannot be supported, then a new hypothesis or different testing methods may be necessary.

Outcomes evaluation and evidence-based practice

Outcomes evaluation is an important component of evidence-based practice, which involves both internal and external research. All treatments are subjected to review to determine if they produce positive outcomes, and policies and protocols for outcomes evaluation should be in place. Outcomes evaluation includes the following:

- **Monitoring** over the course of treatment involves careful observation and record keeping that notes progress, with supporting laboratory and radiographic evidence as indicated by condition and treatment.
- **Evaluating** results includes reviewing records as well as current research to determine if outcomes are within acceptable parameters.
- **Sustaining** involves continuing treatment, but continuing to monitor and evaluate.
- **Improving** means to continue the treatment but with additions or modifications in order to improve outcomes.
- **Replacing** the treatment with a different treatment must be done if outcomes evaluation indicates that current treatment is ineffective.

Facilitation of Learning

Facilitation of learning requires needs assessment and preparation of content that is suited for the receiver in terms of delivery and content. Levels of facilitation of learning include:

- Level 1: This nurse is able to deliver planned educational content that is disease specific but does not have the ability to assess patient readiness to learn or abilities. The patient/family is considered a passive recipient of knowledge.
- Level 3: This nurse is able to individualize treatment according to patient/family needs and has an understanding of different methods of teaching and learning styles. The patient's needs are considered in planning.
- Level 5: This nurse has excellent understanding of teaching methods, learning styles, and assessment for learning readiness and develops an educational plan in cooperation and collaboration with others, including patients, families, and other health and allied professionals.

Development of goals, measurable objectives, and lesson plans

Once a topic for performance improvement education has been chosen, then goals, measurable objectives with strategies, and lesson plans must be developed. A class should stay focused on one area rather than trying to cover many things. For example:

Goal: Increase compliance with hand hygiene standards in ICU.

Objectives:
- Develop series of posters and fliers by June 1.
- Observe 100% compliance with hand hygiene standards at 2 weeks, 1-month, and 2-month intervals after training is completed.

Strategies:
- Conduct 4 classes at different times over a one-week period, May 25-31.
- Place posters in all nursing units, staff rooms, and utility rooms by January 3.
- Develop PowerPoint presentation for class and Intranet/Internet for access by all staff by May 25.
- Utilize handwashing kits.

Lesson plans:
- Discussion period: Why do we need 100% compliance?
- PowerPoint: The case for hand hygiene.
- Discussion: What did you learn?
- Demonstration and activities to show effectiveness
- Handwashing technique.

Approaches to teaching

There are many approaches to teaching, and the nurse educator must prepare, present, and coordinate a wide range of educational workshops, lectures, discussions, and one-on-one instructions on any chosen topic. All types of classes will be needed, depending upon the purpose and material:
- **Educational workshops** are usually conducted with small groups, allowing for maximal participation and are especially good for demonstrations and practice sessions.
- **Lectures** are often used for more academic or detailed information that may include questions and answers but limits discussion. An effective lecture should include some audiovisual support.
- **Discussions** are best with small groups so that people can actively participate. This is a good for problem solving.
- **One-on-one instruction** is especially helpful for targeted instruction in procedures for individuals.
- **Computer/Internet modules** are good for independent learners.

Participants should be asked to evaluate the presentations in the forms of surveys or suggestions, but ultimately the program is evaluated in terms of patient outcomes.

Videos

Videos are a useful adjunct to teaching as they reduce the time needed for one-on-one instruction (increasing cost-effectiveness). Passive presentation of videos, such as in the waiting area, has little value, but focused viewing in which the nurse discusses the purpose of the video presentation prior to viewing and then is available for discussion after viewing can be very effective. Patients and/or families are often nervous about learning patient care and are unsure of their abilities, so they may not focus completely when the nurse is presenting information. Allowing the patients/families to watch a video demonstration or explanation first and allowing them to stop or review the video presentation can help them to grasp the fundamentals before they have to apply them, relieving some of the anxiety them may be experiencing. Videos are much more effective than written materials for those with low literacy or poor English skills. The nurse should always be available to answer questions and discuss the material after the patients/families finish viewing.

Readability

Studies have indicated that learning is more effective if oral presentations and/or demonstrations are supplemented with reading materials, such as handouts. Readability (the grade level of material) is a concern because many patients and families may have limited English skills or low literacy, and it can be difficult for the nurse to assess people's reading level. The average American reads effectively at the 6th to 8th grade level (regardless of education achieved), but many health education materials have a much higher readability level. Additionally, research indicates that even people with much higher reading skills learn medical and health information most effectively when the material is presented at the 6th to 8th grade readability level. Therefore, patient education materials (and consent forms) should not be written at higher than 6th to 8th grade level. Readability index calculators are available on the Internet to give an approximation of grade level and difficulty for those preparing materials without expertise in teaching reading.

Changes in policies, procedures, or working standards

Changes in policies, procedures, or working standards are common and, the quality professional is responsible for educating the staff about changes related to processes, which should be communicated to staff in an effective and timely manner:

- **Policies** are usually changed after a period of discussion and review by administration and staff, so all staff should be made aware of policies under discussion. Preliminary information should be disseminated to staff regarding the issue during meetings or through printed notices.
- **Procedures** may be changed to increase efficiency or improve patient safety often as the result of surveillance and data about outcomes. Procedures changes are best communicated in workshops with demonstrations. Posters and handouts should be available as well.
- **Working standards** are often changed because of regulatory or accrediting requirements and this information should be covered extensively in a variety of different ways: discussions, workshops, handouts so that the implications are clearly understood.

Learning styles

Not all people are aware of their preferred learning style. A range of teaching materials/methods that relates to all 3 learning preferences—visual, auditory, kinesthetic—(and appropriate for different ages) should be available. Part of assessment for teaching involves choosing the right approach based on observation and feedback. Often presenting learners with different options gives a clue to their preferred learning style. Some people have a combined learning style:

Visual learners
- Learn best by seeing and reading:
- Provide written directions, picture guides, or demonstrate procedures. Use charts and diagrams.
- Provide photos, videos.

Auditory learners
- Learn best by listening and talking:
- Explain procedures while demonstrating and have learner repeat.
- Plan extra time to discuss and answer questions.
- Provide audiotapes.

Kinesthetic learners
- Learn best by handling, doing, and practicing:
- Provide hands-on experience throughout teaching.
- Encourage handling of supplies/equipment.
- Allow learner to demonstrate.
- Minimize instructions and allow person to explore equipment and procedures.

Principles of adult learning

Adults have a wealth of life and/or employment experiences. Their attitudes toward education may vary considerably.   There are, however, some principles of adult learning and typical characteristics of adult learners that an instructor should consider when planning strategies for teaching parents, families, or staff:

Practical and goal oriented
- Provide overviews or summaries and examples.
- Use collaborative discussions with problem-solving exercises.
- Remain organized with the goal in mind.

Self-directed
- Provide active involvement, asking for input.
- Allow different options toward achieving the goal.
- Give them responsibilities.

Knowledgeable
- Show respect for their life experiences/ education.
- Validate their knowledge and ask for feedback.
- Relate new material to information with which they are familiar.

Relevancy-oriented
- Explain how information will be applied.
- Clearly identify objectives.

Motivated
- Provide certificates of professional advancement and/or continuing education credit for staff when possible.

Bloom's taxonomy

Bloom's taxonomy outlines behaviors that are necessary for learning, and this can apply to healthcare. The theory describes 3 types of learning:

Cognitive - (Learning and gaining intellectual skills to master 6 categories of effective learning.)
- Knowledge
- Comprehension
- Application
- Analysis
- Synthesis
- Evaluation.

Affective - (Recognizing 5 categories of feelings and values from simple to complex. This is slower to achieve than cognitive learning.)
- Receiving phenomena: Accepting need to learn
- Responding to phenomena: Taking active part in care
- Valuing: Understanding value of becoming independent in care
- Organizing values: Understanding how surgery/treatment has improved life
- Internalizing values: Accepting condition as part of life, being consistent and self-reliant

Psychomotor - (Mastering 7 categories necessary for independence. This follows a progression from simple to complex.)
- Perception: Uses sensory information to learn tasks
- Set: Shows willingness to perform tasks
- Guided response: Follows directions
- Mechanism: Does specific tasks
- Complex overt response: Displays competence in self-care
- Adaptation: Modifies procedures as needed
- Origination: Creatively deals with problems.

Behavior modification and compliance rate

Education, like all interventions, must be evaluated for effectiveness. Two determinants of effectiveness include:

- **Behavior modification** involves thorough observation and measurement, identifying behavior that needs to be changed and then planning and instituting interventions to modify that behavior. An ACNP can use a variety of techniques, including demonstrations of appropriate behavior, reinforcement, and monitoring until new behavior is adopted consistently. This is especially important when longstanding procedures and habits of behavior are changed.
- **Compliance rates** are often determined by observation, which should be done at intervals and on multiple occasions, but with patients, this may depend on self-reports. Outcomes is another measure of compliance; that is, if education is intended to improve patient health and reduce risk factors and that occurs, it is a good indication that there is compliance. Compliance rates are calculated by determining the number of events/procedures and degree of compliance.

Learner outcomes

When the quality professional plans an educational offering, whether it be a class, an online module, a workshop, or educational materials, the professional should identify learner outcomes, which should be conveyed to the learners from the very beginning so that they are aware of the expectations. The subject matter of the educational material and the learner outcomes should be directly related. For example, if the quality professional is giving a class on decontamination of the environment, then a learner outcome might be: "Identify the difference between disinfectants and antiseptics." There may be one or multiple learner outcomes, but part of the assessment at the end of the learning experience should be to determine if, in fact, the learner outcomes have been achieved. A survey of whether or not the learners felt that they had achieved the learner outcomes can give valuable feedback and guidance to the quality professional.

Patient/family education instruction

Both one-on-one instruction and group **instruction** have a place in patient/family education.

- **One-on-one instruction** is the most costly for an institution because it is time intensive. However, it allows the patient and family more interaction with the nurse instructor and allows them to have more control over the process by asking questions or having the instructor repeat explanations or demonstrations. One-on-one instruction is especially valuable when patients and families must learn particular skills, such as managing dialysis, or if confidentiality is important.
- **Group instruction** is the less costly because the needs of a number of people can be met at one time. Group presentations are more planned and usually scheduled for a particular time period (an hour, for example), so patients and families have less control. Questioning is usually more limited and may be done only at the end. Group instruction allows patients/families with similar health problems to interact. Group instruction is especially useful for general types of instruction, such as managing diet or other lifestyle issues.

Readiness to learn

The patient/family's readiness to learn should be assessed because if they are not ready, instruction is of little value. Often readiness is indicated when the patient/family asks questions or shows and interest in procedures. There are a number of factors related to readiness to learn:

- **Physical factors:** There are a number of physical factors than can affect ability. Manual dexterity may be required to complete a task, and this varies by age and condition. Hearing or vision deficits may impact ability. Complex tasks may be too difficult for some because of weakness or cognitive impairment, and modifications of the environment may be needed. Health status, age, and gender may all impact the ability to learn.
- **Experience**: People's experience with learning can vary widely and is affected by their ability to cope with changes, their personal goals, motivation to learn, and cultural background. People may have widely divergent ideas about what constitutes illness and/or treatment. Lack of English skills may make learning difficult and prevent people from asking questions.
- **Mental/emotional status:** The support system and motivation may impact readiness. Anxiety, fear, or depression about condition can make learning very difficult because the patient/family cannot focus on learning, so the nurse must spend time to reassure the patient/family and wait until they are emotionally more receptive.
- **Knowledge/education:** The knowledge base of the patient/family, their cognitive ability, and their learning styles all affect their readiness to learn. The nurse should always begin by assessing what knowledge the patient/family already has about their disease, condition, or treatment and then build form that base. People with little medical experience may lack knowledge of basic medical terminology, interfering with their ability and readiness to learn.

Practice Test

Practice Questions

1. Therapeutic hypothermia is ordered for a patient who was resuscitated from a cardiac arrest associated with ventricular tachycardia. What is the optimal temperature range that should be maintained for therapeutic hypothermia?
    A. 28° C/82.4° F to 30° C/86° F
    B. 30° C/86° F to 32° C/89.6° F
    C. 32° C/89.6° F to 34° C/93.2° F
    D. 34° C/93.2° F to 36° C/96.8° F

2. Which electrolyte imbalance is the most life threatening for patients with renal failure?
    A. hypernatremia
    B. hyponatremia
    C. hypokalemia
    D. hyperkalemia

3. A patient who is undergoing rehabilitation after severe traumatic injuries is depressed about his condition and concerned about his ability to live independently. What is the most effective strategy for the nurse to help improve the patient's motivation?
    A. Provide positive feedback about tasks he is able to complete.
    B. Assist him in developing a list of long-term goals.
    C. Compare his present abilities to his abilities immediately after the injury.
    D. Tell him that everyone feels the same way during therapy.

4. A non-diabetic patient with a Foley catheter develops sudden onset of increased temperature (39° C); a heart rate of 108/min; a respiratory rate of 32/min; peripheral edema with decreased capillary refill; serum glucose of 160 mg/dL; WBC of 16,000; platelet count of 95,000; blood pressure of 86/52 mm Hg; urinary output of 0.2 mL/kg/hr; and flushed skin. The most likely diagnosis is
    A. bacteremia.
    B. pyelonephritis.
    C. sepsis.
    D. kidney failure.

5. A nurse believes that a clinical pathway for treatment of hospitalized asthma patients would help to standardize care and improve patient outcomes. What type of team should be involved in development of the clinical pathway?
    A. nurses and physicians
    B. respiratory therapists and physicians
    C. interdisciplinary team
    D. physicians only

6. Which of the following is an example of a well-written learning objective?
    A. "After attending a workshop about hypertension, the patient will be able to state 4 causes for high blood pressure."
    B. "The patient will understand how to monitor blood sugar."
    C. "The nurse will provide a demonstration on use of the Bi-PAP machine."
    D. "After instruction about infection prevention, the patient will understand infection control procedures."

7. Following brain surgery, a patient's intracranial pressure has increased. What $PaCO_2$ level is optimal to control increased ICP?
    A. 35-38 mm Hg
    B. 38-45 mm Hg
    C. 24-27 mm Hg
    D. 27-32 mm Hg

8. An alert elderly patient has multiple bruises on the chest, back, abdomen, and both arms in various stages of healing and seems fearful and withdrawn when her daughter, who is her caregiver, is present. When questioned about the bruising, the patient states she "fell." The nurse should
    A. question the daughter about the bruising.
    B. report the observations to adult protective services.
    C. ask the hospital social worker to speak with the patient.
    D. report observations to administration.

9. A 38-year-old patient with acute respiratory distress syndrome (ARDS) is placed on mechanical ventilation. The optimal setting for tidal volume for ARDS is usually
    A. 12 mL/kg predicted body weight.
    B. 10 mL/kg predicted body weight.
    C. 6-8 mL/kg predicted body weight.
    D. 4-5 mL/kg predicted body weight.

10. A 36-year-old patient with Guillain-Barré syndrome is hospitalized with ascending paralysis and acute respiratory distress. The patient is stabilized and placed on mechanical ventilation. Which treatment is most indicated to reduce symptoms?
    A. IV Ig or plasmapheresis
    B. corticosteroids
    C. antiviral medications
    D. immunoadsorption

11. A patient with a history of previous myocardial infarction presents with dyspnea and audible basilar rales as well as 2+ peripheral edema. The patient's respiratory rate is 34/min and heart rate is 104/min with lateral displacement of the apical beat. Blood pressure is 162/94 mm Hg. Despite administration of 100% oxygen, the patient's oxygen saturation level is 92% and the patient reports that he feels very short of breath and insists on sitting in tripod position. Which intervention is most indicated to relieve the patient's dyspnea?
    A. morphine sulfate
    B. furosemide IV
    C. CPAP or Bi-PAP
    D. endotracheal intubation with mechanical ventilation

12. A patient who suffered penetrating chest trauma is recovering from surgical repair but complains of increasing chest pain and dyspnea and appears cyanotic. Pulse is 110/min and BP is 80/48 mm HG, and pulsus paradoxus is evident. When auscultating the heart, the nurse notes a mill wheel murmur and shifting tympany when percussing the heart with the patient supine and then sitting upright. Hamman's sign is negative. The most likely cause is
    A. pneumomediastinum.
    B. pneumopericardium.
    C. cardiac tamponade.
    D. pneumothorax.

13. A 68-year-old man with a history of alcoholism has developed sudden onset of severe epigastric pain radiating to the back after eating. The pain is exacerbated when the patient lies flat or walks. He is pale and tachycardic and has nausea and vomiting and a temperature of 39° C. Physical examination shows the upper abdomen is tender but not rigid and without guarding. The most likely cause of these symptoms is
    A. hepatitis.
    B. acute cholecystitis.
    C. small bowel obstruction.
    D. pancreatitis.

14. A patient who is 24-hour postoperative after a pulmonary lobectomy requests pain medication for severe pain, but when the nurse brings the opioid medication a few minutes later, the nurse finds the patient laughing and talking with family. The nurse should
    A. give the patient the opioid medication.
    B. ask the patient if she still needs the pain medication.
    C. withhold the pain medication altogether.
    D. exchange the opioid for acetaminophen.

15. A patient who is restless pulls out his chest tube when trying to get out of bed independently, and no dressing supplies are available at bedside. What immediate action is indicated?
    A. Call for assistance and dressing supplies.
    B. Hold a folded washcloth against the insertion site.
    C. Cover the insertion site with a clean, gloved hand.
    D. Ask the patient to place his hand over insertion site and go for dressings.

16. During the post-surgical period following a bowel resection, a patient develops sudden dyspnea with tachypnea, chest pain, anxiety, fever, and cough. Which of the following tests is most indicated to diagnose pulmonary embolus?
    A. arterial blood gas
    B. D-dimer
    C. CT-PA
    D. chest radiograph

17. A patient with a history of heart failure and supraventricular dysrhythmias has been maintained on digoxin but has developed bradycardia (48 bpm), headache, fatigue, nausea, diarrhea, and green halo vision. The physician has ordered serum digoxin, electrolyte levels, and continuous ECG monitoring. Which of the following electrolyte values would be most concerning?
    A. potassium of 3.2 mEq/L
    B. potassium of 5 mEq/L
    C. sodium 140 mEq/L
    D. magnesium 2 mEq/L

18. Which of the following reactions after a bee sting indicates the patient is at high risk for anaphylaxis?
    A. severe pain at site of sting
    B. itching localized hives about sting site.
    C. swelling extends beyond sting site, involving an entire limb
    D. urticaria, edema, and itching in areas distant from sting

19. A patient is brought to the emergency department with suspected substance abuse. The patient exhibits euphoria, restlessness, hyperactivity, tachycardia, hypertension, dilated pupils, and rhinitis. Which of the following substances did the patient most likely use?
    A. barbiturate (Valium)
    B. heroin
    C. cocaine
    D. amphetamines

20. A patient with paroxysmal supraventricular tachycardia has received IV adenosine in order to slow the heart rate and convert to a sinus rhythm. Following administration of the drug, the nurse should carefully monitor the patient for
    A. ventricular fibrillation.
    B. transient asystole.
    C. premature ventricular contractions.
    D. facial flushing.

21. With chronic kidney disease, potassium-sparing diuretics are recommended for
    A. patients with persistent hypokalemia.
    B. all patients with chronic kidney disease.
    C. patients with hyporeninemic hypoaldosteronism.
    D. patients who cannot tolerate hydrochlorothiazide.

22. A patient has been admitted with unstable angina but without cardiac enzyme elevation. During periods when the patient is pain-free, the nurse notes the following 12-lead ECG changes (Wellens syndrome): slight elevation of ST segments in leads V1 and V3; terminal T-wave inversion in V2 to V3; and intact R waves. This patient is at risk for
    A. ventricular arrhythmias.
    B. acute posterior wall myocardial infarction.
    C. atrial fibrillation.
    D. acute anterior wall myocardial infarction.

23 A patient with valvular diseases has continuous ECG monitoring and shows the following ECG tracing:

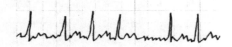

Which of the following best describes this pattern?
A. atrial flutter
B. atrial fibrillation
C. premature ventricular contractions
D. premature atrial contractions

24. A patient has a chest tube in place and all connections are tight, but bubbling is occurring in the water seal container. What initial action is indicated?
A. No initial action is indicated because this is a normal finding.
B. Immediately change drainage system.
C. Clamp the drainage tube close to chest tube and observe water seal.
D. Listen for the sound of hissing.

25. A patient with myasthenia gravis develops sudden exacerbation of these symptoms: extreme weakness, inability to hold up their head, missing gag reflex. The patient is anxious, dyspneic, and tachypneic. Which of the following diagnostic tests is best to differentiate between myasthenic and cholinergic crises?
A. tensilon test
B. MRI
C. ice pack test
D. electromyography

26. A patient with bradyarrhythmia has not responded to pharmaceutical intervention (atropine) and is experiencing hemodynamic instability, so transcutaneous pacing has been initiated. The rate of pacing is usually set at
A. 80 to 90 bpm
B. 70 to 80 bpm
C. 60 to 70 bpm
D. 50 to 60 bpm

27. The most common cause of hospital-associated pneumonia (HAP) is
A. mechanical ventilation.
B. bed rest in a supine position.
C. previous antibiotic therapy.
D. poor hand-washing practices.

28. What precaution should be used when administering IV mannitol solution to patients in order to control increased intracranial pressure?
A. chill solution prior to administration.
B. administer solution through a filter.
C. heat solution prior to administration.
D. administer a test dose to determine response.

29. Which of the following is an indication for intubation and mechanical ventilation for a patient presenting with possible status asthmaticus?
    A. ABGs showing hypocapnia and respiratory alkalosis
    B. pulsus paradoxus of 20 mm Hg
    C. peak expiratory flow rate 38% of predicted
    D. FEV1 25% of predicted

30. The pacing mode that is most commonly used with temporary transvenous pacing is
    A. DDD.
    B. AOO.
    C. VDD.
    D. VVI.

31. A patient with severe urinary tract infection and bacteremia begins to develop petechiae and purpura and is bleeding at the IV site. The patient passes bloody diarrhea. BP is 64/48 mm HG and pulse is 122/min. Recent laboratory findings include increased WBC count, decreased platelet count, and fragmented RBCs. Which further laboratory testing should the nurse anticipate?
    A. liver function tests
    B. kidney function tests
    C. DIC panel
    D. arterial blood gases

32. A 72-year-old man underwent a total knee replacement. Prior to surgery he was alert, responsive, and oriented, but 24 hours after surgery he is having fluctuating periods of confusion with sudden changes in consciousness, inability to sustain attention, disorientation, and visual hallucinations. The most effective pharmaceutical intervention is
    A. lorazepam (Ativan).
    B. benztropine (Cogentin).
    C. chlordiazepoxide (Librium).
    D. paroxetine (Paxil).

33. An older adult who recently traveled in an area endemic to West Nile virus presents with poliomyelitis-like symptoms, including fever, headache, flaccid quadriplegic paralysis, bladder dysfunction, and cranial nerve involvement. What complication should the nurse anticipate most?
    A. heart failure
    B. respiratory failure
    C. disseminated intravascular coagulation
    D. deep vein thrombosis/pulmonary embolism

34. A patient with post-surgical left ventricular failure and low cardiac output has an intra-aortic balloon pump (IABP) inserted. At which point in the cardiac cycle should inflation occur?
    A. end of diastole
    B. beginning of systole
    C. end of systole
    D. beginning of diastole

35. When preparing written materials for patient education, the maximum word length for a sentence should be
  A. 30.
  B. 25.
  C. 20.
  D. 15.

36. A patient with cardiac ischemia develops a hypertensive crisis with blood pressure of 240/130 mm Hg. Which initial pharmaceutical treatment is usually indicated?
  A. sodium nitroprusside
  B. short-acting beta-blockers (labetalol or esmolol)
  C. furosemide
  D. alpha blocker

37. The nurse is reviewing the medication list with a 76-year-old patient who takes multiple drugs for heart disease and COPD, including warfarin and theophylline. Which of the following OTC drugs that the patient reports using regularly is likely to be the most problematic?
  A. acetaminophen
  B. cimetidine
  C. docusate sodium stool softener
  D. topical cortisone cream

38. A patient with a tracheostomy is to receive the Passy-Muir valve to facilitate communication and improve swallowing. What change must be made when placing the valve on the tracheostomy tube?
  A. cuff deflated
  B. cuff inflation increased
  C. no changes necessary
  D. cuff inflation decreased by approximately 50%.

39. A patient who is taking metformin for diabetes mellitus, type 2, is also taking metoprolol for junctional tachycardia and has been prescribed hydrochlorothiazide for persistent elevated blood pressure. What is the primary concern with this drug combination?
  A. increased tachycardia
  B. hyperglycemia
  C. renal failure
  D. muscle cramps

40. A patient with SIRS is at risk for developing MODS. Which organ system is usually the first to fail?
  A. cardiac
  B. renal
  C. hepatic
  D. pulmonary

41. The physician has ordered position therapy for a patient with acute lung injury (ALI) in order to improve oxygenation. Which position is most likely to improve oxygenation and ventilation/perfusion matching and decrease shunting?
    A. supine, flat
    B. supine with head of bed elevated
    C. right or left side lying (most damaged lung in dependent position)
    D. prone

42. If a patient is receiving oxygen therapy with a mask with a reservoir bag and the flow rate is set at 6, what is the estimated FiO_2?
    A. 40%
    B. 50%
    C. 60%
    D. 100%

43. A patient with bronchogenic small (oat) cell carcinoma exhibits lethargy, anorexia, nausea, and vomiting. Urinary output is diminished, and urine specific gravity is increased. Serum sodium is 122 mEq/L, and the patient is beginning to have difficulty concentrating and exhibiting confusion. Based on these observations, the most likely cause is
    A. diabetes insipidus.
    B. hypothyroidism.
    C. renal metastasis.
    D. syndrome of inappropriate secretion of antidiuretic hormone.

44. A patient with a history of COPD and heavy smoking is admitted with respiratory distress, using accessory muscles for breathing. The assessment findings include a heart rate of 122/min; a blood pressure of 86/42 mm Hg; SpO_2 of 80%; diminished lung sounds, especial on the left; tracheal deviation on the right; and increased venous distention. Based on these findings, the most likely cause is
    A. viral pneumonia.
    B. pleural effusion.
    C. aspiration pneumonia.
    D. tension pneumothorax.

45. The three characteristics most often associated with cardiogenic shock include
    A. increased preload, increased afterload, and decreased contractility.
    B. decreased preload, decreased afterload, and decreased contractility.
    C. increased preload, increased afterload, and increased contractility.
    D. increased preload, decreased afterload, and decreased contractility.

46. When auscultating heart sounds, the nurse notes an ejection click, a brief high-pitched sound that occurs immediately after S1. This heart sound is associated with
    A. left ventricular failure.
    B. aortic valve stenosis.
    C. pericarditis.
    D. mitral valve stenosis.

47. An elderly Chinese woman with inoperable metastatic liver cancer believes she has a "liver infection" that will improve with time. Her family members have asked that the patient be shielded from the truth because of her fear of cancer, and the physician has agreed. The best action for the nurse is to
  A. take the issue to the ethics committee.
  B. tell the patient the truth.
  C. respect the family's wishes.
  D. report the physician to administration.

48. A patient with bleeding esophageal varices has undergone balloon tamponade to control sudden onset of bleeding before more definitive therapy can be carried out. What is the maximum period of time that balloon tamponade can be maintained?
  A. 4 hours
  B. 8 hours
  C. 12 hours
  D. 24 hours

49. A patient with atrial fibrillation is to undergo cardioversion. What pharmaceutical intervention is usually prescribed three weeks prior to cardioversion?
  A. digoxin
  B. loop diuretic
  C. anticoagulant
  D. beta blocker

50. A patient receiving total parental nutrition (TPN) exhibits signs of dehydration (dry mucous membranes, decreased ski turgor), increased BUN, and increased urinary specific gravity. The most likely complication resulting in these findings is
  A. hypoglycemia.
  B. hyperammonemia.
  C. azotemia.
  D. deficiency of essential fatty acids.

51. A patient who has undergone open-heart surgery and cardiopulmonary bypass (CPB) has an amylase level of 1100 in the early post-surgical period. This indicates
  A. increased risk of myocardial infarction.
  B. increased risk of hypertensive crisis.
  C. a normal value after CPB.
  D. increased risk of pancreatitis.

52. An 80-year-old patient who lives alone is generally in good health but has shown a steady decline with evidence of malaise, lack of appetite, and weight loss. Laboratory tests and physical examination show no abnormalities other than slight anemia and mild hypertension. The patient is able to carry out ADLs but shows little interest in other activities and has withdrawn from social interactions. Which of the following assessments is most indicated?
  A. Index of Independence of Activities of Daily Living (Katz Index)
  B. Confusion Assessment Method
  C. Palliative Performance Scale
  D. Geriatric Depression Scale

53. When assessing jugular venous pressure, the normal height of the jugular vein pulsation above the sternal angle is less than or equal to
   A. 2 cm.
   B. 4 cm.
   C. 5 cm.
   D. 6 cm.

54. A 50-year-old female patient who has recovered from a recent myocardial infarction is prescribed clopidogrel bisulfate to reduce the risk of thrombus formation. Which statement by the patient indicates the need for further education about the drug?
   A. "I check my skin for signs of bruising when I shower."
   B. "I take acetaminophen for my arthritis pain."
   C. "I take red clover supplement to help reduce hot flashes."
   D. "I can take the pill before or after breakfast."

55. When assisting with insertion of a pulmonary artery catheter, the nurse should inflate the balloon when the catheter
   A. reaches the right atrium.
   B. enters the right ventricle.
   C. enters the pulmonary artery.
   D. reaches the superior vena cava.

56. A patient with alcoholism is admitted after an episode of prolonged binge drinking. He has been a heavy drinker, drinking over a pint of distilled alcoholic beverage daily for over 20 years. His blood alcohol level on admission is 0.3. Which of the following symptoms indicates onset of delirium tremens?
   A. impaired judgment, slurred speech, and unsteady gait
   B. nausea, vomiting, and anxiety
   C. audio and visual hallucinations, agitation, and tremor
   D. global confusion, fever, tachycardia, and, hallucinations

57. A patient with a pulmonary artery catheter in place is restless and moving about. The waveform indicates spontaneous wedging, suggesting that the catheter may have migrated and may result in pulmonary artery infarction. What is the initial intervention?
   A. turn the patient onto the opposite side of the catheter placement.
   B. flush all air from the system.
   C. inflate and deflate the balloon.
   D. withdraw catheter into right atrium.

58. A patient has recently been diagnosed with celiac disease after tests to determine the cause of chronic weight loss, anemia, diarrhea, rash, bone pain, and irregular menses. When discussing dietary interventions, the nurse tells the patient that celiac disease may result in malabsorption of
   A. vitamin B_{12}.
   B. folate and iron.
   C. vitamin C.
   D. vitamin D.

59. Following an automobile accident with abdominal trauma, intra-abdominal pressure is monitored for compartment syndrome. Which of the following intra-abdominal pressures is the minimum pressure that generally indicates the need for surgical decompression?
    A. 5 mm Hg
    B. 13 mm Hg
    C. 20 mm Hg
    D. 26 mm Hg

60. What pressure setting is usually used initially when titrating CPAP?
    A. 1 cm H_2O
    B. 5 cm H_2O
    C. 10 cm H_2O
    D. 20 cm H_2O

61. If a patient's cardiac output is 5.6 L/min and the heart rate is 80/min, the stroke volume is
    A. 0.7 mL
    B. 7 mL
    C. 70 mL
    D. 700 mL

62. A 72-year-old male patient with an acute MI and left ventricular failure has a pulmonary artery catheter in place for hemodynamic monitoring and is developing cardiogenic shock. Hemodynamics include a blood pressure (BP) of 90/60 mm Hg, a heart rate (HR) of 120/min, MAP of 70, SV of 25 mL/min, RAP of 8 mm Hg, PAP of 36/24 mm Hg, PAWP of 20 mm Hg, CO of 3 L/min, CI of 1.5 L/min/m², and SVR of 1626 dynes/sec cm^{-5}. The patient receives oxygen, dobutamine, and nitroprusside. What hemodynamic changes should the nurse expect as a positive response?
    A. increased CO and SV and decreased HR, SVR, and PAWP
    B. decreased HR and increased CO and PAWP
    C. increased CO, SV, SVR, and PAWP and decrease HR
    D. increased HR, CO, SV, and decrease PAWP and SVR

63. A patient is hospitalized with a transmural Q-wave myocardial infarction. In how many hours will the CK level peak?
    A. 3
    B. 14
    C. 27
    D. 45

64. Which of the following changes in fluid intelligence are associated with age?
    A. decreased test anxiety
    B. altered time perception
    C. decreased long-term memory
    D. increased reaction time

65. A patient whose intermittent claudication had progressed to rest pain and had not responded to conservative treatment has undergone a fem-pop bypass. The patient complains of numbness and tingling on the anterior and medial aspect of the leg. This suggests
    A. damage to the femoral nerve.
    B. occlusion of the femoral artery.
    C. normal postoperative sensation.
    D. bypass occlusion.

66. Which of the following drugs puts the patient with diabetes mellitus, type 2, most at risk for episodes of acute hypoglycemia?
    A. metformin (Glucophage)
    B. rosiglitazone (Avandia)
    C. exenatide (Byetta)
    D. glipizide (Glucotrol)

67. A patient with bilateral lung transplants has developed recurrent respiratory infections and increased exercise intolerance with a decline in FEV1. The patient is diagnosed with bronchiolitis obliterans. Which of the follow treatment options is most likely to be taken?
    A. no treatment
    B. increased immunosuppression
    C. decreased immunosuppression
    D. antibiotics

68. A patient who is taking warfarin is scheduled for cardiac catheterization. How long prior to the catheterization should the patient discontinue the warfarin?
    A. 24 hours
    B. two to three days
    C. one week
    D. two weeks

69. A patient has been hospitalized with nausea and vomiting but minimal abdominal distention. The patient has not passed flatus in 14 hours, and abdominal x-ray shows dilated small bowel loops and no colonic or rectal gas. The patient's CBC and electrolytes are within normal limits. Based on these findings, the nurse should suspect that the primary initial intervention will be
    A. contrast studies.
    B. NG suction.
    C. exploratory surgery.
    D. observation.

70. A patient with chronic heart failure develops severe dyspnea, cough with frothy slightly blood-tinged sputum, cyanosis, and diaphoresis. The nurse notes wheezing, rales, and rhonchi throughout the lung fields. Which initial intervention is indicated?
    A. Administer morphine sulfate subcutaneously or IV.
    B. Sit patient upright and administer 100% oxygen with mask.
    C. Provide antibiotic therapy.
    D. Administer furosemide IV.

71. Following percutaneous transluminal coronary angioplasty with right femoral access, the patient complains of right back and flank pain and non-specific complaints of feeling weak and dizzy. Her heart rate increases to 112/min and blood pressure is 78/52 mm Hg. Based on these findings, the nurse should suspect
    A. cardiac tamponade.
    B. allergic reaction.
    C. myocardial infarction.
    D. retroperitoneal hemorrhage.

72. A patient who experienced chest trauma during an automobile accident shows signs of non-hemorrhagic cardiac tamponade and is to undergo pericardiocentesis. What position should the nurse place the patient in for the procedure?
    A. supine, flat
    B. right lateral side lying
    C. upright at 45 degrees
    D. upright at 90 degrees

73. The nurse is conducting stimulation threshold testing for a patient with a temporary pacemaker. Consistent capture is regained at 2 mA. Based on this finding, the output should be set at
    A. 1-2 mA.
    B. 2-3 mA.
    C. 3-4 mA.
    D. 4-6 mA.

74. A patient with Marfan syndrome is admitted with substernal pain, cough, strider, distention of neck veins, and edema of the upper extremities. The most likely cause is
    A. tricuspid regurgitation.
    B. thoracic aortic aneurysm.
    C. pulmonic regurgitation.
    D. aortic stenosis.

75. A patient suffered smoke inhalation when a fire occurred while he was sleeping. Burned materials included wool carpets, furniture with polyurethane foam, and household plastics. The patient is hypotensive and has altered mental status. Physical examination shows evidence of soot in the nares and mouth. Which of the following antidotes is most indicated?
    A. hydroxocobalamin
    B. sodium nitrite
    C. atropine
    D. oxygen therapy

76. A patient with anoxic encephalopathy resulting from fat embolism exhibits flexor (decorticate) posturing. This indicates damage to which part of the brain?
    A. upper pons
    B. brainstem
    C. midbrain
    D. hemispheres

77. A patient with unstable angina has continuous cardiac monitoring. Which of the following findings places the patient at highest risk for fatal or non-fatal myocardial infarction?
    A. appearance of pathologic Q waves
    B. T-wave inversion greater than 0.2 mV
    C. transient ST-segment changes greater than 0.05 mV
    D. slight elevation of Troponin T, between 0.01 and 0.1 ng/mL

78. A patient with valvular disease has right ventricular hypertrophy and exhibits mild cyanosis, angina, dyspnea, heart murmur, and episodes of fainting. These signs and symptoms are characteristic of
    A. pulmonic stenosis.
    B. aortic stenosis.
    C. mitral valve regurgitation.
    D. mitral stenosis.

79. Indications of primary graft dysfunction in lung transplant recipients include
    A. frequent oxygen desaturation.
    B. chest pressure.
    C. fever.
    D. cough.

80. A patient becomes very resistant and uncooperative during dressing changes, often yelling at the nurse, "You're hurting me!" even though the wound care is minimal. What is the best response to the patient?
    A. "I'm being as gentle as I can."
    B. "You had pain medication an hour ago, so you should not be having pain."
    C. "What would you like for me to do differently?"
    D. "Let's talk about how we can work together to make this easier for you."

81. Normal value for mixed venous oxygen saturation (SvO$_2$) is
    A. 96 to 100%.
    B. 60 to 80%.
    C. 45 to 65%.
    D. 75 to 95%.

82. Forty-eight hours after a subtotal gastrectomy, the patient's pulse has increased from a baseline of 72 to 118/min and blood pressure has fallen from 138/88 to 72/48 mm Hg. Urinary output has diminished, and the patient's skin is cold and clammy. The nurse suspects hemorrhage. Which of the following findings is most indicative of extragastric hemorrhage?
    A. abdominal pain
    B. increased bilirubin
    C. melena
    D. clear NG aspirant

83. A patient has undergone a subtotal gastrectomy for gastric cancer and is recovering well and progressing from clear liquids to full liquids and soft foods. What nutritional strategy is most likely to prevent or minimize dumping syndrome?
    A. low fat, high protein, high carbohydrate
    B. high fat, high protein, low carbohydrate
    C. low fat, high protein, low carbohydrate
    D. low fat, low protein, high carbohydrate

84. A patient receiving maintenance lithium at 300 mg three times daily for bipolar disorder has developed vomiting, diarrhea, tinnitus, and tremors. The patient's blood level is 1.8 mEq/L. The initial response should be to
    A. withhold lithium.
    B. increase lithium dosage.
    C. decrease lithium dosage.
    D. maintain lithium dosage and provide an antipsychotic medication.

85. A patient has been receiving unfractionated heparin for five days and has onset of pain in left leg with unilateral edema, erythema, and pain on passive dorsiflexion. Prior to administration of heparin, the patient's platelet count was 160,000 but it is now 104,000 (a 35% reduction). The nurse should expect to
    A. continue unfractionated heparin at same dose.
    B. continue unfractionated heparin at higher dose.
    C. discontinue unfractionated heparin and administer lepirudin or argatroban.
    D. discontinue unfractionated heparin and replace with low-molecular weight heparin.

86. The primary problem with basing research on qualitative data is that qualitative data are
    A. difficult to interpret.
    B. subjective.
    C. uninteresting.
    D. difficult to describe graphically.

87. A patient with an AVM had evidence of reperfusion bleeding during partial embolization, but the patient stabilized. During the postoperative period, the most critical concern is
    A. maintaining blood pressure within established parameters.
    B. monitoring arterial blood gases (ABGs).
    C. monitoring electrolytes.
    D. maintaining fluid balance.

88. A 30-year-old patient is admitted to critical care with second and third degree burns to the right arm (posterior and anterior surfaces), left anterior arm, anterior face, and anterior chest. Utilizing the Rule of 9s, what percentage of total body surface area is injured?
    A. 40.5%.
    B. 22.5%
    C. 36%
    D. 27%.

- 221 -

89. A 40-year-old female patient complains of frequent epistaxis and blood in her urine. Petechial hemorrhages are noted on the lower legs and oral mucosa. A CBC shows that RBCs and WBCs are normal, but the platelet count is 40,000. The patient is diagnosed with idiopathic thrombocytopenia purpura. Based on the patient's symptoms, which of the following treatments is the patient most likely to receive?
   A. observation only
   B. IV Ig immunoglobulin
   C. corticosteroids (oral)
   D. splenectomy

90. A 56-year-old patient with COPD has arterial blood gases done on admission. ABGs are as follows: PaO$_2$ of 88 mm Hg, pH of 7.28, PaCO$_2$ of 48 mm Hg, and HCO$_3$- of 23 mEq/L. Based on this profile, the patient is in
   A. compensated respiratory acidosis.
   B. uncompensated respiratory acidosis.
   C. compensated metabolic acidosis.
   D. uncompensated metabolic acidosis.

91. A patient with diabetic ketoacidosis shows evidence of hypovolemic shock. What IV fluid is utilized initially to reverse dehydration?
   A. 1 to 1.5 L of 0.9% normal saline
   B. 3 to 4 L of 0.9% normal saline
   C. 1 to 2 L of 0.45% sodium chloride
   D. 1 to 2 L of 5% dextrose with 45% sodium chloride

92. Following a craniotomy for removal of a meningioma anterior to the pituitary gland and optic chiasm, the patient develops pronounced diuresis and thirst. Laboratory findings include: serum sodium level of 150, serum osmolality of 304, urine osmolality of 290, and urine specific gravity of 1.004. Based on the patient's condition and laboratory findings, which pharmaceutical intervention is most indicated?
   A. hypertonic saline solution
   B. thiazide diuretics
   C. desmopressin acetate
   D. demeclocycline

93. The primary difference between hyperglycemic hyperosmolar nonketotic syndrome (HHNK) and diabetes ketoacidosis (DKA) is that
   A. treatment options for HHNK and DKA are different.
   B. HHNK does not involve breakdown of fat and DKA does.
   C. HHNK involves overhydration and DKA dehydration.
   D. insulin level is lower in HHNK than in DKA.

94. Which of the following is an example of informal collaboration?
   A. team members discussing the best method of meeting a patient's needs
   B. a nurse reporting a patient's concerns about upcoming surgery to the physician
   C. a nurse asking a nurse on another unit about his experience with a procedure
   D. a nurse asking another team member to assist with moving a patient

95. The nurse is reviewing preoperative laboratory values. The nurse should alert the physician to which of the following values?
    A. glucose level of 98 mg/dL
    B. blood, urea, nitrogen (BUN) level of 26 mg/dL
    C. creatinine level of 0.79 mg/dL
    D. calcium level of 0.2 mg/dL

96. A patient has been stabilized after rupture of a cerebral aneurysm with a grade II subarachnoid hemorrhage and is scheduled for surgical repair within 24 hours of the rupture. However, the patient tells the nurse that he wants to wait until his family arrives from overseas in four days. Which of the following is the best response?
    A. "You should discuss that with your surgeon."
    B. "Delaying surgery could be very dangerous."
    C. "I'm sure your family will understand that you needed to have the surgery."
    D. "The risk of re-bleeding increases every day, putting you at grave risk if you delay."

97. While hospitalized for a stroke, a patient vomited and aspirated some of the gastric contents before the nurse could change the patient's position to prevent aspiration. The initial intervention should be to
    A. administer oxygen.
    B. conduct a bronchoalveolar lavage.
    C. suction the upper airway.
    D. provide prophylactic antibiotics.

98. The first-line treatment for obstructive sleep apnea is
    A. Bi-PAP.
    B. CPAP.
    C. APAP.
    D. Bi-PAP ST.

99. Following a traumatic brain injury, a patient is to have eight-minute apnea testing to aid in the determination of brain death. Four minutes after the ventilator is disconnected, the patient develops cardiac dysrhythmias. What nursing action is indicated?
    A. Obtain a blood sample for ABGs and reconnect the ventilator.
    B. Obtain ECG tracing and continue monitoring for four more minutes.
    C. Obtain a blood sample for ABGs and an ECG tracing and continuing monitoring for four more minutes.
    D. Continue monitoring for four more minutes and then obtain blood sample for ABGs.

100. When asking a patient to sign a consent form for a procedure, the most important factor is the
    A. explanation of the procedure.
    B. patient's ability to give informed consent.
    C. reasons for the procedure.
    D. explanation of possible complications.

101. Which of the following modes of ventilation provides a specified volume of air and rate with no triggering required of the patient and respiratory response decreased through medication (such as pancuronium bromide or morphine)?
    A. synchronized intermittent mandatory ventilation (SIMV)
    B. assist control ventilation (ACV)
    C. pressure support ventilation (PSV)
    D. controlled mandatory ventilation (CMV)

102. A patient who was in a car accident 48 hours ago presents with bilateral periorbital ecchymosis. The patient complains of a salty taste in their mouth. The most likely cause of these symptoms is
    A. eye trauma.
    B. diastatic skull fracture.
    C. Le Fort skull fracture.
    D. basal skull fracture.

103. A patient has been diagnosed with metastatic ovarian cancer with a short life expectancy, but she tells the nurse that she believes that she can cure herself with positive thinking. Which of the following is the best response?
    A. "I've heard that positive thinking has cured some people of cancer."
    B. "The mind can be powerful."
    C. "There's no evidence to support positive thinking as a cure."
    D. "Whatever makes you feel better is ok."

104. Considering ventilator management, in order to avoid toxicity, the fraction of inspired oxygen (FiO_2) should usually be maintained at less than
    A. 21%.
    B. 40%.
    C. 60%.
    D. 80%.

105. An 18-year-old man who identifies as gay is hospitalized under his parents' insurance. The patient insists that his male partner visit him, but his parents have left a note at the nursing desk advising the staff that the partner is not allowed to visit. What is the best action for the nurse?
    A. advise the partner that he cannot visit the patient.
    B. advise the patient that his partner is not allowed to visit.
    C. call the parents and advise them that they cannot prevent visits.
    D. ignore the parents because they have no standing.

106. A patient who sustained a head injury is to have a lumbar puncture to determine if there is CNS bleeding. Which of the following is the most important prior to the lumbar puncture?
    A. CT of the brain
    B. EEG
    C. hemoglobin and hematocrit
    D. coagulation studies

107. In order to avoid protein depletion in trauma patients, how much protein should be provided to the patient each day?
    A. 1.0 to 1.5 g/k
    B. 1.5 to 2.0 g/k
    C. 2.0 to 2.5 g/k
    D. 2.5 to 3.0 g/k

108. Following a subarachnoid hemorrhage, a patient complains of increasing headache and slight nausea and a CTA shows hydrocephalus. The patient remains awake and responsive. The most likely initial treatment is
    A. lumbar puncture for drainage.
    B. serial lumbar punctures for drainage.
    C. observation.
    D. ventriculostomy or ventriculoperitoneal shunt.

109. After an extended stay in the critical care unit, a patient is to be transferred to a general medical-surgical unit. The patient has developed a trusting relationship with her nurse and is upset about the transfer. The patient begs the nurse to intervene so she can stay in the critical care unit. The best solution for the nurse is to
    A. tell the patient that the nurses on the other unit will take good care of her.
    B. tell the patient the nurse will accompany her to the other unit and introduce her.
    C. ask the physician if the patient can stay longer in the critical care unit.
    D. tell the patient that the nurse will stop by every day to visit her.

110. A patient who has been prescribed oral phenytoin (Dilantin) for seizure control should be advised to
    A. limit alcohol intake to two to three drinks daily.
    B. have weekly blood tests.
    C. maintain superior dental care.
    D. stop the drug immediately if adverse effects occur.

111. Following a craniotomy, the patient is carefully monitored for increasing intracranial pressure. Intracranial hypertension occurs when intracranial pressure (ICP) is greater than
    A. 12 mm Hg.
    B. 15 mm Hg.
    C. 20 mm Hg.
    D. 25 mm Hg.

112. A patient receiving continuous renal replacement therapy (CCRT) exhibits increased heart rate, decreased blood pressure, and ECG abnormalities. The nurse should suspect
    A. electrolyte imbalance.
    B. bleeding.
    C. too much or too little dialysate.
    D. problem unrelated to CCRT.

113. The nurse is assessing a patient with suspected ischemic stroke using the NIH stroke scale. The patient speaks only Spanish but no interpreter is available. Only the word list and reading for the assessment are available in Spanish. However, the patient's 13-year-old granddaughter is present and is bilingual. The nurse should
    A. delay the assessment until an interpreter is available.
    B. ask the granddaughter to translate.
    C. omit the sections of the assessment that require verbal directions or responses.
    D. complete the assessment in English using pictures, motions, and pantomime to aid in the patient's comprehension.

114. A patient who has experienced an ischemic stroke arrives at the emergency department in the 3 to 4.5 hour window of time after the stroke. Which of the following would exclude the patient from treatment with recombinant tPA?
    A. age of 81 years
    B. score of 24 on the NIH stroke scale
    C. history of diabetes
    D. history of major surgery 3 months previously

115. Which of the following conditions is most commonly associated with acute renal failure?
    A. respiratory acidosis
    B. respiratory alkalosis
    C. metabolic alkalosis
    D. metabolic acidosis

116. A patient involved in a traumatic motorcycle accident has fractured ribs 9 and 10 on the left side. Injury to which of the following underlying structures is of most concern?
    A. pancreas
    B. spleen
    C. diaphragm
    D. intestines

117. When planning patient education, the nurse realizes that most adults experience low energy in the
    A. early morning.
    B. late morning.
    C. afternoon.
    D. evening.

118. Which of the following defense mechanisms is a patient utilizing if the patient yells at his spouse after receiving bad news from the physician about the his condition?
    A. projection
    B. reaction formation
    C. sublimation
    D. displacement

119. A patient who is legally blind is to use a BiPAP machine when he is discharged. The best method to ensure the patient uses the equipment properly is to
    A. provide instructions in brail or audiotapes.
    B. allow the patient to handle and manipulate the equipment.
    C. teach a family member how to assist the patient.
    D. plan extended training sessions with much repetition.

120. A 20-year-old patient has a severe exacerbation of asthma with pronounced wheezing and dyspnea. The patient is only able to give one- to two-word responses and is using accessory muscles to breathe. The nurse should expect which of the following to be the first-line treatment?
    A. short-acting B_2-Agonist (albuterol) and corticosteroid
    B. theophylline and non-specific B-adrenergic agent (epinephrine)
    C. anticholinergic (ipratropium) and heliox
    D. short-acting B_2-agonist and intravenous magnesium

121. The nurse is aware that a patient is extremely nervous about having an MRI and takes a CD by the patient's favorite singer to the imaging lab so that the patient can listen to the music during the procedure. This is an example of
    A. response to diversity.
    B. collaboration.
    C. patient advocacy.
    D. caring practices.

122. A patient asks the nurse many questions about her medical treatment; but, when the physician is present, the patient becomes very quiet and asks no questions despite the nurse's encouragement to do so. The best solution for the nurse is to
    A. prompt the patient when the doctor is present.
    B. ask the patient why she doesn't ask the doctor questions.
    C. prepare a list of the patient's questions for the physician.
    D. tell the physician that the patient has many questions.

123. A nurse mentors peers new to the profession. Which of the Standards for Acute and Critical Care Nurses under the Standards of Professional Performance does this support?
    A. Quality of care
    B. Education
    C. Collaboration
    D. Collegiality

124. A patient who is critically ill has been "talking" with her husband, who has actually been dead for many years, and describing a beautiful place. The nurse recognizes these as signs of
    A. delirium.
    B. dementia.
    C. impending death.
    D. opioid toxicity.

125. A nurse on the unit states she has no interest in the "politics" of work and just wants to work with the patients and not worry about other departments and institutional problems. This represents
    A. dedication to the nursing profession.
    B. incompetent practice of nursing.
    C. old-fashioned attitude toward the nursing profession.
    D. barrier to systems thinking.

126. A staff nurse repeatedly makes mistakes with electronic charting, insisting that the system is too difficult and inefficient, that the institution made a big mistake in forcing staff to use the computer system, and that most staff agree with this assessment. This is an example of
    A. having an autocratic view.
    B. arriving at weak consensus.
    C. displaying displaced anger.
    D. failing to adapt.

127. Which of the following is the most common cause of hypoxemia?
    A. alveolar hypoventilation.
    B. physiologic shunting.
    C. ventilation/Perfusion (V/Q) mismatch.
    D. intrapulmonary shunting.

128. A patient is admitted with partial obstruction of the airway after aspiration of a metal screw 24 hours earlier. The patient is able to speak with difficulty but is dyspneic and having severe bouts of coughing and complains of chest pain. Which treatment option should the nurse anticipate?
    A. bronchodilator and postural drainage
    B. flexible bronchoscopy
    C. rigid bronchoscopy
    D. bronchotomy

129. A patient with progressive pulmonary arterial hypertension must be monitored for signs of
    A. left ventricular heart failure.
    B. right ventricular heart failure.
    C. ventricular fibrillation.
    D. cardiomyopathy.

130. What is the minimum time period that Heliox should be administered to gain full effects?
    A. 20 minutes
    B. 40 minutes
    C. 60 minutes
    D. 90 minutes

131. Some hospital units are overstaffed, according to patient census, while others are understaffed, requiring nurses to work overtime and resulting in increased costs. While most understaffed units are requesting additional full-time nurses, one unit leader suggests that the hospital switch to acuity-based staffing and increase the number of float nurses from current staff and train them in more than one discipline in order to cut overall costs and meet the needs of multiple units. This suggestion is an example of
    A. divergent thinking.
    B. parallel thinking.
    C. systems thinking.
    D. convergent thinking.

132. When considering the validity of written material, the most important thing to consider is the
    A. source.
    B. author.
    C. date.
    D. statistical evidence.

133. Adhesive atelectasis, caused by surfactant deficiency, is most often associated with
    A. necrotizing pneumonia.
    B. space-occupying lesions.
    C. asbestos exposure.
    D. acute respiratory distress syndrome (ARDS).

134. A patient who underwent a thoracic laminectomy developed increasing dyspnea and hypoxemia with cough, hemoptysis, substernal pain, and subcutaneous emphysema of neck and chest within 4 hours of extubation. The most likely cause is
    A. tracheal perforation.
    B. surgical trauma to chest.
    C. esophageal perforation.
    D. pneumothorax.

135. A patient has undergone bilateral lung volume reduction per video-assisted thoracoscopic surgery (VATS) for severe emphysema. What postoperative complication is most common?
    A. pneumonia
    B. air leaks
    C. aspiration of gastric contents
    D. respiratory failure

136. A patient has suffered blunt chest trauma in an accident with bilateral lung contusions. During what time period should the nurse anticipate possible onset of symptoms of acute respiratory distress syndrome?
    A. 1 to 2 hours
    B. 4 to 12 hours
    C. 12 to 24 hours
    D. 24 to 48 hours

137. A 68-year-old patient with severe asthma is lethargic and somnolent and arouses with difficulty. His PaO_2 has fallen to 58 mm Hg on low-flow oxygen and $PaCO_2$ has increased to 56 mm Hg while the pH is 7.28. Which of the following is the most likely cause of these symptoms?
   A. acute respiratory failure
   B. pulmonary embolism
   C. sepsis
   D. pneumonia

138. A 20-year-old man who had been practicing football in extreme heat is admitted with heat stroke. Which of the following symptoms is typically found with exertional heat stroke as opposed to non-exertional?
   A. anhidrosis
   B. temperature above 41° C/106° F
   C. high risk for rhabdomyolysis
   D. low risk for renal failure

139. An 18-year–old woman comes to the hospital 18 hours after she took "a bottle" of extra-strength acetaminophen. She feels slight nausea but has no other symptoms. At what beginning serum acetaminophen level should N-acetylcysteine (NAC) be administered?
   A. 10 mcg/mL
   B. 50 mcg/mL
   C. 160 mcg/mL
   D. 200 mcg/mL

140. A patient with a history of severe allergic reaction to bananas and kiwis is at risk for allergy to
   A. plastics.
   B. penicillins.
   C. vitamin supplements.
   D. latex.

141. With intrarenal causes of acute renal failure, the expected level of urine sodium is
   A. less than 20 mEq/L.
   B. greater than 20 mEq/L
   C. greater than 30 mEq/L.
   D. greater than 40 mEq/L.

142. Which of the following is the most important factor in delegation?
   A. determining if the task is appropriate based on the person's skills and available time
   B. providing clear instructions, including expected objectives and timeline
   C. monitoring progress and ensuring that tasks were performed correctly
   D. reviewing the final results when the task is completed and recording outcomes

143. A patient who is supposed to be on a low carbohydrate diet has gained weight and reports eating frequent convenience foods that are high in carbohydrates. When questioned, the patient is knowledgeable about the diet, but states that poor vision and arthritis in her hands make food preparation difficult. The most appropriate referral for the patient is
    A. nutritionist.
    B. occupational therapist.
    C. social worker.
    D. home health agency.

144. The nurse must inform the family of a patient that the patient is dying. Which of the following is an effective strategy?
    A. provide the information quickly.
    B. tell the family and then leave and allow them to grieve.
    C. ask the family if they have questions.
    D. advise the family to ask the physician about the patient's condition.

145. The nurse is coaching a new graduate nurse in carrying out a procedure, utilizing a mannequin; however, the graduate nurse makes many errors and appears anxious. What is the best strategy for helping the graduate nurse master the procedure?
    A. point out errors as the nurse makes them.
    B. provide positive feedback, stressing the nurse's correct actions.
    C. suggest the graduate nurse research the procedure and memorize the steps.
    D. remind the graduate nurse that her lack of knowledge could endanger patients.

146. A patient who is dependent on peritoneal dialysis is admitted to the critical care unit with cardiac dysrhythmias. Which renal replacement therapy does the nurse anticipate will be used during hospitalization?
    A. intermittent hemodialysis
    B. continuous venovenous hemofiltration
    C. peritoneal dialysis
    D. continuous arteriovenous hemofiltration

147. A patient is to undergo a left renal biopsy. What is the correct position to place the patient in for the procedure?
    A. prone
    B. upright leaning over bedside table
    C. right side-lying
    D. knee-chest position

148. A patient who is undergoing deep sedation while mechanically ventilated is monitored with the bispectral index system (BSI). Which of the following values indicates that the patient is unconscious with low likelihood of recall?
    A. 50-60
    B. 90-100
    C. 40-50
    D. Less than 20

149. Which of the following drugs used for sedation provides the most prolonged sedation?
    A. diazepam
    B. lorazepam
    C. propofol
    D. midazolam

150. A patient is unconscious with severe generalized tonic-clonic status epilepticus leading to periods of apnea with cause unknown. The patient is administered lorazepam (Ativan) initially and again in 5 minutes when there is no response, but seizures continue. What should the nurse anticipate will be the next step?
    A. administration of another dose of lorazepam
    B. rapid sequence intubation
    C. addition of fosphenytoin
    D. addition of phenobarbital

Answers and Explanations

1. C: The optimal temperature range for therapeutic hypothermia is 32° C/89.6° F to 34° C/93.2° F. Patients may be placed between two cooling blankets, or ice packs may be used to lower temperature. If using ice packs, they should be applied to the femoral area, axillae, and sides of the neck as well as the sides (but not the top) of the chest. Patients must be carefully monitored for oxygen saturation and dysrhythmias. The MAP should be maintained at greater than 80 mm Hg for neuroprotection. The head of bed should be elevated to 30°.

2. D: The electrolyte imbalance that is the most life threatening for patients with renal failure is hyperkalemia (greater than 5.5 mEq/L). Hyperkalemia may cause cardiac abnormalities and ECG changes (peaked or tented T-waves) as well as changes in general condition. Treatment for hyperkalemia includes sodium polystyrene sulfonate (Kayexalate), which can be administered orally or as a retention enema. Kayexalate exchanges sodium ions for potassium ions in the intestines. Unstable patients may receive IV dextrose 50% with insulin and calcium to shift potassium from the blood into the cells. Nebulized albuterol may also lower potassium levels.

3. A: The best method to improve a patient's motivation is to provide positive feedback about tasks the patient is able to complete at the time he is doing the tasks because that helps the patient focus on concrete improvements. Focusing on long-term or even short-term goals may seem overwhelming in the initial stages of rehabilitation, especially if the patient is depressed. Comparing present abilities and initial abilities focuses on the past more than the present and future, and the nurse should never make overgeneralizations that include "everyone" because each person is individual.

4. B: These symptoms are consistent with sepsis and part of the continuum leading to septic shock. The diagnostic criteria for sepsis include many variables. General signs of infection and impending shock are usually present (fever, tachycardia, hypotension, fever) as well as edema and flushing resulting from massive arterial and venous vasodilation in early stages. WBC may be elevated (greater than 12,000) or decreased (less than 4000). Hyperglycemia and coagulopathies are common, and urine output falls because of decreased intravascular volume.

5. C: Clinical pathways should be developed by interdisciplinary teams that include physicians as well as nurses and other healthcare providers who may participate in patient care, such as respiratory and occupational therapists and nutritionists. The team must select the patient group, diagnosis, and procedures based on analysis of evidence through observation, literature review, and interviews. The group should discuss issues and reach consensus and should clearly outline levels of care and days covered by the pathway. Pilot testing and staff education should precede utilization.

6. A: A well-written learning objective should clearly outline expectations of the learning process and usually contains 4 elements: the condition or testing situation ("after attending a workshop about hypertension"); the identity of the learner, not the instructor ("the patient"); the expected behavior ("will be able to state"); and the measurable criterion ("4 causes for high blood pressure").

7. D: Because carbon dioxide acts as a vasodilator, dilating cerebral blood vessels and causing cerebral edema and increased ICP, the optimal $PaCO_2$ level is 27 to 32, which is lower than the normal $PaCO_2$ level of 35 to 45. Ventilation, usually per tracheal intubation, is provided to provide oxygenation and control CO_2 levels although hyperventilation, which constricts cerebral blood

vessels, should be avoided (especially during the first 5 post-operative days) or used only for short periods since it may induce ischemia.

8. B: While state laws may vary somewhat, nurses are mandated reporters for both child abuse and elder abuse, so the nurse should report the observations to adult protective services. Bruises on the parts of the body covered by clothes are characteristic of those inflicted by an abuser who wants to hide evidence of abuse. Arm bruises are often defensive. The nurse should not confront the suspected abuser, as this may put both the nurse and the patient at risk.

9. C: While at one time tidal volume for ARDS was set at 12 mL/kg predicted body weight (PBW), current studies indicate that 6 to 8 mL/kg PBW (low tidal volume ventilation) has a more protective effect on the lungs and reduces mortality rates. PEEP may need to be set higher than usual to prevent atelectasis. Initial settings: tidal volume of 8 mL/kg PBW; respiratory rate of 35/min; PEEP of 5 cm H_2O or higher; FiO_2 less than 70% when possible but high enough to maintain oxygen saturation of 88 to 95%; and tidal volume reduced to 7 mL/kg PBW and then 6 mL/kg PBW over 4 hours or less.

10. A: The two treatments used for GBS are IV Ig or plasmapheresis (plasma exchange). IV Ig may reduce recovery time by 50% by neutralizing myelin antibodies and promoting remyelination although it poses a risk of thromboembolic events, so low doses of heparin may be given. Plasmapheresis may also be used to remove autoantibodies, cytotoxic constituents and immune complexes from serum. There is no advantage to providing both IV Ig and plasmapheresis. Corticosteroids do not improve GBS. Immunoadsorption is still in the trial stage but shows promise.

11. C: This patient is exhibiting typical indications of acute heart failure with dyspnea, orthopnea, basilar rales, lateral displacement of the apical beat (from enlarged left ventricle), peripheral edema, tachycardia, elevated blood pressure, and hypoxia. CPAP or Bi-PAP should be administered since this may increase oxygenation and reduce the need for endotracheal intubation with mechanical ventilation. Nitrates may also be administered to decrease pre-load. While a loop diuretic, such as furosemide, may be indicated, diuretics are no longer considered first-line treatments as they may result in hypotension.

12. B: While many of these symptoms can be found with all of these conditions, two are specific to pneumopericardium: the mill wheel murmur and the shifting tympany. Hamman's sign—a popping or crunching sound heard over the mediastinum—may or may not be present but is more commonly associated with pneumomediastinum. Pneumopericardium can be confirmed CT. Treatment includes needle aspiration and insertion of drainage tube or thoracotomy as well as oxygen therapy. Asymptomatic pneumopericardium may be treated conservatively.

13. D: This pattern of pain—severe epigastric pain radiating to the back—that is exacerbated by lying flat or walking is consistent with pancreatitis. Generally, the upper abdomen is tender but without rigidity or guarding, which may be present with other disorders. Abdominal distention and jaundice may occur in some patients. Fever to 39° C is common as is tachycardia and pallor. Serum amylase and serum lipase may be elevated up to 3 times normal values within 24 hours, and leukocytosis (10,000 to 30,000) may be evident.

14. A: One of the barriers to adequate pain management is nurses' preconceptions about physiological and emotional responses to pain and what a patient in pain should look like. Some patients moan and cry while others show little outward sign of pain, but pain is what the patient says it is, and if a patient requests pain medication for severe pain, then the nurse should give the

opioid. A patient may try to not to show pain to family members or friends even when the patient is very uncomfortable.

15. C: It's very important that an impermeable covering be placed over the insertion site until the chest tube can be reinserted to prevent air from sucking into the pleural cavity. If no plastic or petroleum gauze dressing is available, the nurse can cover the insertion site with a clean gloved hand while calling for assistance. The physician must be notified as soon as the insertion site is secured. The patient's arterial blood gases should be assessed as soon as possible.

16. B: The CT-PA is most diagnostic for PE. D-dimer is almost always elevated with PE as endogenous fibrinolysis results in decreased levels of fibrinogen and increased D-dimer as the body attempts to digest the clot. A normal D-dimer generally can rule out PE, but an abnormal D-dimer is common in hospitalized patients and not diagnostic alone. Usually both the D-dimer and CT-PA are used. While hypoxemia and hypocapnia are common with PE, arterial blood gas values may alter for other reasons and remain within normal range even with pulmonary emboli. Pulmonary angiogram is rarely used, and chest radiograph is not diagnostic.

17. A: A potassium level of 3.2 mEq/L indicates hypokalemia, which increases the risk of digoxin toxicity. Immediate treatment includes withholding digoxin (the number of doses or the need for reduction in dosage depends on the severity of the reaction as well as the cause). With hypokalemia, potassium supplement should be administered as well as supportive therapy, such as acetaminophen for headache and an antidiarrheal. The digoxin antidote, digoxin immune Fab, is not routinely given but may be administered if indicated, usually because of severe toxicity with hyperkalemia, severe cardiac dysrhythmias, or digoxin overdose.

18. D: Pain and local swelling, erythema, and itching are common after bee sting and may extend to an entire limb or extended area, but urticaria, edema, and itching occurring in areas distant from the sting site suggest a systemic reaction leading to anaphylaxis. Patients may feel lightheaded and nauseated and may have tightness in the chest, dyspnea, and lingual edema as well as generalized hives because of vasodilation and edema. Hypotension, bronchospasm, laryngospasm, and loss of consciousness may lead to respiratory and cardiac arrest.

19. C: Cocaine: euphoria, restlessness, hyperactivity, tachycardia, hypertension, dilated pupils, and rhinitis (from sniffing cocaine). Patients may show damage to the nasal septum and may develop severe cardiac problems, including myocardial infarction. Peak effect occurs in 2 to 30 minutes and persists 30 to 60 minutes. Barbiturate (such as Valium): relaxed state, lack of inhibition, inability to concentrate, drowsiness, slurred speech, and sleepiness. Heroin: euphoria, lethargy, constricted/pinpoint pupils, drowsiness, and lack of motivation. Amphetamines: hyperactivity, agitation, euphoria, inability to sleep, and loss of appetite.

20. B: The patient receiving adenosine should be carefully monitored for transient asystole since the drug slows AV node conduction, sometimes resulting in heart block and development of new dysrhythmias, including atrial fibrillation. Facial flushing is a common side effect and is short-lived (usually only lasting one to two minutes) as the drug is very fast acting with a half-life of less than 10 seconds. Other adverse effects can include dizziness, numbness and tingling in the arms, headache, nausea, and dyspnea.

21. A: Because potassium-sparing diuretics markedly increase the risk of hyperkalemia in patients with chronic kidney disease, they are usually used only with patients who have persistent hypokalemia or hypertension. Risk is highest in patients whose glomerular filtration rate is less

than 30 mL/min/1.73 m² and are also receiving ACEI or ARBs. Dosages should begin low and be increased slowly. Electrolyte levels must be monitored frequently. Hyporeninemic hypoaldosteronism is a contraindication for the use of potassium-sparing diuretics.

22. D: Wellens syndrome can occur in patients with unstable angina, indicating marked stenosis of the left anterior descending coronary artery and impending acute anterior wall myocardial infarction. Cardiac enzymes are usually within normal range or show only slight elevation. This is an emergency situation that requires immediate cardiac catheterization for angioplasty or stent placement before complete occlusion occurs. The R waves remain intact because the myocardial infarction has not yet taken place. ST segments (V1 and V3) may be normal or show slight elevation, and terminal T-wave inversion occurs (V2-V3) during pain-free periods.

23. B: This pattern is consistent with atrial fibrillation. Atrial fibrillation results in ineffective beats that do not adequately empty the atria so that blood begins to pool, increasing the risk of thrombus formation and emboli. While stroke volume decreases, the ventricular rate increases to compensate but the decreased cardiac output can result in myocardial ischemia. Treatment may include cardioversion (per electrical cardioversion or pharmaceutical), ventricular pacing, and anticoagulant therapy if the atrial fibrillation lasts more than 24 hours.

24. C: If bubbling occurs in the water seal container, this indicates that there is an air leak somewhere in the system. The first step is to check the chest tube by clamping the drainage tube just below the chest tube. If this stops the bubbling, then the leak is superior to the clamp from the chest tube or the patient's chest. If bubbling continues after clamping, then the leak is in the system below the clamp, so the drainage system should be changed.

25. A: Myasthenic crisis (usually due to too little medication) and cholinergic crisis (due to too much medication) both present with similar symptoms—profound weakness, respiratory distress, anxiety—and the Tensilon test (also used to diagnose myasthenia gravis) is used to differentiate the two. The Tensilon (edrophonium) test consists of administration of small doses (up to a total of 10 mg) of edrophonium. A positive response (improvement in muscle strength) indicates myasthenic crisis and a negative response (no improvement) indicates a cholinergic crisis.

26. C: With transcutaneous pacing, the rate is usually set at 60 to 70 bpm with the current increased slowly until capture, after which the current is slowly lowered if possible. Electrodes (gel-covered paddles/pads) are usually placed on the left chest and left back so that the heart is between them. Leads connect to a computerized ECG and defibrillator, which is synchronized so the electrical current is delivered during QRS (ventricular depolarization). It's important that the current be delivered at the correct time or ventricular tachycardia or ventricular fibrillation may occur.

27. A: While all of these are risk factors for hospital-associated pneumonia (HAP), 80% of HAP is the result of ventilator-associated pneumonia (VAP), a subgrouping of HAP that may occur 48 or more hours after initiation of ventilation per endotracheal tube or tracheostomy. When patients are receiving mechanical ventilation, they have depressed epiglottal and cough reflexes, increased secretions, and decreased cilia activity, all increasing the risk of aspiration and colonization of bacteria in the lungs. Two common pathogens associated with HAP are *Pseudomonas aeruginosa* and *Staphylococcus aureus*.

28. B: Mannitol tends to form crystals at low temperatures, so it should always be administered through a filter. Crystals are more likely to form with concentrations of over 15%. Mannitol solutions may be kept in a warming device to prevent crystal formation but should be cooled to

body temperature prior to administration. Test doses are indicated for patients with renal impairment. Mannitol is usually administered over a 30- to 60-minute period while the patient is carefully monitored for changes in ICP and cerebral perfusion.

29. C: With status asthmaticus, indications for intubation and mechanical ventilation include peak expiratory flow rate less than 40% of predicted as well as FEV1 less than 20% of predicted. On initial presentation, hyperventilation usually results in ABGs showing hypocapnia and respiratory alkalosis, but if the patient's condition worsens, hypoxemia and hypercapnia develop, resulting in respiratory and metabolic acidosis. Patients may exhibit decreased level of consciousness, diminished or absent breath sounds, inability to breathe in supine position, and pulsus paradoxus greater than 25 mm Hg.

30. D: The pacing mode that is most commonly used with temporary transvenous pacing is VVI. The electrode is placed in the ventricle and paces the ventricle first, senses ventricular activity, and inhibits ventricular output when it senses intrinsic ventricular depolarization. This is the fastest type of pacing to use in emergency situations because it is more difficult to position and maintain a temporary atrial lead. VVI is also the pacing mode often used with epicardial leads after cardiac surgery, especially in the presence of third-degree AV block.

31. C: These symptoms are consistent with disseminated intravascular coagulation, so a DIC panel is indicated to determine if factors necessary for clotting are decreased and if clotting times are prolonged (if so, these findings may confirm DIC). DIC occurs as secondary to another disorder, such as bacteremia or sepsis, trauma, necrotizing enterocolitis, cancer, malaria, and placenta abruptio. With DIC, both excess clotting and hemorrhage may occur at the same time. Identifying and treating the underlying cause is critical to treatment.

32. A: The two most commonly used drugs to treat delirium are lorazepam and haloperidol. Anticholinergics, such as benztropine, may trigger delirium, especially in older adults. Delirium has similar symptoms as dementia; but with delirium the symptoms tend to fluctuate, so patients may have both periods of lucidity and profound confusion. Delirium may be triggered by many conditions, such as trauma, depression, surgery, untreated pain, and electrolyte imbalance. A patient's attention deficit may be noted if the patient is unable to count backward from 1 to 20 or spell his first name backward.

33. B: Patients who develop West Nile virus flaccid paralysis are at high risk for respiratory failure, which may require mechanical ventilation and is the primary cause of mortality. WNV flaccid paralysis is similar to poliomyelitis with damage to anterior horn cells. It may involve paralysis of one limb or all four limbs. A similar manifestation is WVN-associated Guillain-Barré syndrome. Patients may also develop WNV meningitis and/or encephalitis. Treatment is supportive and depends on symptoms, as no specific medication is available for WNV.

34. D: Inflation must be timed exactly to the beginning of diastole at the dicrotic notch. Inflation and deflation must be coordinated with the patient's cardiac cycle to achieve hemodynamic stability. If inflation occurs too early, it may force the aortic valve to close prematurely, impairing ejection. If inflation occurs too late, the assistive function is shortened (although this does not directly cause harm to the patient). The balloon should deflate at the end of diastole just prior to the aortic upstroke.

35. C: To increase reading ease for patients, the maximum word length for a sentence should be 20 words, keeping in mind that a word count of 13 to 20 is approximately equivalent to a seventh-

- 237 -

grade reading level, 7 to 12 equivalent to sixth-grade reading level, and 3 to 6 equivalent to a fifth-grade reading level. Complex sentence structures should be avoided and materials presented in active voice and second person (you). Language should be simple and conversational, avoiding technical terms.

36. A: Sodium nitroprusside is often given initially to treat hypertensive crisis related to cardiac ischemia because it provides very fast-acting vasodilation. Treatment must be given immediately to lower blood pressure and prevent damage to vital organs because a diastolic BP greater than 120 mm Hg is considered a hypertensive emergency. The goal is usually not to lower BP to normal levels, and a decrease in 10% to 15% may reduce symptoms. With hypertensive urgency, when organs are not in immediate danger, the goal is one-third reduction in six hours, one third in the next 24 hours, and one-third over 2-4 days.

37. B: Cimetidine carries a high risk of drug interactions, especially in older adults, because it binds hepatic enzymes that metabolize many different drugs. Cimetidine inhibits oxidation of the drugs and may raise blood concentrations. It is especially a concern with drugs, such as warfarin and theophylline, which have a narrow therapeutic index. Cimetidine, like all H_2 antagonists, may inhibit absorption of drugs that require an acidic gastric environment. Cimetidine is the oldest H_2 antagonist, and newer drugs, such as famotidine, have far fewer drug interactions.

38 A: When the Passy-Muir valve is placed on a tracheostomy tube, the cuff must be completely deflated. If mechanical ventilation is used, the tidal volume should also be increased. The Passy-Muir valve is a one-way valve that opens on inhalation so that air can enter the lungs and closes on exhalation, forcing the air over the vocal chords and out the mouth instead of out the tracheostomy tube. The valve may be used to help the patient regain normal breathing patterns, improve swallowing, and decrease the risk of aspiration.

39. B: The primary concern with combining these drugs is that hydrochlorothiazide can interfere with the action of antidiabetic agents, decreasing hypoglycemic effects; so patients may develop hyperglycemia and should be advised to careful monitor their blood glucose levels when beginning treatment since the dosage for the antidiabetic agent may need to be increased. Patients should also be advised to avoid licorice, which may cause increased potassium loss, and alcohol, which may cause orthostatic hypotension.

40. D: Because the lungs are especially sensitive to the inflammatory changes that occur with SIRS, the pulmonary system is often the first to fail and the subsequent lack of oxygen causes other systems to fail as well. While there is much variation in the manner in which systems fail, some sequentially and others failing at the same time, the most common progression is from the lungs to the liver, the GI system, the kidneys, and the heart. MODS may be primary from direct injury or secondary, such as from SIRS.

41. D: Prone positioning is used with ALI to improve oxygenation to the less damaged parts of the lungs and to improve ventilation/perfusion matching and decrease intrapulmonary shunting. Prone positioning should improve PaO_2 by more than 10 mm Hg within 30 minutes, although no minimum or maximum time period for prone positioning has been established, and the treatment is usually reserved for those with life-threatening conditions because of the difficulty in positioning patients and preventing pressure. Special frames, such as the Vollman Prone Positioner, or pillows must be used so that the abdomen hangs free so the diaphragm descent is not impaired.

42. C: When oxygen is delivered via a mask with a reservoir bag, the estimated FiO_2 is 10 times the setting: 6 is equal to 60% estimated FiO_2. The flow rate should be set from 6 to 10. With a nasal cannula or catheter, the base setting of a flow rate of 1 is FiO_2 of 24 and each increase in the flow rate increases the FiO_2 by 4 percentage points: 1—24%, 2—28%, 3—32%, 4—36%, 5—40%, 6—44%. With an oxygen mask, each increase in flow rate increases the FiO_2 by 10%: 5-6 is 40%, 6-7 is 50%, and 7-8 is 60%.

43. D: Syndrome of inappropriate secretion of antidiuretic hormone (SIADH) can be triggered by many different disease processes and many medications, but a common cause is bronchogenic small (oat) cell carcinoma because these abnormal cells synthesize and release ADH. The initial symptoms (lethargy, anorexia, nausea, and vomiting) result from dilutional hyponatremia; however, as the sodium level falls to critical levels (below 120 mEq/L), neurological symptoms become more evident as the patient becomes increasingly confused and unable to concentrate. Without treatment, the patient will progress to seizures, coma, and death. The first-line treatment is fluid restriction.

44. D: These findings are consistent with tension pneumothorax, which will require insertion of a chest tube on the left side. Tension pneumothorax can occur in COPD patients with rupture of lung bullae and also may occur in patients on mechanical ventilation. Patients are usually in severe respiratory distress with tachycardia and tachypnea. Classic signs include tracheal shift, decreased lung expansion, increased percussion notes, decreased breath sounds, and distended jugular veins, although many patients do not exhibit all of these signs.

45. A: The three characteristics most often associated with cardiogenic shock include increased preload, increased afterload, and decreased contractility. These characteristics combine to cause decreased cardiac output and increased systemic vascular resistance as a compensatory measure to protect internal organs. Tissue perfusion and coronary artery perfusion decrease as cardiac output falls. Because the left ventricle cannot adequately pump the blood, the fluid backs up, causing pulmonary edema and right ventricular failure. Patients exhibit hypotension, tachycardia, decreased heart sounds, chest pain, basilar rales, tachypnea, pallor, and cool clammy skin.

46. B: The ejection click (brief high-pitched sound that occurs immediately after S1) is associated with aortic valve stenosis. Gallop rhythms include S3, which occurs after S3 and may indicate left ventricular failure in older adults, although it may be a normal finding in children and young adults; and S4, which occurs before S1 and may indicate ventricular hypertrophy, coronary artery disease, or aortic valve stenosis. The opening snap, an unusual high-pitched sound that occurs immediately after S2, is associated with mitral valve stenosis. The friction rub, which is a harsh grating sound during systole and diastole, is associated with pericarditis.

47. C: At one time, patients were routinely shielded from bad news, but the pendulum has swung in the opposite direction and now it is generally believed that patients should always be told the truth. This is a cultural belief more common in the West than the East. In some culture, such as Asian cultures, people are often not told that they are dying or have cancer, especially if no cure is possible. In this case, the nurse should respect the family's wishes.

48. D: While balloon tamponade can be maintained for up to 24 hours, it should be left in place for the shortest period possible because of the risk of serious complications, such as airway obstruction, esophageal injury, and aspiration (especially if the gastric balloon ruptures and the tube migrates upward or if the patient is confused and pulls on the tube). When removing the tube,

the esophageal tube is deflated first and the patient observed for bleeding for a few hours prior to deflation of the gastric balloon.

49. B: Atrial fibrillation is often treated with cardioversion, a timed electrical shock to the heart to convert a tachydysrhythmia to a sinus rhythm. An anticoagulant, such as warfarin, is usually prescribed 3 weeks prior to the procedure in order to reduce the risk of emboli. Patients on digoxin must discontinue the drug at least two days prior to the procedure. In some cases, antiarrhythmics, such as diltiazem hydrochloride (Cardizem) or amiodarone hydrochloride (Cordarone) may be prescribed prior to the cardioversion to slow the heart rate.

50. C: Azotemia: dehydration, increased BUN, and increased urinary specific gravity. Management includes decreasing amino acids in PN formula or changing to Nephramine. Hypoglycemia: decreased serum glucose, diaphoresis, pallor, lethargy, confusion, and weakness. Management includes stopping insulin and increasing concentration of dextrose as well as slowing infusion rate and evaluating for sepsis. Hyperammonemia: lethargy, change in mental status, asterixis. Management includes decreasing protein concentration in PN formula and evaluating for hepatic insufficiency. EFA deficiency: dry skin, thrombocytopenia. Management includes increasing lipid intake (at least 2 times weekly), oral fats (if possible), and topical fats.

51. B: Amylase levels are often elevated after CPB, but only 3% or fewer patients develop pancreatitis; however, levels over 1000 UI/L indicate increased risk, so patients must be monitored carefully. The increased amylase level may develop because of decreased renal excretion. Patients may exhibit nausea, anorexia, and ileus. Treatment is primarily supportive. If pancreatitis develops, it typically results from necrosis associated with lengthy CPB and prolonged decreased cardiac output. Patients with a history of alcoholism are at increased risk.

52. D: These nonspecific signs and symptoms of decline are characteristic of failure to thrive, which is commonly associated with depression in older adults, so the Geriatric Depression Scale should be administered. GDS is a simple 15-question questionnaire that requires only "yes" or "no" answers with a score of greater than 5 "yes" answers indicating depression. Failure to thrive may result from medications (anticonvulsants, antidepressants, opioids, SSRIs, neuroleptics, diuretics, beta-blockers, anticholinergics, alpha-antagonists, and benzodiazepines), chronic illness, socioeconomic factors, and abuse or neglect.

53. B: The normal height of the jugular vein pulsation above the sternal angle is 4 cm or less. If the measurement is greater than 4 cm, this can indicate increased pressure in the right atrium and right heart failure. However, pericarditis and tricuspid stenosis may also increase pressure as well as laughing or cough (which can trigger the Valsalva response). The jugular venous pressure is a non-invasive method of estimating central venous pressure although the procedure is usually not accurate with heart rate of over 100/min.

54. C: Red clover is contraindicated with clopidogrel because it increases the risk of bleeding. NSAIDs and salicylates also increase risk of bleeding and should be avoided or monitored carefully. Clopidogrel is an antiplatelet inhibitor (adenosine diphosphate inhibitor). It inhibits platelet aggregation and forming of a clot by changing the membrane so that it can no longer receive the signal to aggregate. Adverse effects include bleeding, chest pain, hypertension, edema, flu-like symptoms, abdominal pain, indigestion, diarrhea, epistaxis, rash, pruritus, bradycardia, dizziness, edema, leg and pelvic pain, and chills.

55 A: The balloon for a pulmonary artery catheter is usually inflated when the catheter tip reaches the right atrium, allowing it to float through the right ventricle and into the right pulmonary artery. The balloon should be inflated to a maximum of 1.5 mL of air. The waveforms and pressures should be recorded as the catheter passes from the right atrium into the pulmonary artery where it occludes the vessel in position for recording of pulmonary artery wedge pressure (PAWP). Once the PAWP is obtained, the balloon is deflated and the catheter secured.

56. D: Patients with delirium tremens (onset usually greater than 48 hours after drinking cessation) frequently exhibit global confusion, hallucinations, delusions, fever, tachycardia, and hypertension. Patients may become very aggressive and violent as they respond to feelings of paranoia and fear. Many patients feel as though something is crawling on their skin and may believe they are dying. DTs occur in about 5% of patients undergoing alcohol withdrawal and can be fatal without prompt treatment. Patients may progress from alcohol intoxication to alcohol withdrawal, to DTs.

57. A: Spontaneous wedging can occur if the catheter becomes displaced, often from the patient moving about or from warming of the catheter. The first action should be to try to dislodge the catheter by turning the patient onto the opposite side of the catheter placement. Other interventions include asking the patient to raise or straighten the arm or turn the head and gently cough. If this does not resolve the problem, then the catheter may need to be repositioned.

58. B: Celiac disease results in malabsorption of folate and iron, so patients are often anemic. Additionally, damage to the lining of the small intestines from gluten sensitivity interferes with absorption of fats and calcium, so patients may exhibit osteomalacia and bone pain and steatorrhea. Celiac disease is an autoimmune disorder in which antibodies to gluten in the diet cause inflammation and damage to intestinal villi. Patients must be maintained on a strict gluten-free diet. Gluten is found in some grains, such as wheat.

59. D: An intra-abdominal pressure of more than 25 mm Hg indicates the need for immediate surgical decompression to prevent cardiovascular and renal damage. Normal intra-abdominal pressures range from 0 to 5 mm Hg, but perfusion of internal organs may be impaired with pressures above 13 mm Hg. Below 25 mm Hg, treatment usually includes hypervolemic therapy to expand volume and improve perfusion. If decompression is indicated, crystalloids are usually administered first to prevent too rapid reperfusion, which can cause acidosis and cardiac arrest.

60. B: CPAP is titrated at bedtime after the patient has participated in a demonstration of the equipment and usually begins with the pressure set at low at about 5 cm H_2O until the patient falls asleep after which the pressure is slowly increased by 1 cm H_2O every 15 minutes with the patient carefully observed until relief of symptoms occurs. During titration, the patient is usually placed in supine position. The pressure may be adjusted up and down until optimal pressure is achieved.

61. C: In order to calculate the stroke volume, the patient's cardiac output and heart rate must be known. If the cardiac output is 5.6 L/min, this equals 5600 mL. If the heart rate is 80, then the calculation is: CO/HR = SV, 5600/80 = 70 mL. Normal cardiac output ranges from 4 to 6 L per minute. Normal SV is 60 to 70 mL per heartbeat.

62. A: Oxygen should help relieve hypoxemia. Inotropes, such as dobutamine, improve contractility of the heart, increasing the CO (normal 4-6 L/min) and SV (normal 60-70 mL/beat). Vasodilators, such as nitroprusside, should decrease the SVR and PAWP. Combined action should decrease the heart rate and improve the blood pressure, which should in turn increase the MAP, which is barely

within normal range (70 to 110 mm Hg). MAP of at least 60 mm Hg is required for adequate perfusion.

63. C: Characteristics of a Q-wave myocardial infarction include peak CK levels at 27 hours (compared to 12 to 13 hours for non-Q-wave MI). Infarction of the coronary artery is usually prolonged with coronary occlusion complete in 80 to 90%. Most but not all Q-wave MIs are transmural. As the tissue damage approaches the full-thickness of the heart muscle, Q waves (wide and deep) begin to appear on the ECG, especially early in the morning because of adrenergic activity. The mortality rate for Q-wave MI is about 10%.

64. B: Fluid intelligence is the ability to see relationships, reason, and think abstractly—all qualities needed to facilitate learning. Older adults tend to have altered time perception so that time seems to pass more quickly than when they were younger, so they may focus more on the here and now rather than on future needs. Other changes include increased test anxiety, decreased short-term (rather than long-term) memory, increased processing and reaction time, and persistence of stimuli (confusing older learning with newer).

65. A: The femoral nerve may become damaged during the fem-pop bypass procedure, resulting in numbness and tingling in the anterior and medial aspects of the thigh. The femoral nerve activates muscles used to extend the leg and move the hips, so damage may impair mobility (depending upon the degree). The damage may occur as direct injury or from compression related to edema and inflammation. The symptoms may recede over time, although some patients will need physical therapy to strengthen muscles.

66. D: The two types of drugs most commonly implicated in acute hypoglycemia are insulins and sulfonylureas, including glipizide (Glucotrol), which stimulates beta cells in the pancreas to produce more insulin. The hypoglycemic effect of sulfonylureas may be potentiated by other medications that compete for binding sites on albumin. Patients with sulfonylurea-induced hypoglycemia and altered mental status require hospitalization, IV glucose, and careful monitoring, since oral ingestion of carbohydrates alone may not prevent relapses, which may occur for days.

67. B: Because bronchiolitis obliterans is a progression of allograft rejection, the usual treatment approach is to increase immunosuppression, often initially with methylprednisolone, although there is little evidence this actually improves the condition, and it may further increase risk of infection. Bronchiolitis obliterans results in inflammation of the small airways and fibrosis with development of intraluminal polyps and hyperplasia that obstructs the bronchioles and may extend into the alveolar ducts and distal alveoli. Prognosis is poor.

68. A: Because warfarin decreases the clotting time, warfarin should be discontinued two to three days prior to the procedure and the INR should be under 2. Vitamin K or fresh frozen plasma may be administered to reverse the effects of warfarin if necessary. Aspirin and other antiplatelet medications are usually given before cardiac catheterization. Heparin therapy can be continued during cardiac catheterization but discontinued for removal of the sheath.

69. C: These signs and symptoms are characteristic of complete small bowel obstruction (especially not passing flatus for more than 12 hours), the dilated loops of small bowel, and the lack of air in the colon and rectum; so the initial intervention is likely to be exploratory surgery since the risk for ischemia is high. If the blockage is in the proximal part of the small bowel, abdominal distention may not be evident. Laboratory studies, such as the complete blood count and electrolytes, may be normal or abnormal, depending on many factors.

70. B: These signs and symptoms are consistent with acute pulmonary edema; and since the client is dyspneic and cyanotic, the nurse should immediately sit the patient upright and administer 100% oxygen per mask to relieve the patient's hypoxemia and achieve a PO_2 above 60%. Some patients may require Bi-PAP or endotracheal intubation and mechanical ventilation. Morphine sulfate (2 to 8 mg) may be administered subcutaneously or intravenously in severe cases. Other treatments include loop diuretics to promote venous dilation and diuresis, nitrates, bronchodilators, digoxin (if tachycardia present), and ACE inhibitors to reduce afterload.

71. D: Signs and symptoms of retroperitoneal hemorrhage may be nonspecific, especially at first, but as blood accumulates, back and flank pain may occur. Pulse rate increases and blood pressure will fall as the patient becomes increasingly hypotensive. Hemoglobin may show an abrupt decrease. A CT scan of the abdomen should show the mass. This is a medical emergency, and the patient must be transferred immediately back to the cath lab for angiography to locate the site of perforation and leakage. A vascular closure device may be used, and/or a balloon inflated over the bleeding site to control bleeding.

72. C: When undergoing pericardiocentesis, the patient should be positioned upright at 45 degrees because this allows good visualization and easy access and brings the heart closer to the chest wall. Patients often receive atropine before the procedure to prevent vasovagal reactions. A nasogastric tube may need to be inserted if the patient has abdominal distention. After the needle is inserted, the obturator is removed and a syringe attached to aspirate blood or fluid. A sterile alligator clamp is attached from the needle to a precordial lead of the ECG for monitoring to ensure that the ventricle is not punctured.

73. D: Stimulation threshold testing is conducted to determine the minimum output necessary to consistently capture the heart. Once the output for consistent capture is determined, the output should be set at 2 to 3 times this level, so if threshold testing shows consistent capture at 2 mA, the output should be set at 4 to 6 mA. The procedure for sensitivity testing is: first, verify paced rhythm, increasing rate temporarily if necessary to override intrinsic rhythm; then watch monitor while slowly decreasing output and not when loss of capture occurs; gradually increase output until 1:1 capture resumes; and set output.

74. B: The symptoms are consistent with thoracic aortic aneurysm. Patients with Marfan syndrome are at risk for thoracic aortic aneurysms and should be monitored carefully to prevent rupture. Surgery is indicated for aneurysms of 5 cm or more. With MFS, the aneurysm usually occurs at the sinuses of Valsalva (aortic root) and in most cases is ascending with type A dissection. It the aneurysm is in the ascending aorta or arch, open surgical repair is indicated and carries a higher risk than repairs in the descending aorta. Beta-blockers may slow aneurysm dilation.

75. A: Wool, plastics, and polyurethane foam produce cyanide gas when burned, so the patient is at risk for cyanide poisoning and should receive hydroxocobalamin as the antidote of choice. It is usually administered with sodium thiosulfate, which potentiates the effects. Hydroxocobalamin combines chemically with cyanide to form vitamin B_{12}, which can be excreted through the kidneys. Sodium nitrite can also be used for cyanide poisoning but has more adverse effects and is contraindicated with severe smoke inhalation.

76. D: Flexor (decorticate) posturing indicates hemispheric damage. Brainstem damage results in flaccidity and areflexia while midbrain and upper pons damage results in extensor (decerebrate) posturing. Anoxic encephalopathy can occur within 5 minutes if the brain is without oxygenation.

Absence of pupillary responses and elicited eye movements indicates severe brain damage. If there is damage to the frontal or occipital areas of the brain but the midbrain and pons are intact, horizontal movement of the eyes may be evident.

77. C: Patients are at high risk for fatal or non-fatal MI if they have unstable angina and the following findings: ECG changes including transient ST-segment changes greater than 0.05 mV, persistent VT, and BBB; troponin T elevated to greater than 0.1 ng/mL; increased ischemic symptoms in previous 48 hours; rest pain longer than 20 minutes; pulmonary edema, new or increased MR murmur, S3 or increased rales; decreased BP; bradycardia or tachycardia; and advanced age (over 75). T-wave inversion, pathologic Q waves, and slight elevation of Troponin T (<0.1 ng/mL) are moderate risk factors.

78. A: Pulmonic stenosis constricts blood flow from the right ventricle to the lungs, resulting in right ventricular hypertrophy as the pressure increases in the right ventricle. Respiratory symptoms develop as pulmonary blood flow is decreased, including dyspnea and mild cyanosis. Depending on the degree of stenosis, some patients may be asymptomatic, or symptoms may develop slowly and not be evident until adulthood. Treatment includes balloon valvuloplasty to separate valve cusps in younger children and pulmonary valvotomy for adults and older children.

79. A: Primary graft dysfunction (reperfusion injury) is a major cause of illness and death in lung recipients with symptoms and treatment similar to ARDS. Indications include frequent oxygen desaturation, general malaise, increased dyspnea and work associated with the act of breathing, and intolerance to activity. Causes may include increased capillary permeability, interrupted lymphatic drainage, edema, and mismatch in compliance and vascular resistance between donor and recipient. Treatment includes high oxygen concentrations, decreased tidal volumes, PP ventilation for those intubated, and increased oxygen supplementation and pulmonary toileting for those extubated.

80. D: The best approach is to attempt to collaborate with the patient, allowing the patient to feel more in control: "Let's talk about how we can work together to make this easier for you." There can be many reasons why patients are uncooperative and have an exaggerated response to pain. The patient may simply be frustrated, or the patient may be tired or fearful. It's possible that the pain medication isn't adequate, but the nurse needs to really listen to the patient to try to determine the best solution.

81. B: SvO_2 measures oxygen saturation in mixed venous blood via a catheter in the pulmonary artery. Normal value is 60 to 80%. SaO_2 measures oxygen saturation in arterial blood with a gas analyzer. Normal value is 96 to 100%. SpO_2 measures oxygen saturation with a pulse oximeter. Normal value is also 96 to 100%. $ScvO_2$ measures oxygen saturation in mixed venous blood from the head, neck, arms and upper thorax per a fiber-optic catheter or central venous catheter. Normal value is greater than 70% and is usually 5 to 10% higher than SvO_2 value.

82. D: Extragastric hemorrhage most often occurs 24 to 48 hours after surgery and may present with sudden onset of hypotension, tachycardia, and diminished urinary output. Peritoneal drains may show some bloody or blood-tinged discharged while NG aspirant remains essentially clear. Symptoms may mimic myocardial infarction. CT scan is used for diagnosis. Causes of bleeding include lacerated spleen, liver injury (from retractors), pancreatic bed hemorrhage, and improperly secured vessels. If blood transfusions do not stabilize the patient, then exploratory laparotomy is indicated.

83. B: A high-fat, high-protein, and low-carbohydrate diet is recommended for patients after gastric surgery to prevent or minimize dumping syndrome. Carbohydrates are absorbed more quickly than fats or proteins, increasing dumping symptoms. Additionally, a high-carbohydrate diet may exacerbate the postprandial hypoglycemia that often occurs two to three hours after a patient eats because of the sudden bolus of high carbohydrates that enters the small intestine and triggers release of insulin. Lying down after eating helps to slow the movement of food through the GI tract, decreasing symptoms.

84. A: The patient is exhibiting signs of mild lithium toxicity. Symptoms of mild toxicity are evident with levels 1.5 to 2.5 mEq/L. The therapeutic level of lithium for maintenance therapy is 0.6 to 1.2 mEq/L and 1.0 to 1.5 mEq/L for acute episodes of mania. Lithium has a narrow therapeutic index and levels should be monitored weekly initially and then monthly with patients educated about signs of toxicity. More severe life-threatening symptoms (ECG abnormalities, seizures, coma) can occur with blood levels above 2.5 mEq/L.

85. C: Although the patient's platelet count remains above 100,000, a reduction of 30% to 50% with evidence of thrombi and vascular occlusion is indicative of heparin-induced thrombocytopenia Type II, which is an immune-mediated response to heparin. While most often associated with unfractionated heparin, it can also be caused by low-molecular-weight heparin, so the intervention is to immediately discontinue the heparin and administer lepirudin or argatroban. HIT Type II can be confirmed with the functional assays heparin-induced platelet aggregation (HIPA) and serotonin release assay (SRA). ELISA can be used to identify presence of HIT antigen.

86. B: The primary problem with basing research on qualitative data is that the data are subjective and objective data have more validity for research. However, both may provide valuable information. Qualitative data are usually described verbally or in graphic form. Gathering qualitative data can require considerable time because it may involve interviewing numerous participants. Quantitative data, which are described statistically, may be derived from surveys, questionnaires, and other methods of obtaining numerical data.

87. A: The most critical concern after AVM repair (surgery or embolization) is reperfusion bleeding, so strict control of BP to prevent it from exceeding the maximum established (usually 140 systolic) must be maintained. As feeder arteries are occluded, blood is diverted into vessels that are maximally dilated and tissues that have often suffered from chronic ischemia, so the increased pressure from additional blood flow may cause leakage of blood from the vessels. To prevent reperfusion bleeding, AVM repair is often done in two to four stages with partial embolization or excision done at each stage.

88. D: The patient has burns covering approximately 27% of his body. The Rule of 9s is used to estimate total body surface area burned in order to calculate the need for fluid replacement and other treatments. Rule of 9s: each arm 9%--4.5% anterior and 4.5% posterior; each leg 18%--9% anterior and 9% posterior; groin area 1%; upper chest 9%; abdomen 9%; upper back 9%; lower back/buttocks 9%; head 9%--4.5% anterior and 4.5% posterior.

89. C: While idiopathic thrombocytopenia purpura is often self-limiting, because the patient is exhibiting symptoms, this puts her at risk for more serious complications (such as intracerebral hemorrhage), so the usual initial treatment is a course of oral corticosteroids, which usually results in an increase of the platelet count to normal level within 2 to 6 weeks. If symptoms are severe, then IV Ig may be used to suppress the antibody response. High-dose IV methylprednisolone may

also be administered. Following IV Ig or methylprednisolone, platelet transfusions are recommended. If no response to medical treatment, splenectomy may be considered.

90. B: The patient is in uncompensated respiratory acidosis, indicating hypoventilation: PaO_2 of 88 mm Hg (normal value 80 to 100) indicates the patient is not hypoxemic; pH of 7.28 (normal value 7.35 to 7.45) indicates acidosis since it is greater than 7.4; $PaCO_2$ of 48 mm Hg (normal value 35 to 45) represents respiratory acidosis resulting from hypoventilation since the value if greater than 45 (less than 35 would represent respiratory alkalosis); HCO_3- of 23 mEq/L (normal value 22 to 26) remains normal. Because both the pH and the $PaCO_2$ are abnormal, this indicates uncompensated ABGs, since the pH has not returned to normal level.

91. A: Usually for severe dehydration related to DKA, 1 to 1.5 L of 0.9% normal saline with insulin is administered at the rate of 1 L/hour, after which serum sodium levels should be determined. If the serum sodium is low, IVs and insulin are continued with 0.9% normal saline at the rate of 4 to 14 mL/kg, but if sodium is normal or high, the IV fluids are switched to 0.45% sodium chloride at the rate of 4 to 14 mL/kg until serum glucose reaches 250 mg/dL. Then IV fluid is changed to 5% dextrose with 0.45% sodium chloride (150-250 mL/hr.).

92. C: These laboratory values are consistent with diabetes insipidus. Desmopressin acetate is used to increase water resorption in the nephron. Central DI often develops secondary to neurosurgery, traumatic brain injury, meningitis, and encephalitis. Inadequate amounts of vasopressin are secreted, resulting in dilute urine with decreased osmolality and specific gravity with frequent urination while serum osmolality and serum sodium increase, resulting in increased thirst. Thiazide diuretics are used with nephrogenic DI and hypertonic saline solution and demeclocycline with severe SIADH.

93. B: The primary difference between HHNK and DKA is that HHNK does not involve breakdown of fats (into ketones) and DKA does because some insulin production remains with HHNK although it is inadequate to prevent hyperglycemia (greater than 600 mg/dL). HHNK is a disease that occurs in those with diabetes and insulin resistance, leading to persistent hyperglycemia and osmotic diuresis. As fluid shifts from intracellular to extracellular spaces, glucosuria and dehydration cause hypernatremia and increased serum osmolality (greater than 350 mOsm/L). Treatment is similar to DKA: insulin and IV fluids.

94. C: Asking a nurse on another unit about his experience with a procedure is an example of informal collaboration because the collaboration does not stem from established organization or protocol, such as teams or hierarchical structures. When members of a team help each other, this represents formal collaboration because that is the purpose of a team. Collaboration is a continuous process in nursing, occurring almost every time a healthcare provider interacts with other healthcare providers, patients, or family members. Both informal and formal collaboration may be equally valuable.

95. B: All of the laboratory values are within normal limits except for the BUN, which is elevated to 26 from a normal of 7 to 17 mg/dL (reference values may vary somewhat). While this is outside the normal range, it is usually evaluated with creatinine to determine if there is kidney damage, and the creatinine level is normal. BUN values may be elevated by dehydration and some commonly-used drugs, such as acetaminophen and ibuprofen.

96. D: The best response is the one that provides the reason for early surgery: "The risk of re-bleeding increases every day, putting you at grave risk if you delay." Approximately 4% of patients

experience re-bleeding during the first 24 hours with a 1 to 2% chance of re-bleeding every day for at least a month. Re-bleeding carries a mortality rate of approximately 70%. Surgical repair, which may include clipping or embolization, is usually scheduled within 48 hours for grades I and II and for some grade III SAH.

97. C: The immediate intervention for directly observed aspiration is suction of the upper airway to prevent further aspiration by removing remaining gastric contents. Following this, oxygen should be administered as needed while the patient awaits bronchoscopy for removal of large particles. Bronchoalveolar lavage poses the risk of disseminating the aspirant throughout the lung fields, causing more damage. The most common sites for aspiration infiltration are the right middle lobe and lower lobes, but this can vary depending on the patient's position and volume of aspirant.

98. B: The first-line treatment for obstructive sleep apnea (OSA) is CPAP. OSA occurs when the pharynx collapses during sleep because of narrow or restricted airway. It is most common in those who are overweight, especially middle-aged males. It is characterized by heavy snoring with apneic periods that may last up to one minute, usually at least 30 times per night. CPAP delivers pressurized room air to a nasal or oral interface/mask and allows for adjusting of airflow and expels carbon dioxide through a vent or valve. Most machines can provide pressures ranging from 2 to 20 cm H_2O.

99. A: If dysrhythmias occur during apnea testing, the nurse should obtain a blood sample for ABGs and reconnect the ventilator, since the testing should not be the cause of death. Apnea testing includes disconnecting the ventilator and administering 100% oxygen at 6L/min per endotracheal tube. The patient is observed closely for respiratory movements and a blood sample obtained for ABGs after 8 minutes. Then, the patient is reconnected to the ventilator. During the test, the patient's core body temperature should be maintained at 36.5° C or higher with a systolic BP at 90 mm Hg or higher. Euvolemia and eucapnia ($PaCO_2$ about 40 mm Hg) should be established.

100. B: The most important factor in having a patient sign a consent form is the patient's ability to give informed consent. This means that the patient must have the legal right by age or emancipation and must be able to comprehend. If a patient is cognitively impaired because of dementia, sedation, or condition, this can pose a problem because patients cannot legally give consent if they are unable to understand. If patients don't speak English, a translator should be provided.

101. D: Controlled mandatory ventilation (CMV): This mode provides a specified volume of air and rate with no triggering required of the patient and respiratory response decreased through medication. Synchronized intermittent mandatory ventilation (SIMV): This mode provides a specified tidal volume that is synchronized with the patient's breathing. Assist control ventilation (ACV): This mode is triggered by the patient's own breathing, but if apneic periods occur, the machine will initiate respirations at a specified tidal volume. Pressure support ventilation (PSV): This mode requires the patient to initiate all breaths, which are supplemented by positive pressure.

102. D: While bilateral periorbital ecchymosis (Raccoon's eyes) may indicate eye trauma (as well as multiple myeloma and disseminated neuroblastoma), it is likely that the patient has a basilar skull fracture because of the previous car accident. Raccoon's eyes may not be evident for two to three days after an injury, but the "salty" taste in the patient's mouth suggests leakage of cerebrospinal fluid. In some cases Battles sign—ecchymosis in the mastoid area behind the ear—may be present as well.

103. A: While it's very unlikely that a miracle cure will occur as a result of positive thinking, patients often need to hold onto hope to cope with dying, and thinking positively may help them to find some peace, so the nurse should be supportive without making false claims, dismissing the idea, or trying to dissuade the person with reason: "The mind can be powerful." Additionally, positive thinking may increase the release of endorphins, which may help to alleviate some discomfort.

104. B: For ventilator management, the fraction of inspired oxygen (FiO$_2$) should be maintained below 40% (0.4) to avoid oxygen toxicity although the patient may initially need a higher concentration of oxygen. Normal room air provides 21% (0.2). The flow rate will vary depending on the type of oxygen delivery system used. For example, with a nasal cannula at flow rate of 5 L/min, FiO$_2$ is 40%. With a Venturi mask and flow rate of 8 L/min, FiO$_2$ is 35 to 40%.

105. D: The best and only legal action is to ignore the parents, as they have no standing. Rights go with the individual patient, not the one for paying for insurance. Because the patient is 18 years old and legally an adult, he has the right to decide who visits or not, and the parents should have been advised of this. The nurse cannot legally contact the parents about the patient without his permission. He should be advised of the parents' action so that he can deal with the issue.

106. A: Because the patient sustained a head injury and is at risk for increased intracranial pressure, the patient should have a CT of the brain prior to the procedure so it can be reviewed for signs of a brain shift that may indicate ICP. With increased ICP, when pressure is suddenly relieved by withdrawing of cerebral spinal fluid, the brain structures may herniate through the foramen magnum, compressing the brainstem, which is critical for regulation of cardiac and respiratory function.

107. A: Trauma patients should be provided 1 to 1.5 g/k/day of protein. Higher amounts show no benefit. Trauma results in increased breakdown of protein because of catabolism in addition to protein losses that may have occurred with blood loss. Patients may lose as much as 10% of lean body mass within 10 days. When 25% or more of lean body mass is lost, protein malnutrition is severe and can result in increased mortality. Protein is more critical than total calories and the increased catabolic rate resists protein supplementation although synthesis of protein increases with infusions of amino acids.

108. C: About 25% of those with subarachnoid hemorrhage develop hydrocephalus as a late complication because blood that has been absorbed by arachnoid villi may result in villi obstruction and decreased absorption of cerebrospinal fluid. In about half of these cases, the condition is self-limiting and resolves without intervention, so if patients remain awake and responsive and do not have severe symptoms, observation for 24 hours is the usual initial intervention. If the patient's condition worsens, then in some cases serial lumbar punctures are done to drain fluid, but the most common treatment is ventriculostomy or ventriculoperitoneal shunt.

109. B: Patients often establish close relationships with nurses caring for them and begin to develop dependency, so the best solution is for the nurse to make the transfer as easy as possible is by accompanying the patient to her new room and introducing her to staff, ensuring that the patient is settled into her new unit without difficulty. The nurse should not make unrealistic promises (such as daily visits) that she may not be able to keep.

110. C: Phenytoin may cause gingival hyperplasia, so patients should be advised to carefully maintain dental care and to see dentists regularly. Patients may have monthly blood tests initially but once stabilized blood tests are usually done every six months. Patients should be advised to

- 248 -

avoid alcohol entirely when taking any anticonvulsant drug. Stopping anticonvulsant drugs abruptly may trigger rebound seizures, so if adverse effects occur, the patient should be advised to immediately contact the physician for guidance in withdrawing the drug if necessary.

111. C: Intracranial hypertension occurs with intracranial pressure greater than 20 mm Hg. Normal intracranial pressure ranges from 7 to 15 mm Hg. Because of the constraints of the skull, the volume in the brain is fixed and has 3 components: blood, tissue, and cerebrospinal fluid. According to the Kelli-Moore hypothesis, an increase in one component requires a compensating decrease in another component. The brain may accommodate some increase in volume with little increase in ICP, but when the brain's volume limit is reached, even a small increase in volume may result in a significant increase in ICP.

112. A: When patients receiving CCRT exhibit increased heart rate, decreased blood pressure and ECG abnormalities, the nurse should suspect electrolyte imbalance. Electrolyte levels must be carefully monitored and output values checked at least every hour. Hypotension may also decrease the ultrafiltration rate as blood flow through lines decreases. Fluid volume must also be monitored since too much or too little fluid may result in changes in mentation and increased or decreased CVP or PAOP.

113. B: While in most cases it is inappropriate to use family members—especially children—to interpret, the granddaughter can be asked to assist because the directions for the test are relatively simple ("How old are you? What is the date today?"). In all cases, the nurse may use some type of pantomime to assist the patient, such as demonstrating how to show the teeth when scoring facial palsy. The patient's first response should be recorded. The granddaughter should be asked not to coach the patient in any way or give hints.

114. A: The usual contraindications to recombinant tPA apply to people who have had strokes and appear for treatment within the 3-hour window after the stroke, but additional exclusions apply to those who appear in the 3- to 4.5-hour window. This patient is excluded from treatment because he is over 80 years old. Other exclusions include a history of both stroke and diabetes, score on the NIH stroke scale of more than 25, and any current use of oral anticoagulants.

115. D: Metabolic acidosis is associated with acute renal failure because the impaired kidneys are unable to excrete increased levels of acids due to decreased excretion of phosphates and other organic acids and because the tubules are unable to excrete ammonia or reabsorb sodium bicarbonate. Characteristics of metabolic acidosis include low (acidic) pH level and decreased bicarbonate. Symptoms may vary, but with chronic renal failure, the patient may remain asymptomatic until the bicarbonate level falls to 15 mEq/L or less.

116. B: With fractures of ribs 8 and above on the right side, the primary concern is injury to the spleen. Fractured ribs are usually the results of severe blunt trauma, so underlying injuries are common. With fractures of ribs 8 and above on the left side, the primary concern is injury to the liver. Fractures of the upper two ribs (either one side or both) pose a risk of injury to the trachea, bronchi, and great vessels. If three or more adjacent ribs are fractured both anteriorly and posteriorly, a flail chest results.

117. C: Studies show that most adults experience a period of low energy in the afternoon (the reason for afternoon naps). About 55% of adults are most alert and work and study best in the early morning while about 28% do best in the evening, so group education is probably best planned for

morning while individual education should be more flexible according to the patient's preference whenever possible. Most people are aware whether they are "morning" or "evening" people.

118. D: Displacement: The patient directs anger at other individuals (the wife in this case) rather than directing it at the person (physician), who is the actual source of bad news (threat). Projection: The patient believes that others are exhibiting the patient's own unacceptable characteristics (seeing in others what the person cannot recognize in himself/herself). Reaction formation: The patient behaves or expresses the opposite of how the patient actually feels. Sublimation: The patient converts repressed feelings into actions that are socially acceptable.

119. B: Patients who are legally blind often have developed the ability to compensate for lack of vision with increased acuity in other senses, including the sense of touch, smell, hearing, and taste. Patients who are blind should be encouraged to handle and manipulate equipment while the nurse explains, using as much verbal description as possible. Patients may have developed improved memory skills that allow them to learn quickly from spoken words. Family members may want to learn about the equipment as well, but the focus should be on teaching the patient to use it independently.

120. A: The first-line treatment for acute exacerbations of asthma is short-acting B_2-agonsit, such as nebulized albuterol and a corticosteroid, such as oral prednisone or IV methylprednisolone. While corticosteroids will not have immediate effect, it is important to administer the drug early to maintain control. Nonspecific B-adrenergic agents, such as epinephrine, are usually reserved for treatment before intubation for patients unresponsive to other treatments. Anticholinergic medications, such as ipratropium bromide, may be added to albuterol. Theophylline has many side effects so is often avoided. IV magnesium and heliox are usually given only if patients do not respond to other treatments.

121. D: The nurse provided the CD for the patient to help relieve the patient's anxiety and to show caring. This is an example of caring practice in which the nurse carries out acts of kindness and provides a supportive caring relationship for the patient. Caring practices require the nurse to take a creative approach to care and to look at the needs of the whole person. The nurse makes a choice to take action for the benefit of the patient, often beyond that which is required.

122. C: Many patients are afraid of their doctors or don't want to "bother" them, so prompting the patient or telling the physician that the patient has questions may still not elicit them. The best method is to prepare a list of the patient's questions for the physician and to explain the patient's reluctance to ask the physician the questions directly. The patient may not be able or willing to articulate the reasons for not asking questions directly.

123. D: Collegiality: interacting with others and contributing to professional development of peers and other healthcare providers. Quality of care: evaluating the quality of care in a systematic manner. Education: acquiring and maintaining both current knowledge and competencies necessary to provide care to the critically ill. Collaboration: working together with patients, families, and health care providers to provide excellence in patient care. Ethics: making decisions and acting in an ethical manner. Individual practice evaluation: reflecting knowledge of professional and legal standards, laws, and regulations. Research: using clinical inquiry. Resource utilization: considering safety, effectiveness, and cost.

124. C: Talking to people who aren't there and who have died is often a sign of impending death. Patients nearing death may also say they must prepare for a trip and may describe a place they

appear to be able to see. Some patients express awareness that they are dying. The role of the nurse is to remain supportive to the patient and the family and provide as much comfort care as possible. When treatments are no longer necessary or effective because the patient is dying, the nurse should request discontinuation of the treatments.

125. D: There are three barriers to systems thinking here. Identifying with professional role instead of purpose: looking only at one's own role and needs and not considering the roles of others and the institution as a whole. Feeling victimized: blaming others (institution, administration, other healthcare professional) for own shortcomings and believing nothing can be done to improve situations. This feeling may become institutionalized, making changes difficult. Relying on past experience: persisting in trying to apply old solutions to new problems.

126. D: There are four barriers to systems thinking here. Failing to adapt: feeling very threatened by changes, such as the switch to electronic charting. Some may feel they cannot learn new procedures and may react angrily or withdraw. Having an autocratic attitude: believing that only their perceptions or practices are the correct one and focusing on narrow views and short-term outcomes. Arriving at weak consensus: superficially solving problems without really delving into all issues. Displaying displaced anger: directing anger at someone or something other than the cause of the problem.

127. C: V/Q mismatch, which occurs when well-ventilated alveoli lack adequate perfusion while poorly-ventilated alveoli have adequate perfusion, is the most common cause of hypoxemia. This is true because many common respiratory disorders can result in V/Q mismatch, including asthma, COPD, pulmonary embolus, pneumonia, and pulmonary hypertension. With V/Q mismatch, administration of 100% oxygen should increase oxygen saturation because oxygen improves uptake of oxygen in areas with poor ventilation. Dead space occurs when there is ventilation but no perfusion (such as in the trachea), and a shunt occurs where there is perfusion but no ventilation.

128. C: Rigid bronchoscopy is the treatment option of choice for removal of foreign bodies from the respiratory tract because the larger diameter makes retrieval less difficult. In some cases, flexible bronchoscopy may be used first to isolate the location of the foreign body, but the diameter is generally too small to withdraw foreign objects and attempting to grasp the object at the end of the scope and remove it in that manner may result in significant tissue damage. Bronchotomy is indicated if removal per bronchoscopy is unsuccessful. Bronchodilators and postural drainage is useful in only a small number of asymptomatic cases.

129. B: A patient with progressive pulmonary arterial hypertension must be monitored for signs of right ventricular heart failure, a common complication. With PAH, the pulmonary vascular bed becomes obstructed or damaged so that it cannot dilate adequately for increased blood flow, so this blood then increases pulmonary artery pressure, which in turn increases pulmonary vascular resistance. This requires increased workload for the right ventricle, leading to hypertrophy and failure. The patient may begin to have peripheral edema, ascites, liver engorgement, crackles, distended jugular veins, and heart murmur.

130. A: Heliox should be administered for at least 20 minutes in order for the patient to gain the full effects. Heliox is usually administered in mixtures of 80% He/20% O_2 or 70% He/30% O_2. The 70/30 mixture is indicated for patients with hypoxemia, so this mixture is more commonly used. Heliox is used to reduce airway resistance in order to increase oxygenation. Recent studies indicate that evidence is insufficient to recommend use of Heliox for acute asthma or COPD exacerbations, although it is frequently ordered.

131. C: The nurse who suggested the switch to acuity-based staffing is exercising systems thinking by looking at the organization as a whole and determining what best serves the organization and the patients rather than looking at only the needs of the unit. Systems thinking requires an understanding of interrelationships and structures as well as the ability to anticipate outcomes and understand how different actions affect outcomes. The nurse has applied a practical solution to a systems problem.

132. A: While all of these are important considerations when evaluating the validity of written material, the source of the material is the primary concern followed by the author's credentials. Articles printed in the popular press must meet different standards than articles printed in juried journals (such as *The New England Journal of Medicine*). The Internet has few rules, so much that is found on websites may look authentic but have no validity whatsoever. Wikipedia, while often helpful, cannot ever be used for evidence.

133. D: Adhesive atelectasis, caused by surfactant deficiency is most often associated with acute respiratory distress syndrome because surfactant production, which is critical to maintaining alveolar surface tension, is reduced, so alveoli collapse. With ARDS, alveolar collapse occurs widely throughout both lungs rather than in isolated areas, such as may occur with other causes of atelectasis. PEEP must be adequate to prevent further alveolar collapse in order to improve oxygenation.

134. A: Increasing dyspnea and hypoxemia with cough, hemoptysis, substernal pain, and subcutaneous emphysema of neck and chest are consistent with perforation of the trachea, which is a complication of endotracheal intubation. Perforation, especially in the posterior trachea, can occur during intubation or extubation. With this surgery, repositioning after surgery could also increase risks. Slight perforations may heal spontaneously with artificial airway that seals the perforation, but many, especially those who have cardiovascular instability, cannot adequately ventilate the lungs, or have tears greater than 4 cm, will require thoracotomy to repair.

135. B: Air leaks are a very common complication following bilateral lung volume reduction regardless of the surgical approach (VATS or median sternotomy). Patients return from surgery with two chest tubes in each hemithorax, and these are usually placed immediately in water seal drainage. Other complications include pneumonia, cardiac dysrhythmias, and infection. A small number of patients may go into respiratory failure and require reintubation. Adequate pain control is important to allow the patient to clear secretions and to encourage movement.

136. D: While onset of symptoms varies depending on many factors, including the severity of injury, usual signs and symptoms of acute respiratory distress syndrome (the most common complication of lung contusion) usually occur within 24 to 48 hours when hypoxemia becomes more obvious. Contusion results in pulmonary edema because of torn capillaries and micro-hemorrhage. Alveoli collapse and atelectasis are common. Inflammation occurs, increasing risk of respiratory failure. Ventilation/perfusion mismatch decreases oxygen saturation. Damage from chest contusion may not be visible on chest radiograph for a number of hours. CT scans or ultrasounds are more accurate.

137. A: These symptoms (decreased PaO_2 less than 60 mm Hg, increased $PaCO_2$ greater than 45 mm Hg, and decreased pH) are consistent with acute respiratory failure, type II, which is usually the result of alveolar hypoventilation and hypoxemia. With chronic respiratory failure, which usually develops over a period of days, the pH is closer to normal because of compensation. Patients with

- 252 -

hypoventilation should be positioned in semi-erect position. Treatment includes oxygen, ventilation, bronchodilators, steroids, sedatives, and analgesics, nutritional support, correction of acidosis, and monitoring for complications.

138. C: Patients with exertional heat stroke (EHS) are at high risk for rhabdomyolysis, DIC, and renal failure, while these are rare with non-exertional heat stroke (NEHS). Because patients with EHS can still sweat and exhibit diaphoresis, temperatures tend to be well below the highs (over 41° C/106° F) seen with NEHS, which is associated with anhidrosis. CNS system manifestations may be similar at times. Those with EHS often suffer syncope and loss of consciousness while those with NEHS may exhibit very mild irritability to deep coma.

139. C: The 72-hour protocol for N-acetylcysteine (NAC) is provided with serum levels greater than 150 mcg/mL. Patients often show no symptoms or only slight gastrointestinal upset for the first 24 hours after ingestion of acetaminophen, but evidence of hepatic damage usually is evident by the second day. Toxic dosages are greater than 140 mg/kg in one dose or greater than 7.5 g in 24 hours. Serum levels should always be done because patients often overestimate or underestimate the amount of drugs taken.

140. D: Patients who are allergic to bananas, kiwis, avocados, and chestnuts are at increased risk of allergy to latex because of cross reactivity and should be maintained in a latex-free environment. Reactions may occur with 5 types of exposure: inhalational, contact, mucous membrane, internal (surgical, invasive procedures), intravascular (IV). Other patients at higher risk include those with multiple surgeries, those with neural tube defects, those with congenital urogenital disorders, and those who work in the rubber industry, and those with allergies to anesthetics.

141. D: Sodium levels vary according to the underlying cause of acute renal failure. Prerenal causes: Urine sodium is decreased to below 20 mEq/L with urine osmolality increased to 500 mOsm. Urine specific gravity is increased. Intrarenal causes: Urine sodium is increased to more than 40 mEq/L, while urine osmolality is usually about 350 mOsm. Urine specific gravity is low normal. Postrenal causes: Urine sodium varies but is usually decreased to 20 mEq/L or less. Urine osmolality also varies but may be equal to or more than the serum level. Urine specific gravity also varies.

142. A: While all of these are important, assigning a task to someone who does not have the necessary skills or time to complete the task can result in the task not being completed correctly or even danger to the patient, so the first thing the nurse must do is determine if the task is appropriate for the person to whom it is delegated. This must be followed by clear instructions, monitoring progress, reviewing the final results, and recording outcomes as the responsibility for the task remains with the delegating nurse.

143. B: The most appropriate referral for the patient is an occupational therapist who can help the patient develop strategies and skills needed to compensate for poor vision and arthritis and provide information about adaptive equipment that the patient can use to prepare food. The occupational therapist can help the patient establish goals for independent food preparation and help the patient modify tasks. The occupational therapist may also help the patient learn how to better manage her arthritis to minimize symptoms.

144. C: Providing sensitive information to patients or family members should be done slowly rather than quickly so that they have time to digest the information. The nurse should ask if they have questions and should avoid technical jargon and consider psychosocial implications and well as cultural differences. It's important to respond to people's feelings and discuss follow-up. The nurse

should exercise patience, understanding that people respond to bad news in very different ways, including both anger and silence.

145. B: The best strategy when coaching another nurse is usually to provide positive feedback, stressing the nurse's correct actions rather than focusing on errors because the latter may increase the graduate nurse's anxiety and result in more errors. The nurse may use questioning to help the graduate nurse recognized problem areas. The nurse should provide a demonstration and encourage the graduate nurse to ask questions. The primary objective should be to help the learner gain both confidence and skills.

146. C: Most patients who are maintained of peritoneal dialysis at home should continue to receive PD after admission to a critical care unit unless there are specific contraindications, which include recent abdominal surgery, significant pulmonary disease, peritonitis, and need for rapid removal of fluid. The most common complications of PD are peritonitis and infection of exit site, so the nurse must carefully monitor laboratory values and patient condition for signs of infection. Patients usually are very knowledgeable about the amount and type of dialysate to be infused and the frequency of infusion.

147. A: The patient undergoing a renal biopsy should be placed in prone position because the biopsy is done from the posterior aspect. A small pillow may be placed under the patient's abdomen. The procedure is done under a local anesthetic (1% lidocaine). After removal of the biopsy needle, pressure should be applied. After the site is bandaged, the patient should be placed in supine position for 6 to 8 hours, and the patient should be observed for at least 12 hours to ensure bleeding does not go undetected.

148. A: The bispectral index system (BIS) can be used to both monitor the degree of consciousness for those who are receiving deep sedation and response to analgesia. BIS applies an algorithm to EEG activity and displays the result as a number (0 to 100) rather than a tracing. A value of 50 to 60 is usually the goal for deep sedation in which the patient is unconscious with low likelihood of recall. With values over 70, the patient is probably aware, while a score above 95 indicates an awake state. Brain waves are suppressed with values under 20.

149. A: Diazepam: Onset is 2 to 5 minutes, but the half-life ranges from 20 to 120 hours with prolonged sedation. Lorazepam: Onset is 5 to 20 minutes, and half-life is 8 to 15 hours with prolonged sedation. Propofol: Onset is 1 to 2 minutes with a half-life of 2 to 8 minutes when used for short-term sedation. If administered continuously, the sedative effect may last for 26 to 32 hours. Midazolam: Onset of action is rapid (2 to 5 minutes) and half-life ranges from 3 to 11 hours. Sedative effect is prolonged with continuous administration.

150. B: Because of the risk that periods of apnea associated with severe seizures can lead to respiratory failure and death, if a patient with status epilepticus does not respond to the first two doses of the benzodiazepine anticonvulsant medication, the next step is usually rapid sequence intubation so the patient can be ventilated while treatment continues. Fosphenytoin and phenobarbital may be added, but this may cause apnea, so intubation is necessary prior to administration of the drugs.

Secret Key #1 - Time is Your Greatest Enemy

Pace Yourself

Wear a watch. At the beginning of the test, check the time (or start a chronometer on your watch to count the minutes), and check the time after every few questions to make sure you are "on schedule."

If you are forced to speed up, do it efficiently. Usually one or more answer choices can be eliminated without too much difficulty. Above all, don't panic. Don't speed up and just begin guessing at random choices. By pacing yourself, and continually monitoring your progress against your watch, you will always know exactly how far ahead or behind you are with your available time. If you find that you are one minute behind on the test, don't skip one question without spending any time on it, just to catch back up. Take 15 fewer seconds on the next four questions, and after four questions you'll have caught back up. Once you catch back up, you can continue working each problem at your normal pace.

Furthermore, don't dwell on the problems that you were rushed on. If a problem was taking up too much time and you made a hurried guess, it must be difficult. The difficult questions are the ones you are most likely to miss anyway, so it isn't a big loss. It is better to end with more time than you need than to run out of time.

Lastly, sometimes it is beneficial to slow down if you are constantly getting ahead of time. You are always more likely to catch a careless mistake by working more slowly than quickly, and among very high-scoring test takers (those who are likely to have lots of time left over), careless errors affect the score more than mastery of material.

Secret Key #2 - Guessing is not Guesswork

You probably know that guessing is a good idea - unlike other standardized tests, there is no penalty for getting a wrong answer. Even if you have no idea about a question, you still have a 20-25% chance of getting it right.

Most test takers do not understand the impact that proper guessing can have on their score. Unless you score extremely high, guessing will significantly contribute to your final score.

Monkeys Take the Test

What most test takers don't realize is that to insure that 20-25% chance, you have to guess randomly. If you put 20 monkeys in a room to take this test, assuming they answered once per question and behaved themselves, on average they would get 20-25% of the questions correct. Put 20 test takers in the room, and the average will be much lower among guessed questions. Why?

1. The test writers intentionally write deceptive answer choices that "look" right. A test taker has no idea about a question, so picks the "best looking" answer, which is often wrong. The monkey has no idea what looks good and what doesn't, so will consistently be lucky about 20-25% of the time.
2. Test takers will eliminate answer choices from the guessing pool based on a hunch or intuition. Simple but correct answers often get excluded, leaving a 0% chance of being correct. The monkey has no clue, and often gets lucky with the best choice.

This is why the process of elimination endorsed by most test courses is flawed and detrimental to your performance- test takers don't guess, they make an ignorant stab in the dark that is usually worse than random.

$5 Challenge

Let me introduce one of the most valuable ideas of this course- the $5 challenge:

You only mark your "best guess" if you are willing to bet $5 on it.
You only eliminate choices from guessing if you are willing to bet $5 on it.

Why $5? Five dollars is an amount of money that is small yet not insignificant, and can really add up fast (20 questions could cost you $100). Likewise, each answer choice on one question of the test will have a small impact on your overall score, but it can really add up to a lot of points in the end.

The process of elimination IS valuable. The following shows your chance of guessing it right:

If you eliminate wrong answer choices until only this many remain:	Chance of getting it correct:
1	100%
2	50%
3	33%

However, if you accidentally eliminate the right answer or go on a hunch for an incorrect answer, your chances drop dramatically: to 0%. By guessing among all the answer choices, you are GUARANTEED to have a shot at the right answer.

That's why the $5 test is so valuable- if you give up the advantage and safety of a pure guess, it had better be worth the risk.

What we still haven't covered is how to be sure that whatever guess you make is truly random. Here's the easiest way:

Always pick the first answer choice among those remaining.

Such a technique means that you have decided, **before you see a single test question**, exactly how you are going to guess- and since the order of choices tells you nothing about which one is correct, this guessing technique is perfectly random.

This section is not meant to scare you away from making educated guesses or eliminating choices- you just need to define when a choice is worth eliminating. The $5 test, along with a pre-defined random guessing strategy, is the best way to make sure you reap all of the benefits of guessing.

Secret Key #3 - Practice Smarter, Not Harder

Many test takers delay the test preparation process because they dread the awful amounts of practice time they think necessary to succeed on the test. We have refined an effective method that will take you only a fraction of the time.

There are a number of "obstacles" in your way to succeed. Among these are answering questions, finishing in time, and mastering test-taking strategies. All must be executed on the day of the test at peak performance, or your score will suffer. The test is a mental marathon that has a large impact on your future.

Just like a marathon runner, it is important to work your way up to the full challenge. So first you just worry about questions, and then time, and finally strategy:

Success Strategy

1. Find a good source for practice tests.
2. If you are willing to make a larger time investment, consider using more than one study guide- often the different approaches of multiple authors will help you "get" difficult concepts.
3. Take a practice test with no time constraints, with all study helps "open book." Take your time with questions and focus on applying strategies.
4. Take a practice test with time constraints, with all guides "open book."
5. Take a final practice test with no open material and time limits

If you have time to take more practice tests, just repeat step 5. By gradually exposing yourself to the full rigors of the test environment, you will condition your mind to the stress of test day and maximize your success.

Secret Key #4 - Prepare, Don't Procrastinate

Let me state an obvious fact: if you take the test three times, you will get three different scores. This is due to the way you feel on test day, the level of preparedness you have, and, despite the test writers' claims to the contrary, some tests WILL be easier for you than others.

Since your future depends so much on your score, you should maximize your chances of success. In order to maximize the likelihood of success, you've got to prepare in advance. This means taking practice tests and spending time learning the information and test taking strategies you will need to succeed.

Never take the test as a "practice" test, expecting that you can just take it again if you need to. Feel free to take sample tests on your own, but when you go to take the official test, be prepared, be focused, and do your best the first time!

Secret Key #5 - Test Yourself

Everyone knows that time is money. There is no need to spend too much of your time or too little of your time preparing for the test. You should only spend as much of your precious time preparing as is necessary for you to get the score you need.

Once you have taken a practice test under real conditions of time constraints, then you will know if you are ready for the test or not.
If you have scored extremely high the first time that you take the practice test, then there is not much point in spending countless hours studying. You are already there.

Benchmark your abilities by retaking practice tests and seeing how much you have improved. Once you score high enough to guarantee success, then you are ready.

If you have scored well below where you need, then knuckle down and begin studying in earnest. Check your improvement regularly through the use of practice tests under real conditions. Above all, don't worry, panic, or give up. The key is perseverance!

Then, when you go to take the test, remain confident and remember how well you did on the practice tests. If you can score high enough on a practice test, then you can do the same on the real thing.

General Strategies

The most important thing you can do is to ignore your fears and jump into the test immediately- do not be overwhelmed by any strange-sounding terms. You have to jump into the test like jumping into a pool- all at once is the easiest way.

Make Predictions

As you read and understand the question, try to guess what the answer will be. Remember that several of the answer choices are wrong, and once you begin reading them, your mind will immediately become cluttered with answer choices designed to throw you off. Your mind is typically the most focused immediately after you have read the question and digested its contents. If you can, try to predict what the correct answer will be. You may be surprised at what you can predict.

Quickly scan the choices and see if your prediction is in the listed answer choices. If it is, then you can be quite confident that you have the right answer. It still won't hurt to check the other answer choices, but most of the time, you've got it!

Answer the Question

It may seem obvious to only pick answer choices that answer the question, but the test writers can create some excellent answer choices that are wrong. Don't pick an answer just because it sounds right, or you believe it to be true. It MUST answer the question. Once you've made your selection, always go back and check it against the question and make sure that you didn't misread the question, and the answer choice does answer the question posed.

Benchmark

After you read the first answer choice, decide if you think it sounds correct or not. If it doesn't, move on to the next answer choice. If it does, mentally mark that answer choice. This doesn't mean that you've definitely selected it as your answer choice, it just means that it's the best you've seen thus far. Go ahead and read the next choice. If the next choice is worse than the one you've already selected, keep going to the next answer choice. If the next choice is better than the choice you've already selected, mentally mark the new answer choice as your best guess.

The first answer choice that you select becomes your standard. Every other answer choice must be benchmarked against that standard. That choice is correct until proven otherwise by another answer choice beating it out. Once you've decided that no other answer choice seems as good, do one final check to ensure that your answer choice answers the question posed.

Valid Information

Don't discount any of the information provided in the question. Every piece of information may be necessary to determine the correct answer. None of the information in the question is there to throw you off (while the answer choices will certainly have information to throw you off). If two seemingly unrelated topics are discussed, don't ignore either. You can be confident there is a relationship, or it wouldn't be included in the question, and you are probably going to have to determine what is that relationship to find the answer.

Avoid "Fact Traps"

Don't get distracted by a choice that is factually true. Your search is for the answer that answers the question. Stay focused and don't fall for an answer that is true but incorrect. Always go back to the question and make sure you're choosing an answer that actually answers the question and is not just a true statement. An answer can be factually correct, but it MUST answer the question asked. Additionally, two answers can both be seemingly correct, so be sure to read all of the answer choices, and make sure that you get the one that BEST answers the question.

Milk the Question

Some of the questions may throw you completely off. They might deal with a subject you have not been exposed to, or one that you haven't reviewed in years. While your lack of knowledge about the subject will be a hindrance, the question itself can give you many clues that will help you find the correct answer. Read the question carefully and look for clues. Watch particularly for adjectives and nouns describing difficult terms or words that you don't recognize. Regardless of if you completely understand a word or not, replacing it with a synonym either provided or one you more familiar with may help you to understand what the questions are asking. Rather than wracking your mind about specific detailed information concerning a difficult term or word, try to use mental substitutes that are easier to understand.

The Trap of Familiarity

Don't just choose a word because you recognize it. On difficult questions, you may not recognize a number of words in the answer choices. The test writers don't put "make-believe" words on the test; so don't think that just because you only recognize all the words in one answer choice means that answer choice must be correct. If you only recognize words in one answer choice, then focus on that one. Is it correct? Try your best to determine if it is correct. If it is, that is great, but if it doesn't, eliminate it. Each word and answer choice you eliminate increases your chances of getting the question correct, even if you then have to guess among the unfamiliar choices.

Eliminate Answers

Eliminate choices as soon as you realize they are wrong. But be careful! Make sure you consider all of the possible answer choices. Just because one appears right, doesn't mean that the next one won't be even better! The test writers will usually put more than one good answer choice for every question, so read all of them. Don't worry if you are stuck between two that seem right. By getting down to just two remaining possible choices, your odds are now 50/50. Rather than wasting too much time, play the odds. You are guessing, but guessing wisely, because you've been able to knock out some of the answer choices that you know are wrong. If you are eliminating choices and realize that the last answer choice you are left with is also obviously wrong, don't panic. Start over and consider each choice again. There may easily be something that you missed the first time and will realize on the second pass.

Tough Questions

If you are stumped on a problem or it appears too hard or too difficult, don't waste time. Move on! Remember though, if you can quickly check for obviously incorrect answer choices, your chances of guessing correctly are greatly improved. Before you completely give up, at least try to knock out a couple of possible answers. Eliminate what you can and then guess at the remaining answer choices before moving on.

Brainstorm

If you get stuck on a difficult question, spend a few seconds quickly brainstorming. Run through the complete list of possible answer choices. Look at each choice and ask yourself, "Could this answer the question satisfactorily?" Go through each answer choice and consider it independently of the other. By systematically going through all possibilities, you may find something that you would otherwise overlook. Remember that when you get stuck, it's important to try to keep moving.

Read Carefully

Understand the problem. Read the question and answer choices carefully. Don't miss the question because you misread the terms. You have plenty of time to read each question thoroughly and make sure you understand what is being asked. Yet a happy medium must be attained, so don't waste too much time. You must read carefully, but efficiently.

Face Value

When in doubt, use common sense. Always accept the situation in the problem at face value. Don't read too much into it. These problems will not require you to make huge leaps of logic. The test writers aren't trying to throw you off with a cheap trick. If you have to go beyond creativity and make a leap of logic in order to have an answer choice answer the question, then you should look at the other answer choices. Don't overcomplicate the problem by creating theoretical relationships or explanations that will warp time or space. These are normal problems rooted in reality. It's just that the applicable relationship or explanation may not be readily apparent and you have to figure things out. Use your common sense to interpret anything that isn't clear.

Prefixes

If you're having trouble with a word in the question or answer choices, try dissecting it. Take advantage of every clue that the word might include. Prefixes and suffixes can be a huge help. Usually they allow you to determine a basic meaning. Pre- means before, post- means after, pro - is positive, de- is negative. From these prefixes and suffixes, you can get an idea of the general meaning of the word and try to put it into context. Beware though of any traps. Just because con is the opposite of pro, doesn't necessarily mean congress is the opposite of progress!

Hedge Phrases

Watch out for critical "hedge" phrases, such as likely, may, can, will often, sometimes, often, almost, mostly, usually, generally, rarely, sometimes. Question writers insert these hedge phrases to cover every possibility. Often an answer choice will be wrong simply because it leaves no room for exception. Avoid answer choices that have definitive words like "exactly," and "always".

Switchback Words

Stay alert for "switchbacks". These are the words and phrases frequently used to alert you to shifts in thought. The most common switchback word is "but". Others include although, however, nevertheless, on the other hand, even though, while, in spite of, despite, regardless of.

New Information

Correct answer choices will rarely have completely new information included. Answer choices typically are straightforward reflections of the material asked about and will directly relate to the question. If a new piece of information is included in an answer choice that doesn't even seem to relate to the topic being asked about, then that answer choice is likely incorrect. All of the information needed to answer the question is usually provided for you, and so you should not have to make guesses that are unsupported or choose answer choices that require unknown information that cannot be reasoned on its own.

Time Management

On technical questions, don't get lost on the technical terms. Don't spend too much time on any one question. If you don't know what a term means, then since you don't have a dictionary, odds are you aren't going to get much further. You should immediately recognize terms as whether or not you know them. If you don't, work with the other clues that you have, the other answer choices and terms provided, but don't waste too much time trying to figure out a difficult term.

Contextual Clues

Look for contextual clues. An answer can be right but not correct. The contextual clues will help you find the answer that is most right and is correct. Understand the context in which a phrase or statement is made. This will help you make important distinctions.

Don't Panic

Panicking will not answer any questions for you. Therefore, it isn't helpful. When you first see the question, if your mind goes blank, take a deep breath. Force yourself to mechanically go through the steps of solving the problem and using the strategies you've learned.

Pace Yourself

Don't get clock fever. It's easy to be overwhelmed when you're looking at a page full of questions, your mind is full of random thoughts and feeling confused, and the clock is ticking down faster than you would like. Calm down and maintain the pace that you have set for yourself. As long as you are on track by monitoring your pace, you are guaranteed to have enough time for yourself. When you get to the last few minutes of the test, it may seem like you won't have enough time left, but if you only have as many questions as you should have left at that point, then you're right on track!

Answer Selection

The best way to pick an answer choice is to eliminate all of those that are wrong, until only one is left and confirm that is the correct answer. Sometimes though, an answer choice may immediately look right. Be careful! Take a second to make sure that the other choices are not equally obvious. Don't make a hasty mistake. There are only two times that you should stop before checking other answers. First is when you are positive that the answer choice you have selected is correct. Second is when time is almost out and you have to make a quick guess!

Check Your Work

Since you will probably not know every term listed and the answer to every question, it is important that you get credit for the ones that you do know. Don't miss any questions through careless mistakes. If at all possible, try to take a second to look back over your answer selection and make sure you've selected the correct answer choice and haven't made a costly careless mistake (such as marking an answer choice that you didn't mean to mark). This quick double check should more than pay for itself in caught mistakes for the time it costs.

Beware of Directly Quoted Answers

Sometimes an answer choice will repeat word for word a portion of the question or reference section. However, beware of such exact duplication – it may be a trap! More than likely, the correct choice will paraphrase or summarize a point, rather than being exactly the same wording.

Slang

Scientific sounding answers are better than slang ones. An answer choice that begins "To compare the outcomes…" is much more likely to be correct than one that begins "Because some people insisted…"

Extreme Statements

Avoid wild answers that throw out highly controversial ideas that are proclaimed as established fact. An answer choice that states the "process should be used in certain situations, if…" is much more likely to be correct than one that states the "process should be discontinued completely." The first is a calm rational statement and doesn't even make a definitive, uncompromising stance, using a hedge word "if" to provide wiggle room, whereas the second choice is a radical idea and far more extreme.

Answer Choice Families

When you have two or more answer choices that are direct opposites or parallels, one of them is usually the correct answer. For instance, if one answer choice states "x increases" and another answer choice states "x decreases" or "y increases," then those two or three answer choices are very similar in construction and fall into the same family of answer choices. A family of answer choices is when two or three answer choices are very similar in construction, and yet often have a directly opposite meaning. Usually the correct answer choice will be in that family of answer choices. The "odd man out" or answer choice that doesn't seem to fit the parallel construction of the other answer choices is more likely to be incorrect.

Additional Bonus Material

Due to our efforts to try to keep this book to a manageable length, we've created a link that will give you access to all of your additional bonus material.

Please visit http://www.mometrix.com/bonus948/ccrnadult to access the information.